DIFFERENTIAL DIAGNOSIS IN DERMATOLOGY

SECOND EDITION

DIFFERENTIAL DIAGNOSIS IN DERMATOLOGY

SECOND EDITION

KLAUS F HELM MD

Professor of Dermatology and Pathology
Department of Dermatology
Pennsylvania State University College of Medicine
Hershey, Pennsylvania
USA

GALEN T FOULKE MD

Assistant Professor of Dermatology
Department of Dermatology
Pennsylvania State University College of Medicine
Hershey, Pennsylvania
USA

JAMES G MARKS Jr MD

Professor
Department of Dermatology
Pennsylvania State University College of Medicine
Hershey, Pennsylvania
USA

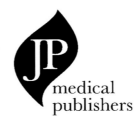

JP
medical
publishers

London • New Delhi • Panama City

© 2018 JP Medical Ltd.
Published by JP Medical Ltd, 83 Victoria Street, London, SW1H 0HW, UK
Tel: +44 (0)20 3170 8910   Fax: +44 (0)20 3008 6180
Email: info@jpmedpub.com   Web: www.jpmedpub.com

The right of Klaus F Helm, Galen T Foulke and James G Marks to be identified as the authors of this work have been asserted by them in accordance with the Copyright, Designs and Patents Act 1988.

All rights reserved. No part of this publication may be reproduced, stored or transmitted in any form or by any means, electronic, mechanical, photocopying, recording or otherwise, except as permitted by the UK Copyright, Designs and Patents Act 1988, without the prior permission in writing of the publishers. Permissions may be sought directly from JP Medical Ltd at the address printed above.

All brand names and product names used in this book are trade names, service marks, trademarks or registered trademarks of their respective owners. The publisher is not associated with any product or vendor mentioned in this book.

Medical knowledge and practice change constantly. This book is designed to provide accurate, authoritative information about the subject matter in question. However, readers are advised to check the most current information available on procedures included and check information from the manufacturer of each product to be administered, to verify the recommended dose, formula, method and duration of administration, adverse effects and contraindications. It is the responsibility of the practitioner to take all appropriate safety precautions. Neither the publisher nor the authors assume any liability for any injury and/or damage to persons or property arising from or related to use of material in this book.

This book is sold on the understanding that the publisher is not engaged in providing professional medical services. If such advice or services are required, the services of a competent medical professional should be sought.

Every effort has been made where necessary to contact holders of copyright to obtain permission to reproduce copyright material. If any have been inadvertently overlooked, the publisher will be pleased to make the necessary arrangements at the first opportunity.

ISBN: 978-1-909836-19-8

British Library Cataloguing in Publication Data
A catalogue record for this book is available from the British Library

Library of Congress Cataloging in Publication Data
A catalog record for this book is available from the Library of Congress

Publisher:	Richard Furn
Development Editor:	Gavin Smith
Editorial Assistant:	Katie Pattullo
Design:	Designers Collective Ltd

Preface

While our primary objective in writing *Differential Diagnosis in Dermatology* – enabling healthcare providers to accurately diagnose skin diseases – remains unchanged, we have expanded and enhanced the book in a number of ways.

Firstly, the design of the algorithms and the layout of each chapter have been improved to help the logical flow of the content stand out. We have added short 'Disease discussion' sections at the end of each chapter to provide management guidance on commonly encountered diseases. Lastly, we have included a self-assessment chapter to enable readers to test themselves on the physical signs of cutaneous disease.

Aside from these changes, *Differential Diagnosis in Dermatology 2nd Edition* continues to provide what we hope is a unique and invaluable system of presenting both common and uncommon dermatologic differential diagnoses in a problem-oriented manner. Unlike other text-atlases that catalog diseases in a purely descriptive manner, this book is organized in a way that enables clinicians to work through the diagnostic dilemmas they are likely to encounter in clinical practice.

A templated approach to evaluating skin diseases is the unifying theme. Firstly, diagnostic algorithms at the start of each chapter help the reader to arrive at a shortlist of differential diagnoses. Next, highly structured sets of 'compare and contrast' tables and clinical photographs enable the reader to refine the shortlist still further. The overarching goal is to provide a roadmap that helps the clinician arrive at the correct diagnosis.

While the first edition of *Differential Diagnosis in Dermatology* limited itself to the discussion of differential diagnoses, we have added succinct discussions of the commonest disorders described in the algorithms and tables. These cover etiology, clinical features and recommended treatment. Combined with the unique approach to working through the differential diagnosis of skin lesions, we hope the inclusion of this management information enhances the book's value to primary care providers and dermatologists by helping them diagnose and treat the many patients they see with cutaneous skin disorders.

Klaus F Helm
Galen T Foulke
James G Marks Jr
October 2017

Contents

Preface — v

PART 1: LOCALIZED RASHES

Chapter 1
Scalp — 1

Chapter 2
Face — 27

Chapter 3
Oral mucosa — 49

Chapter 4
Hands and feet — 65

Chapter 5
Nails — 79

Chapter 6
Legs — 89

Chapter 7
Genitalia — 111

PART 2: GENERALIZED RASHES

Chapter 8
Papulosquamous diseases — 129

Chapter 9
Excoriations — 157

Chapter 10
Vesicular and bullous diseases — 171

Chapter 11
Macular and urticarial rashes — 193

Chapter 12
Generalized pustular eruptions — 205

PART 3: NEOPLASMS

Chapter 13
Epidermal growths · 215

Chapter 14
Pigmented growths · 253

Chapter 15
Benign dermal neoplasms · 281

Chapter 16
Malignant dermal neoplasms · 299

PART 4: SELF ASSESSMENT

Chapter 17
Self-assessment · 317

Index · 337

Section 1

LOCALIZED RASHES

Chapter 1 Scalp

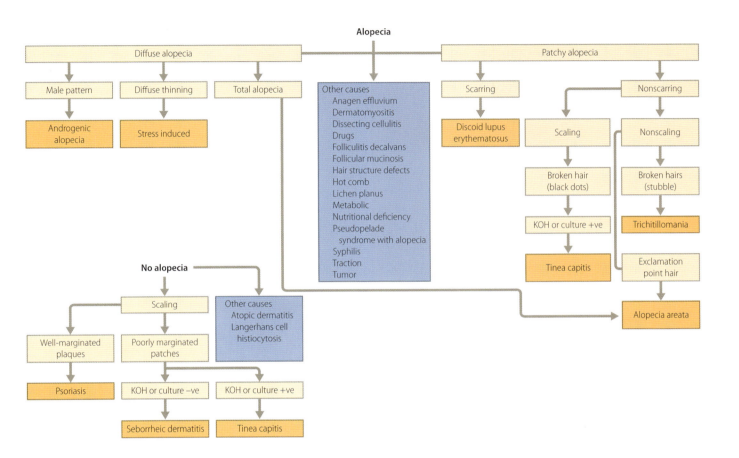

INTRODUCTION

The average scalp contains more than 100,000 hairs in a mixture of different growth phases. Eighty-five percent are in an active growing phase (anagen), 5% are in a transitional phase (catagen), and 10% are in a resting phase (telogen). The average number of hairs shed daily is approximately 100. The hair grows approximately 1 cm each month. In the adult, there are two types of hair: *vellus* (fine, usually light colored, fuzzy hair) and *terminal* (coarse, thick, usually pigmented hair).

Disorders of the hair and scalp are fairly frequent presenting complaints. The physical examination is often the most critical component in the evaluation of these patients. However, a detailed history and, on occasion, laboratory tests or a scalp biopsy may also be required to establish a definitive diagnosis. Initially, the examination should determine whether there is hair loss. Diseases such as psoriasis, seborrheic dermatitis, and diffuse tinea capitis present as inflammatory conditions of the scalp usually without associated hair loss. When alopecia (hair loss) is present, it is helpful to observe the pattern—diffuse or patchy. *Diffuse alopecia* may occur in a typical distribution involving the frontal and vertex regions of the scalp, characteristic of androgenic or male/female pattern baldness. Diffuse, thinning, or total alopecia can be seen in alopecia areata, following physically or mentally stressful events (telogen effluvium), or secondary to a metabolic disorder, drug reactions, or a dietary deficiency. In patients with *patchy alopecia*, the presence or absence of scarring is important in the differential diagnosis. Discoid lupus erythematosus is the prototype of the scarring form of alopecia. Nonscarring patchy alopecia can be seen in alopecia areata, trichotillomania, and tinea capitis. Additionally, scarring is an important prognostic sign, since destruction of the hair follicle results in permanent loss of hair, whereas nonscarring alopecia may be a temporary phenomenon.

1. TINEA CAPITIS VERSUS ALOPECIA AREATA

■ Features in common: nonscarring patches of hair loss

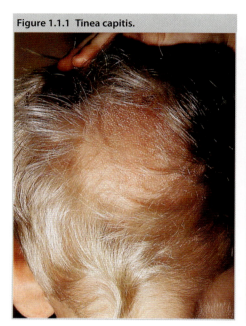

Figure 1.1.1 Tinea capitis.

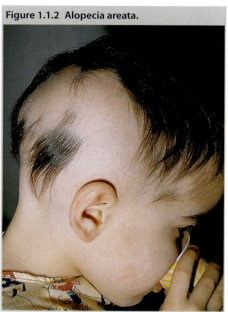

Figure 1.1.2 Alopecia areata.

■ Distinguishing features

	Tinea capitis	Alopecia areata
Physical examination		
Morphology	Scaling Inflammation Kerion: boggy, crusted, purulent plaque Broken hair: black dot No exclamation point hairs	No scaling No or slight inflammation No kerion No broken hair Exclamation point hairs
Distribution	Scaling patches scattered on face, trunk, extremities	Alopecia elsewhere on face, trunk, extremities
History		
Symptoms	Family member or friend with tinea Pet with tinea	Family history positive
Exacerbating factors	None	None
Associated findings	Cervical lymphadenopathy Nail dystrophy No autoimmune disease	No lymphadenopathy Nail pits and dystrophy Vitiligo, thyroiditis, anemia
Epidemiology	Epidemic among inner-city school children	Sporadic
Biopsy	Usually not done Fungal structures	Usually not necessary Dystrophic hair with lymphocytic infiltrate around hair bulb
Laboratory	No blood work KOH and/or culture positive	Complete blood count Thyroid-stimulating hormone KOH and/or culture negative
Outcome	Curable	Variable and unpredictable
KOH, potassium hydroxide.		

Differential diagnosis of patchy alopecia

- Nonscarring
  - Trichotillomania
  - Secondary syphilis
  - Bacterial infection
- Scarring
  - Discoid lupus erythematosus
  - Lichen planus
  - Malignant tumor

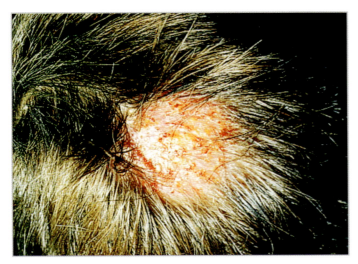

Figure 1.1.3 Tinea capitis. *Clue to diagnosis:* boggy, crusted, scaling plaque with alopecia (kerion).

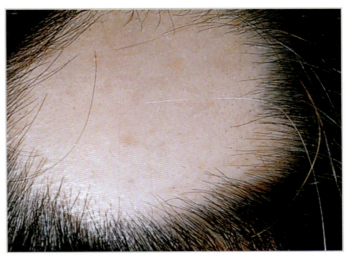

Figure 1.1.4 Alopecia areata. *Clue to diagnosis:* smooth patch of alopecia with exclamation point hairs in the periphery.

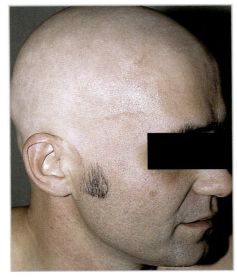

Figure 1.1.5 Alopecia areata: almost total loss of scalp hair is termed alopecia totalis.

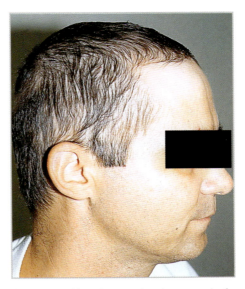

Figure 1.1.6 Alopecia areata showing regrowth of hair after treatment.

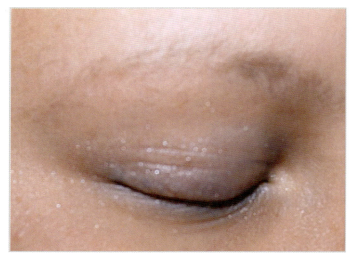

Figure 1.1.7 Alopecia areata showing loss of eyebrow and eyelashes.

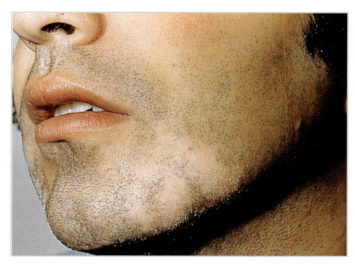

Figure 1.1.8 Alopecia areata showing patches of alopecia in the beard.

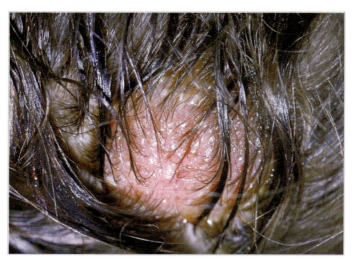

Figure 1.1.9 Tinea capitis kerion.

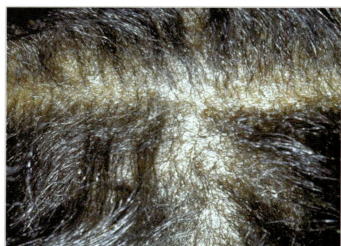

Figure 1.1.10 Tinea capitis.

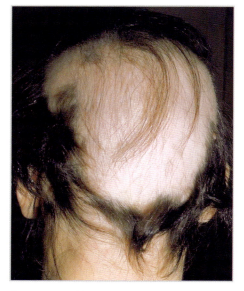

Figure 1.1.11 Alopecia areata.

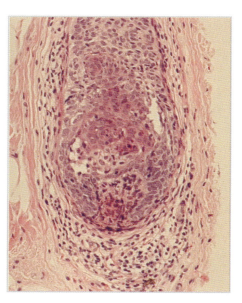

Figure 1.1.12 Alopecia areata showing lymphocytic infiltrate around the hair bulb.

2. SEBORRHEIC DERMATITIS VERSUS TINEA CAPITIS

Features in common: scaling patches without hair loss

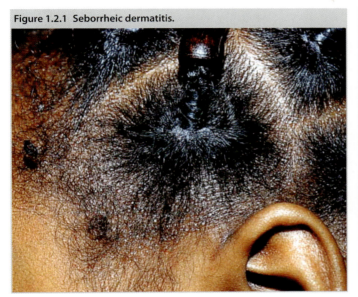

Figure 1.2.1 Seborrheic dermatitis.

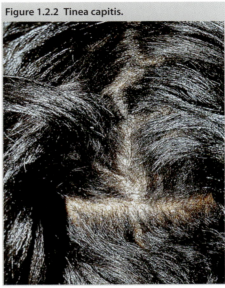

Figure 1.2.2 Tinea capitis.

Distinguishing features

	Seborrheic dermatitis	Tinea capitis
Physical examination		
Morphology	Yellow or white scaling No hair loss No broken hair	White scaling No hair loss or possible hair loss Broken hair – black dot
Distribution	Eyebrows, eyelids, nasolabial folds, ears, chest	Scaling patches scattered on face, trunk, extremities
History		
Symptoms	Mild itching No one else affected	Mild itching Family member or friend with tinea Pet with tinea
Exacerbating factors	Poor hygiene	None
Associated findings	AIDS, Parkinson's disease	Cervical lymphadenopathy
Epidemiology	5% of healthy adults affected 33% of AIDS patients affected	Epidemic among inner-city school children
Biopsy	Not done Nonspecific dermatitis No fungal structures	Usually not done Fungal structures
Laboratory	KOH and/or culture negative HIV testing in severe or treatment-resistant cases	KOH and/or culture positive No HIV testing
Outcome	Chronic	Curable

AIDS, acquired immunodeficiency syndrome; HIV, human immunodeficiency virus; KOH, potassium hydroxide.

Differential diagnosis of nonscarring, scaling scalp patches without hair loss

- Psoriasis
- Langerhans cell histiocytosis
- Atopic dermatitis

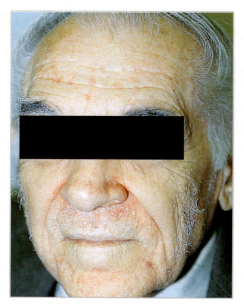

Figure 1.2.3 Seborrheic dermatitis. *Clue to diagnosis:* scaling patches involving eyebrows and nasolabial fold.

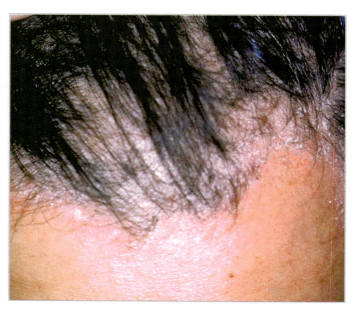

Figure 1.2.4 Seborrheic dermatitis.

3. TRICHOTILLOMANIA VERSUS TINEA CAPITIS

Features in common: patchy alopecia with broken hairs

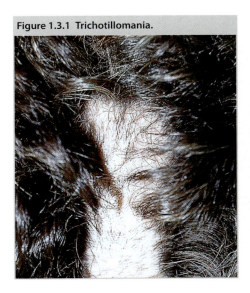

Figure 1.3.1 Trichotillomania.

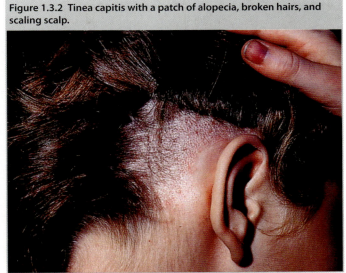

Figure 1.3.2 Tinea capitis with a patch of alopecia, broken hairs, and scaling scalp.

Distinguishing features

	Trichotillomania	Tinea capitis
Physical examination		
Morphology	No scaling No inflammation Hairs unequal lengths – stubble No kerion "Friar Tuck" sign – rim of normal hair in periphery of scalp	Scaling Inflammation Broken hair – black dot Kerion
Distribution	Loss of eyebrows and eyelashes – plucked	Scaling patches elsewhere on face, trunk, extremities No loss of eyebrows or eyelashes
History		
Symptoms	No itching Emotional distress No one else affected	Mild itching Family member or friend with tinea Pet with tinea
Exacerbating factors	Stress	None
Associated findings	No cervical lymphadenopathy Psychiatric or emotional problems	Cervical lymphadenopathy No emotional problems
Epidemiology	Sporadic Children and women	Epidemic among inner-city school children
Biopsy	Often not required No fungal structures Empty hair shafts	Usually not done Fungal structures No empty hair shafts
Laboratory	KOH and/or culture negative	KOH and/or culture positive
Outcome	Chronic Children – usually self limited Adults – resistant to psychotherapy	Curable

KOH, potassium hydroxide.

Differential diagnosis of patchy alopecia without scarring

- Alopecia areata
- Secondary syphilis

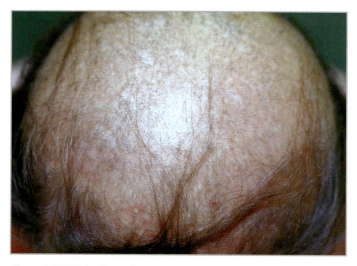

Figure 1.3.3 Trichotillomania.

4. TRICHOTILLOMANIA VERSUS ALOPECIA AREATA

■ Features in common: patchy alopecia without scarring

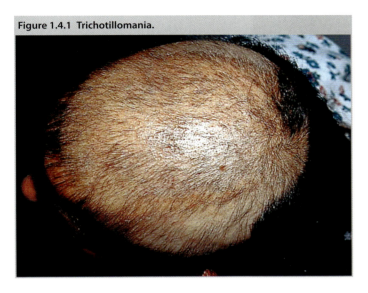

Figure 1.4.1 Trichotillomania.

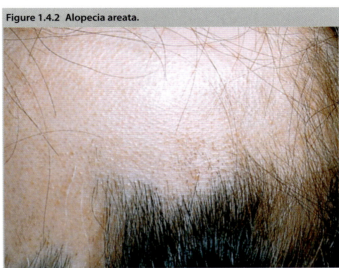

Figure 1.4.2 Alopecia areata.

■ Distinguishing features

	Trichotillomania	Alopecia areata
Physical examination Morphology	No inflammation No exclamation point hairs; hairs unequal lengths – stubble	No or slight inflammation Exclamation point hairs; hairs same length
Distribution	'Friar Tuck' sign – rim of normal hair in periphery of scalp Loss of eyebrows and eyelashes – plucked	Alopecia elsewhere on face, trunk, extremities
History Symptoms	Family history negative	Family history positive
Exacerbating factors	Stress	None
Associated findings	No nail pits or dystrophy No autoimmune diseases Psychiatric or emotional problems	Nail pits and dystrophy Vitiligo, thyroiditis, anemia No psychiatric problems
Epidemiology	Sporadic Children and women	Sporadic All ages
Biopsy	Often not required Empty hair shafts	Usually not necessary Dystrophic hair with lymphocytic infiltrate around hair bulb
Laboratory	None	Complete blood count Thyroid-stimulating hormone
Outcome	Chronic Children – usually self-limited Adults – resistant to psychotherapy	Variable and unpredictable

Differential diagnosis of patchy alopecia without scarring

- Tinea capitis
- Secondary syphilis

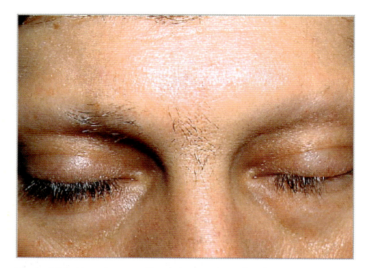

Figure 1.4.3 Alopecia areata. *Clue to diagnosis:* Loss of eyebrows and eyelashes. Examination of scalp confirms the diagnosis.

5. DISCOID LUPUS ERYTHEMATOSUS VERSUS ALOPECIA AREATA

Features in common: patchy alopecia without scarring

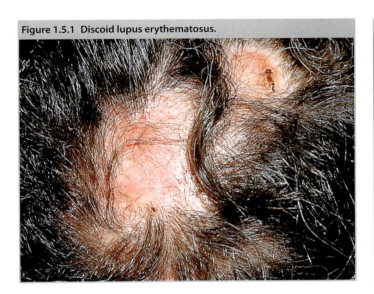

Figure 1.5.1 Discoid lupus erythematosus.

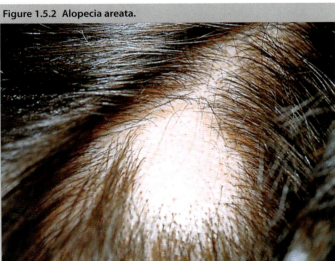

Figure 1.5.2 Alopecia areata.

Distinguishing features

	Discoid lupus erythematosus	Alopecia areata
Physical examination		
Morphology	Scarring Inflammation Scaling	Nonscarring No or slight inflammation No scaling
Distribution	No exclamation point hairs Sun-exposed areas	Exclamation point hairs Not in sun-exposed areas
History		
Symptoms	May itch Family history negative	No itching Family history positive
Exacerbating factors	Sunlight may cause flare-up	None
Associated findings	No nail changes Systemic lupus erythematosus in 5% to 10%	Nail pits and dystrophy Vitiligo, thyroiditis, anemia
Epidemiology	Sporadic	Sporadic
Biopsy	Yes – hyperkeratosis with follicular plugging, vacuolar degeneration of basal cell layer, perivascular and perifollicular inflammation	Usually not necessary Dystrophic hair with lymphocytic infiltrate around hair bulb
Laboratory	Complete blood count Platelet count Urinalysis Antinuclear antibody testing	Complete blood count Thyroid-stimulating hormone
Outcome	Chronic – spontaneous remission in 50%	Variable and unpredictable

SCALP

■ Differential diagnosis of patchy alopecia

- Nonscarring
  - Trichotillomania
  - Secondary syphilis
  - Tinea capitis
  - Alopecia areata
- Scarring
  - Lichen planus
  - Malignant tumor
  - Folliculitis decalvans
  - Dissecting cellulitis
  - Discoid lupus erythematosus

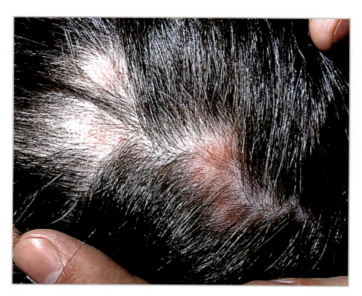

Figure 1.5.3 Discoid lupus erythematosus. *Clue to diagnosis:* Scarring discoid plaques.

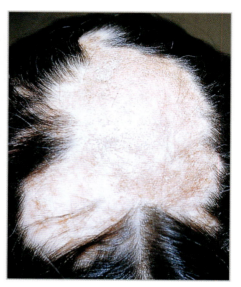

Figure 1.5.4 Discoid lupus erythematosus: old burned-out discoid lupus erythematosus.

6. STRESS-INDUCED ALOPECIA (TELOGEN EFFLUVIUM) VERSUS ANDROGENIC ALOPECIA

■ Features in common: nonscarring diffuse alopecia

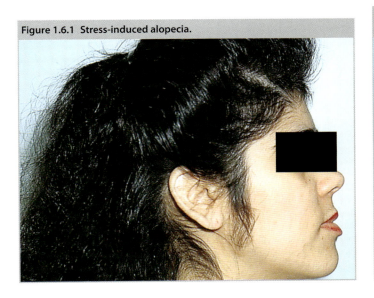

Figure 1.6.1 Stress-induced alopecia.

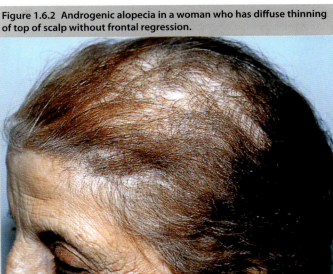

Figure 1.6.2 Androgenic alopecia in a woman who has diffuse thinning of top of scalp without frontal regression.

■ Distinguishing features

	Stress-induced alopecia (telogen effluvium)	Androgenic alopecia
Physical examination Morphology	No obvious alopecia	Obvious alopecia
Distribution	Diffuse	Frontotemporal and vertex – men No frontal recession – women
History Symptoms	Acute onset Hair comes out by 'handfuls' after shampooing, combing	Gradual onset Asymptomatic
Exacerbating factors	Stressful event No androgens, progesterones	No stressful event Androgens, progesterones
Associated findings	Drug-induced – heparin, coumadin, retinoids, β-blockers, oral contraceptives	Women with androgen excess – acne, hirsutism, clitoromegaly
Epidemiology Biopsy	Sporadic Not done	Family history positive Not done
Laboratory	None	Usually none In females suspected to have androgen excess – free and total testosterone, dehydroepiandrosterone sulfate testing
	Hair pull – greater than 5 hairs	Hair pull – 1–2 hairs
Outcome	Resolves	Chronic

Differential diagnosis of nonscarring diffuse hair loss

- Alopecia areata
- Systemic lupus erythematosus
- Metabolic (thyroid) disorders
- Drug induced disorders
- Nutritional deficiency

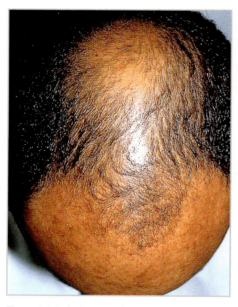

Figure 1.6.3 Androgenic alopecia in a man. *Clue to diagnosis:* Frontal and vertex regression.

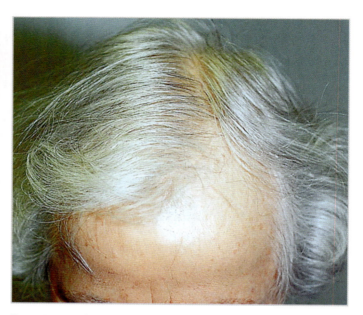

Figure 1.6.4 Androgenic alopecia in a woman with recent onset of frontal regression: the patient had a testosterone-producing ovarian tumor.

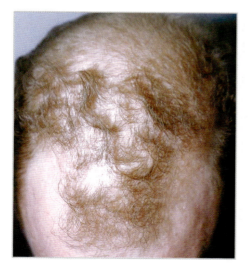

Figure 1.6.5 Androgenic alopecia.

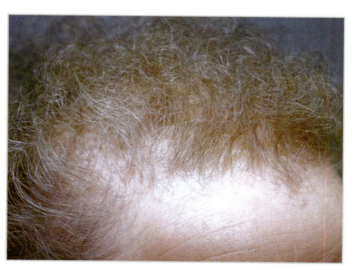

Figure 1.6.6 Androgenic alopecia in a woman, characterized by diffuse thinning without frontal regression.

7. PSORIASIS VERSUS SEBORRHEIC DERMATITIS

■ Features in common: scaling patches without alopecia

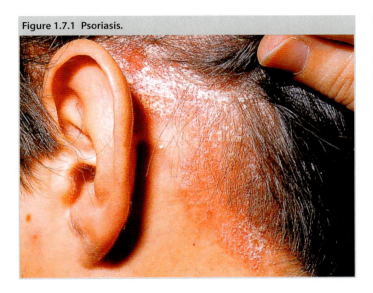

Figure 1.7.1 Psoriasis.

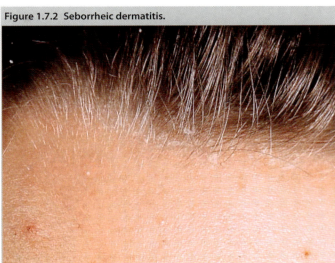

Figure 1.7.2 Seborrheic dermatitis.

■ Distinguishing features

	Psoriasis	Seborrheic dermatitis
Physical examination		
Morphology	Well-demarcated patches/plaques Silvery scaling	Poorly demarcated patches Yellow or white scaling
Distribution	Elbows, knees, nails, elsewhere	Eyebrows, eyelids, nasolabial folds, ears, chest
History		
Symptoms	Moderate itching	Mild itching
Exacerbating factors	Trauma Physical or emotional stress/illness Medications – β-blockers, lithium	No trauma Poor hygiene
Associated findings	Arthritis Nail dystrophy	No arthritis AIDS Parkinson's disease No nail changes
Epidemiology	Positive family history	No family history 5% of healthy adults affected 33% of AIDS patients affected
Biopsy	Not done Hyperkeratosis, acanthosis, neutrophils in epidermis, dermal capillary proliferation, perivascular inflammation	Not done Nonspecific dermatitis
Laboratory	None	HIV testing in severe or treatment-resistant cases
Outcome	Chronic	Chronic

Differential diagnosis of scaling scalp patches without alopecia

- Tinea capitis
- Langerhans cell histiocytosis
- Atopic dermatitis

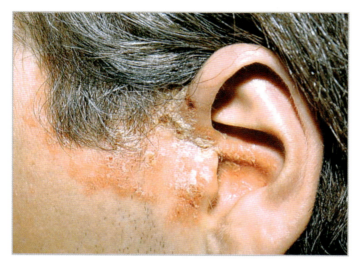

Figure 1.7.3 Psoriasis. *Clue to diagnosis:* Poorly-defined margins, inflamed, scaling plaque.

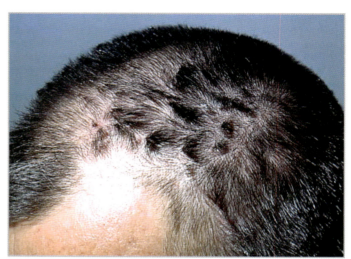

Figure 1.7.4 Psoriasis. *Clue to diagnosis:* Hair clumps together in tentlike configuration ('tent sign').

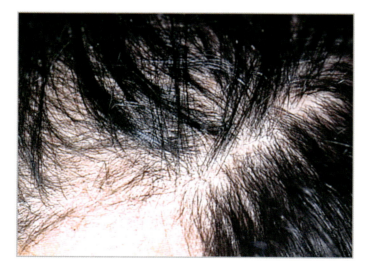

Figure 1.7.5 Seborrheic dermatitis. *Clue to diagnosis:* Patches with poorly-defined margins.

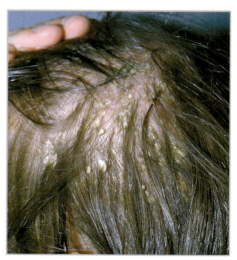

Figure 1.7.6 Psoriasis.

8. ALOPECIA/NO ALOPECIA

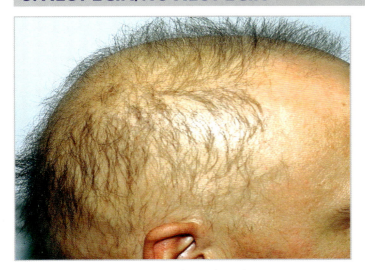

Figure 1.8.1 Anagen effluvium secondary to chemotherapy.

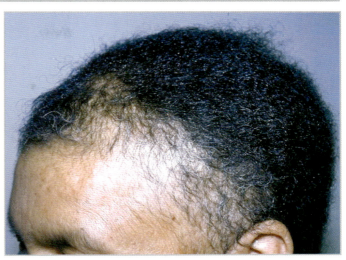

Figure 1.8.2 Traction alopecia.

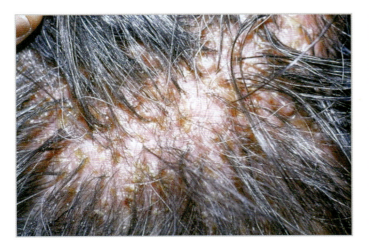

Figure 1.8.3 Langerhans cell histiocytosis

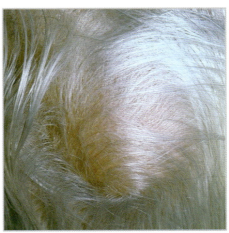

Figure 1.8.4 Plasmacytoma.

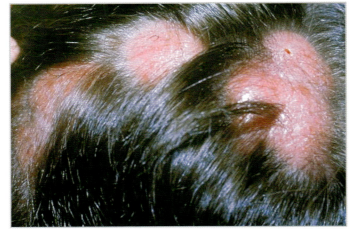

Figure 1.8.5 Lymphoma.

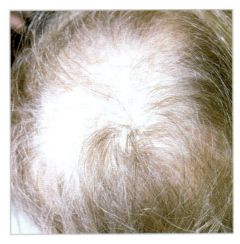

Figure 1.8.6 Conradi–Hünermann syndrome.

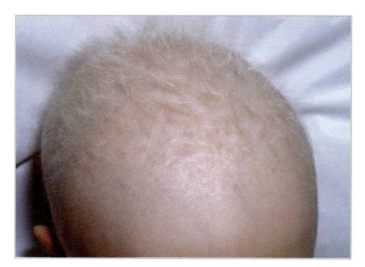

Figure 1.8.7 Ectodermal dysplasia.

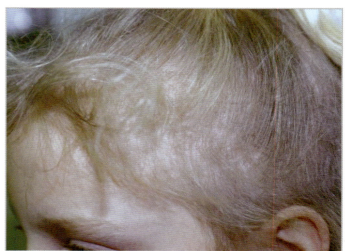

Figure 1.8.8 Loose anagen syndrome.

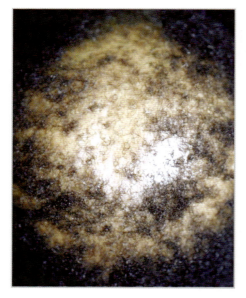

Figure 1.8.9 Central centrifugal cicatricial alopecia

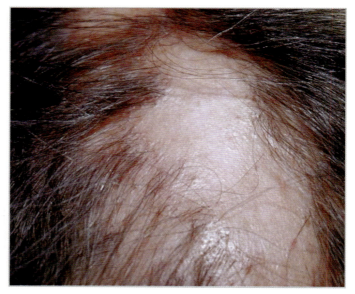

Figure 1.8.10 Lichen planopilaris.

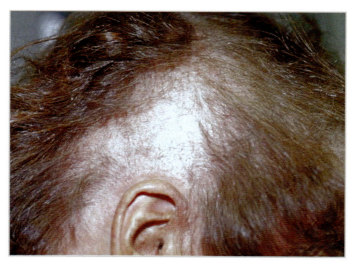

Figure 1.8.11 Dermatomyositis.

9. OTHER EXAMPLES

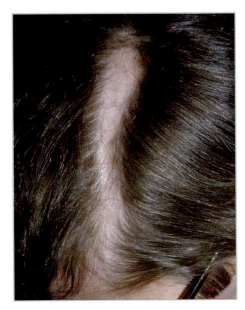

Figure 1.9.1 Linear scleroderma.

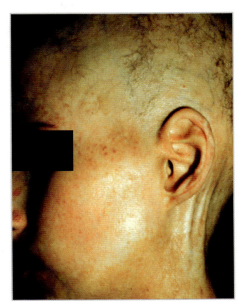

Figure 1.9.2 Graft vs host disease.

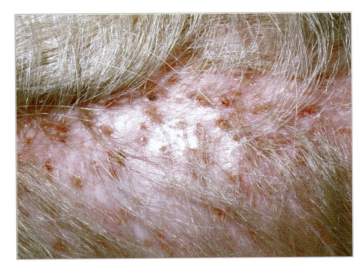

Figure 1.9.3 Folliculitis decalvans.

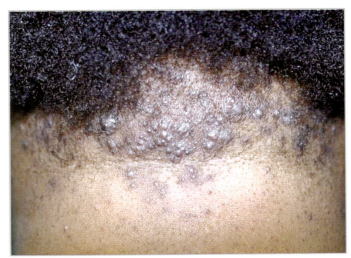

Figure 1.9.4 Keloidal folliculitis.

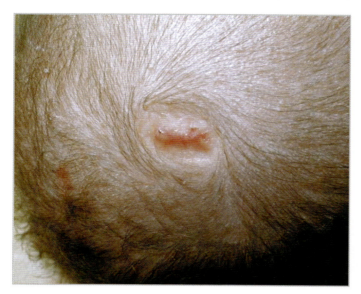

Figure 1.9.5 Aplasia cutis.

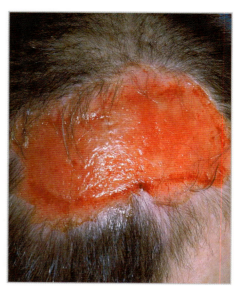

Figure 1.9.6 Epidermolysis bullosa acquisita.

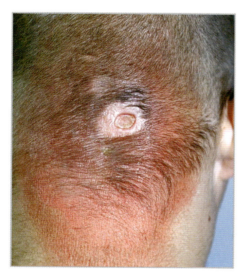

Figure 1.9.7 Factitial.

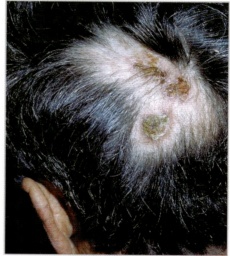

Figure 1.9.8 Traumatic alopecia secondary to prolonged compression of the scalp during surgery.

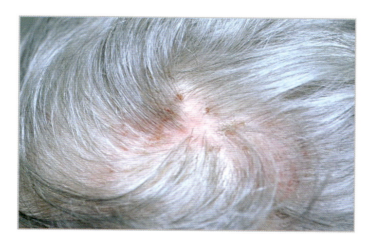

Figure 1.9.9 Cicatricial pemphigoid.

DISEASE DISCUSSION

Androgenic alopecia

Definition and etiology

Androgenic alopecia, or common baldness, is the nonscarring replacement of dark terminal hairs by vellus hairs and atrophic follicles. This hair loss is androgen dependent and involves the vertex and frontotemporal regions of the scalp in genetically predisposed men and women.

Clinical features

Common baldness is an androgen-dependent inherited condition that begins in late adolescence or early adulthood. The onset and progression are gradual and highly variable. It affects almost 100% of whites, whereas in other ethnic groups, such as native Americans and Asians, it is uncommon.

Initially, the young man or woman may notice increased hair shedding after washing or combing with subsequent thinning of the hair in the frontotemporal and vertex regions of the scalp. The coarse dark terminal hairs are replaced by finer depigmented vellus hairs. These vellus hairs then become atrophic, leaving a smooth shiny scalp with few or no follicular orifices. Characteristically, the posterior and lateral margins of the scalp are spared. In men, there is bitemporal hair recession and balding of the vertex, which can progress to complete baldness. In women, the frontal hairline remains intact, but there is mild to moderate diffuse thinning over the top of the scalp. This rarely results in total baldness. Although thinning continues throughout life, it is most prominent between the ages of 30 and 50 years.

The diagnosis is usually straightforward and made without difficulty in men. In women, a hormonal abnormality should be considered if frontal recession develops together with other signs of androgen excess such as acne, hirsutism, or menstrual irregularities. A skin biopsy is rarely done. In women in whom androgen excess is suspected, serum-free and total testosterone and dehydroepiandrosterone sulfate tests are ordered to screen for pituitary, adrenal, or ovarian disorders.

Treatment (Table 1.1)

A 5% minoxidil (Rogaine) foam applied twice a day is somewhat effective in growing hair in areas that were previously bald. Men are more responsive than women. Additionally, minoxidil may stop or retard the progression of baldness, but it must be used continuously to preserve growth. Finasteride 1 mg daily may be prescribed for men only and has a similar response to topical minoxidil. Surgical treatment involving hair transplants remains an important therapeutic option. Baldness can also be covered with a hairpiece or wig.

Table 1.1 Treatment of androgenic alopecia

Treatment	Precautions
Mild/moderate disease	
Minoxidil 5% foam bid	None
Finasteride 1 mg daily	Contraindicated in women
Severe disease	
Hair transplant	Select appreciate candidate
Wig	None

Alopecia areata

Definition and etiology

Alopecia areata is an idiopathic disorder that causes round or oval patches of nonscarring alopecia.

Clinical features

Alopecia areata affects both children and adults but most often occurs in early adulthood. Both sexes are affected equally. The emotional stress that accompanies alopecia areata appears to be reactive rather than causative. Although the pathogenesis of alopecia areata is poorly understood, an immunologic process is probable. Occasionally, autoimmune disease such as Hashimoto's thyroiditis and pernicious anemia have been associated with alopecia areata. In approximately 25% of patients, a family history of the disorder is found.

The clinical findings include round or oval patches of complete hair loss. The underlying skin is smooth without any evidence of scarring. Closer inspection may reveal the presence or absence of follicular orifices. In the absence of orifices, regrowth of the hair will not occur. In the periphery of the patches of alopecia, 'exclamation point' hairs occur. These are so named because of their resemblance to this punctuation mark – the diameter of the distal hair is greater than that of the proximal segment. In some cases the hair loss can involve the entire scalp; this is referred to as *alopecia totalis*. If it occurs over the entire body, it is referred to as *alopecia universalis*. Erythema and slight tenderness may be present early in the course of the disease. Subsequently, the scalp may become slightly depressed. Fine stippling and pitting of the nails are infrequent associated findings.

The differential diagnosis of nonscarring forms of alopecia includes trichotillomania, secondary syphilis, and tinea capitis. Although a skin biopsy is not usually necessary, biopsy findings will reveal small dystrophic hair structures with an infiltrate of lymphocytes surrounding the hair bulbs of anagen hairs like a swarm of bees. For extensive alopecia areata, a complete blood count, glucose, and thyroid-stimulating hormone assay are done to rule out associated autoimmune diseases.

Treatment (Table 1.2)

A variety of treatments have been tried, but topical, and intralesional

Table 1.2 Treatment of alopecia areata

Treatment	Precautions
Mild/moderate disease	
Clobetasol solution 0.5% bid	Atrophy with chronic application
Triamcinolone 10 mg/mL intralesional every 4–6 weeks	Atrophy
Irritants – anthralin, retinoids	Severe irritation
Severe disease	
Squaric acid sensitization	Severe allergic contact dermatitis Urticaria
Prednisone (short course)	Hyperglycemia, hypertension, insomnia, mood change, weight gain, infection, osteoporosis
Hydroxychloroquine	Periodic eye exam
PUVA (psoralen plus ultra violet light A)	Eye protection

corticosteroids are used most often. Other therapeutic modalities include topical anthralin, topical minoxidil, topical retinoic acid, and immunotherapy with contact irritants and allergens. None of these treatments is uniformly successful. The majority of patients with alopecia areata will experience a spontaneous recovery and therefore need no treatment. Relapses, however, are not uncommon. Extensive hair loss and disease duration of more than 1 year are poor prognostic signs. The patient needs to be aware that alopecia areata has a variable and often unpredictable course.

Discoid lupus erythematosus

Definition and etiology

Discoid lupus erythematosus is an autoimmune disorder that causes scarring alopecia of the scalp.

Clinical features

Discoid lupus erythematosus causes scarring plaques on the scalp, head, trunk, and extremities. The preferential distribution is in sun-exposed areas. Five to ten per cent of patients with discoid lupus erythematosus also have systemic disease.

The examination reveals oval scarring patches of alopecia, with an active erythematous border and white atrophic center. Within the plaques, prominent keratin-filled hair follicles and telangiectasia are present.

The differential diagnosis of scarring alopecia includes lichen planus and malignant tumor. It should be fairly easy to differentiate discoid lupus erythematosus from nonscarring types of alopecia, such as alopecia areata. Biopsy findings, usually diagnostic for discoid lupus erythematosus, reveal an atrophic epidermis and dystrophic hair follicles without hair shafts. A lymphocytic infiltrate characteristically occurs at the dermal/ epidermal junction, where hydropic degeneration of the basal cells occurs. The infiltrate is also distributed in a patchy manner around dermal vessels and hair follicles. In addition to general history and physical examination, a complete blood count, platelet count, urinalysis, complete metabolic profile and antinuclear antibody testing are done to rule out systemic lupus erythematosus.

Treatment (Table 1.3)

The initial treatment of discoid lupus erythematosus is application of a potent topical or intralesional corticosteroid. When this fails to control the inflammatory process, the use of antimalarials such as hydroxychloroquine is indicated.

Table 1.3 Treatment of discoid lupus erythematosus

Treatment	Precautions
Universal	
Sun protection – sunscreens, hat	None
Mild/moderate disease	
Clobetasol solution 0.5% bid	Atrophy
Triamcinolone 10 mg/ml intralesional	Atrophy
Tacrolimus ointment 0.1% bid	Burning sensation
Severe disease	
Hydroxychloroquine 200 mg bid	Periodic eye exam
Immunosuppressants: azathioprine, methotrexate, mycophenolate mofetil, thalidomide	Numerous

Psoriasis

Definition and etiology

Psoriasis is an inflammatory disease characterized by increased proliferation of the epidermis. The cause of psoriasis is unknown, but abnormal epidermal kinetics as well as activation of the immune system within the skin must be taken into account.

Clinical features

Approximately one-third of patients have a family history positive for psoriasis. This is a relatively common skin disease affecting approximately 2-5% of the population of the United States. The most common time of onset is in the third decade of life, but it can present at any time. The major precipitating or aggravating factors include streptococcal pharyngitis, trauma to the skin, emotional stress, and use of drugs such as β-blocking agents and lithium. The examination reveals sharply demarcated, erythematous, silvery, scaling plaques without associated alopecia. The extensor surfaces of the elbows and knees are typically involved, and dystrophic nail changes occur as well. The differential diagnosis of psoriasis of the scalp includes seborrheic dermatitis, tinea capitis, histiocytosis X, and atopic dermatitis. Usually, a skin biopsy is not necessary. If a biopsy is done, however, characteristic findings will include hyperkeratosis, parakeratosis, acanthotic epidermis, inflammatory infiltrate in the dermis, and neutrophils migrating into the epidermis, forming microabscesses.

Treatment (Table 1.4)

Psoriasis of the scalp is more difficult to treat than it is elsewhere because delivery of the therapeutic agent is more difficult. Treatment modalities include topical preparations (solution or foam) containing steroids, tars, and anthralin. For thick, scaling plaques, fluocinolone 0.05% oil (Derma-smooth FS oil) is used to remove the scale. Severe cases are treated with systemic/ biologic agents.

Seborrheic dermatitis

Definition and etiology

Seborrheic dermatitis is a common chronic eczematous process predominantly affecting the scalp, eyebrows, face, and, to a lesser extent, other hairy regions of the body. The cause is thought to be an inflammatory reaction to the lipid-loving yeast, *Pityrosporum ovale*.

Clinical features

Seborrheic dermatitis has a waxing and waning course with a variable amount of pruritus. It occurs in infancy and after puberty when the sebaceous glands secrete sebum, which encourages the growth of *Pityrosporum ovale*. Seborrheic dermatitis has been associated with Parkinson's disease and acquired immunodeficiency syndrome (AIDS). Rarely, seborrheic dermatitis can be generalized, resulting in exfoliative dermatitis.

Physical examination demonstrates the predilection of seborrheic dermatitis for the hairy, sebaceous-gland-rich regions of the body. Characteristically, the scalp, eyebrows, eyelids, nasolabial creases, ears, and chest are involved. This distribution is distinctive and helps to differentiate this disease from other scaling or eczematous eruptions. Patches of seborrheic dermatitis are characterized by ill-marginated borders, mild to moderate erythema, and yellow or white, greasy, fine scaling. Alopecia does not occur. The mildest form of seborrheic dermatitis without inflammation is the fine, white scaling of dandruff.

Table 1.4 Treatment of psoriasis

Treatment	Precautions
Mild disease	
Moisturizers	None
Tars, anthralin	Stain, irritation
Hydrocortisone cream/ointment 1% bid	Rarely causes allergic contact dermatitis
Pimecrolimus cream 1% bid	Burning sensation
Moderate disease	
Ultra violet light – nUVB 2–3 times/week	Burn, skin cancer
Triamcinolone cream/ointment 0.1% bid	Atrophy with chronic application
Tacrolimus ointment 0.1% bid	Burning sensation
Calcipotriene cream/ointment	None/slight irritation
Fluocinolone 0.05% oil (Derma-smooth FS oil)	None
Apremilast 30 mg bid	Weight loss, diarrhea, nausea, headache, depression
Severe disease	
Clobetasol cream/ointment 0.5%	Atrophy with chronic application
Ultra violet light – nUVB 2–3 times/week	Burn, skin cancer
Acitretin 25 mg daily	Dry skin, hair loss, elevated serum lipids, birth defects, check periodic liver function tests
Methotrexate 10–20 mg once a week	Bone marrow suppression, liver toxicity/cirrhosis, nausea /diarrhea,
Biologics (etanercept, adalimumab, infliximab, ustekinumab, secukinumab)	Infection, possible increase in lymphoma, injection site reactions, etc.

Table 1.5 Treatment of seborrheic dermatitis

Treatment	Precautions
Universal	
Shampoo – zinc pyrithione 1%, selenium sulfide 1% or 2.5%, ketoconazole 1% or 2%	None
Mild disease	
Hydrocortisone cream/ointment 1% bid	Rarely causes allergic contact dermatitis
Pimecrolimus cream 1%	Burning sensation
Moderate/severe disease	
Triamcinolone cream/ointment 0.1% bid Clobetasol cream/ointment/solution 0.5% bid	Atrophy with chronic application
Tacrolimus ointment 0.1%	Burning sensation
Short course of oral antifungal such as itraconazole	Follow for liver toxicity, drug interactions

The differential diagnosis of seborrheic dermatitis of the scalp includes psoriasis, tinea capitis, Langerhans cell histiocytosis , and atopic dermatitis. Usually, the ill-marginated patches and disease distribution (involving the face) make the diagnosis of seborrheic dermatitis straightforward. Biopsy is rarely performed because it reveals only nonspecific dermatitis.

Treatment (Table 1.5)

Use of an antiseborrheic shampoo containing zinc pyrithione, selenium sulfide, or ketoconazole is the treatment of choice. For patients with a form of disease that is more inflammatory and more pruritic, a topical steroid is added.

Stress-induced alopecia (telogen effluvium)

Definition and etiology

An alteration in the normal hair cycle that results in excessive loss of telogen (resting) hairs is characteristic of stress-induced alopecia. It is also referred to as *telogen effluvium*. This alteration of the hair cycle is precipitated by marked emotional or physiologic stress.

Clinical features

The onset of stress-induced alopecia occurs 2–3 months after the causative stressful event, which may be high fever, childbirth, major surgery, or a severe emotional disorder. The growing anagen hairs are prematurely converted to resting telogen hairs, which are then shed. These patients are distressed because their hair is coming out by the 'handful' after shampooing and combing.

Close physical examination reveals diffuse mild thinning of the hair that may not be readily apparent to the health professional. The scalp is normal without inflammation or scaling. A hair pull test, which is accomplished by gently pulling 2–3 dozen hairs, will result in the loss of more than five hairs, when normally only 1 or 2 hairs pull out. A loss of 400 to 500 hairs daily is not uncommon (Fewer than 100 is normal).

The differential diagnosis of stress-induced alopecia includes alopecia areata, systemic lupus erythematosus, abnormal thyroid function, drug-induced disease, androgenic alopecia, and nutritional deficiencies involving essential fatty acids, biotin, or zinc. Although a biopsy is usually not done, biopsy findings will show that more than 25% of the hairs are telogenic. Appropriate laboratory studies and history taking will rule out other causes of diffuse alopecia.

Treatment (Table 1.6)

For most patients with stress-induced alopecia, the stressful event is short-lived, and reassurance is all that is required.

Tinea capitis

Definition and etiology

Tinea capitis is a superficial fungal infection of the scalp caused by dermatophytes – usually *Trichophyton tonsurans* and *Microsporum canis*. *Trichophyton tonsurans* is the most common cause of tinea capitis in the United States, particularly in urban black children, thought to be a result both of geography and ethnicity, probably owing in part to structural differences in the hair. *Microsporum canis* is the most common causative organism worldwide.

Table 1.6 Treatment of stress-induced alopecia

Treatment	Precautions
Reassure not going bald	Do not miss a systemic cause: thyroid dysfunction, drug-induced, diffuse alopecia areata
Minoxidil 5% foam bid	May get unwanted hair growth, irritation

Clinical features

Human to human spread of *Trichophyton tonsurans* results in epidemics of tinea capitis. The fungus can be cultured from hairs and scales found on combs, hats, and brushes. *Microsporum canis* is spread from cats and dogs to humans and is sporadic in occurrence.

The clinical appearance of tinea capitis varies. Sometimes it may appear as a mild to moderate, diffuse, scaling, seborrheic-like dermatitis with minimal inflammation. At other times, there may be inflamed, scaling patches of alopecia containing broken hair shafts (black dots) and indurated, boggy, purulent plaques of alopecia referred to as *kerion*. Prominent cervical adenopathy is commonly associated with inflammatory tinea capitis.

The differential diagnosis of tinea capitis includes seborrheic dermatitis, alopecia areata, trichotillomania, psoriasis, and bacterial scalp infection. Results of a potassium hydroxide (KOH) preparation or fungal culture confirm the diagnosis of tinea capitis.

Treatment (Table 1.7)

Effective treatment of tinea capitis requires oral antifungal agents. Topical preparations are inadequate. For children, griseofulvin, 20–25 mg/kg daily for 6–8 weeks, is usually effective. Additionally, shampooing with ketoconazole and selenium sulfide several times a week is helpful in reducing the number of viable fungal spores. An alternative medication is oral terbinafine. In some instances, asymptomatic family members should also be treated because they may be carriers of *T. tonsurans*. Household pets should also be examined for the presence of a dermatophyte infection.

Trichotillomania

Definition and etiology

Trichotillomania is a self-induced traumatic alopecia that results from pulling, plucking, and breaking one's own hair.

Clinical features

Trichotillomania affects children and adults, predominantly female, who have emotional or psychiatric problems. In children, sibling rivalry, mental retardation, hospitalization, or discord at home or in school can trigger trichotillomania. In adults, it is usually a sign of a personality disorder, sometime severe.

Coarse-feeling broken hairs or stubble are characteristic of trichotillomania. The scalp is normal without inflammation or scarring.

Table 1.7 Treatment of tinea capitis

Treatment (confirm diagnosis with fungal culture)	Precautions
Ketoconazole shampoo 1% or 2% Selenium shampoo 2.5%	None
Terbinafine: 62.5 mg for less than 20 kg, 125 mg for 20–40 kg, 250 mg for greater than 40 kg, daily for 6–8 weeks	Rare hepatic toxicity. CBC and liver function tests at baseline
Griseofulvin 20–25 mg/kg daily for 6–8 weeks	Rare hepatic toxicity
CBC, complete blood count	

Table 1.8 Treatment of trichotillomania

Treatment
Mild/moderate disease
Supportive emotionally
Severe disease
Psychiatric referral – clomipramine, SSRI's

Ill-marginated, irregularly shaped patches of alopecia are the most common presentation. In some individuals, however, almost all the scalp hair has been pulled, plucked, or broken, resulting in a rim of normal hair in the periphery referred to as the 'Friar Tuck' sign. The eyebrows and eyelashes may also be plucked.

The differential diagnosis includes tinea capitis, alopecia areata, and secondary syphilis. The clinical examination is usually enough to establish the diagnosis, but occasionally a biopsy is required. Examination reveals normally growing hairs, empty hair follicles in a noninflamed dermis, and traumatized follicles with broken or no hair and perifollicular hemorrhage.

Treatment (Table 1.8)

Treatment is generally supportive. Insight into the self-induced nature of the disorder should be provided. In children, the condition is usually self-limited. In adults, however, trichotillomania may be a sign of a severe emotional or mental disturbance requiring a psychiatric referral. Clomipramine, a tricyclic antidepressant, or selective serotonin-reuptake inhibitors appear to have a role in the short-term treatment of this obsessive–compulsive disorder.

Chapter 2 Face

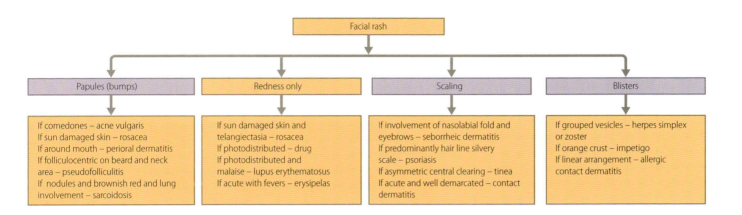

INTRODUCTION

Of the many locations affected by dermatologic diseases, from a patient's and a cosmetic perspective, facial rashes are most important. Patients frequently ignore or are content not to treat inconspicuous cosmetic rashes like tinea pedis, but may be distressed by even a single pimple on the face. The face is involved in many different dermatologic diseases because it contains numerous sebaceous glands and is constantly exposed to the environment. Diseases involving the follicular-sebaceous gland apparatus include seborrheic dermatitis, acne vulgaris, pseudofolliculitis barbae, and acne rosacea. Exposure to sunlight can result in photodistributed rashes such as polymorphous light eruption, photocontact dermatitis, and lupus erythematosus. Exposure to chemicals found in cosmetics and other products can produce contact dermatitis.

1. ACNE VULGARIS VERSUS ACNE ROSACEA

■ Features in common: red papules and pustules

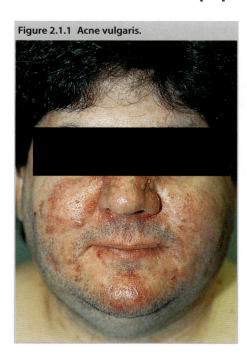

Figure 2.1.1 Acne vulgaris.

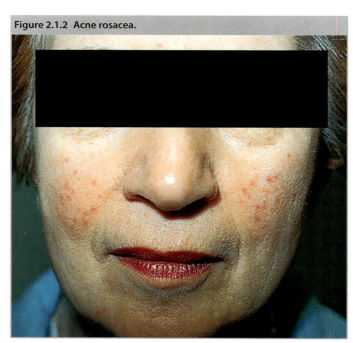

Figure 2.1.2 Acne rosacea.

■ Distinguishing features

	Acne vulgaris	Acne rosacea
Physical examination Morphology	Primary lesion is comedo Telangiectasias not prominent Nodular-cystic lesions may be present No background erythema No rhinophyma	Comedones rarely found Telangiectasias often prominent No cystic lesions Mainly erythema and easy blushing Rhinophyma in advanced cases
Distribution	Involves face, back, chest	Affects face, eyelids, rarely axilla
History Symptoms Exacerbating factors	No history of easy blushing Cosmetics and chemicals Medications: androgens, lithium, corticosteroids	Occasionally history of easy blushing Sunlight, spicy foods, heat, cold, steroid creams
Associated findings	None, occasionally signs of androgen excess: hirsutism, oily skin	Conjunctivitis
Epidemiology	Primarily affects teenagers and young adults Family history of acne may be present	Primarily affects adults Frequently found in fair-skinned patients of Celtic origin
Biopsy	Follicular plugging	Perivascular and perifollicular mixed inflammatory infiltrate, telangiectatic blood vessels
Laboratory	None In case of suspected androgen excess: testosterone, free testosterone, dehydroepiandrosterone testing	None Frequently demodex organisms within hair follicles
Outcome	Chronic; end result of severe acne may be depressed icepick-like scars	Chronic; end result of severe rosacea in men is rhinophyma

Differential diagnosis of acneiform eruption

Common causes
- Acne rosacea
- Acne vulgaris
- Drug-induced acne
  - Androgens
  - Corticosteroids
  - Dilantin
  - Epidermal growth factor inhibitors
  - Halogenoderma
  - Lithium
  - Isoniazid
  - Braf inhibitors and Mek inhibitors
- Perioral dermatitis
- Pseudofolliculitis barbae
- Tinea faciei

Rarer causes and mimickers
- Adenoma sebaceum (tuberous sclerosis)
- Androgen excess (due to tumors or genetic factors)
- Favre–Racouchot disease (actinic comedones)
- Fibrous papule
- Haber's syndrome
- Lupus miliaris disseminatum faciei (may be variant of rosacea)
- Nevus comedonicus
- Pyoderma faciale
- Sebaceous hyperplasia
- Sycosis barbae
- Trichodiscomas
- Trichoepitheliomas

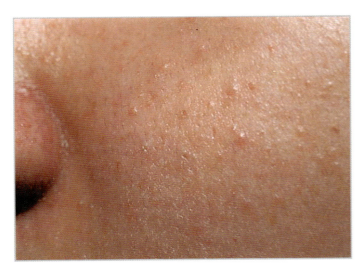

Figure 2.1.3 Acne vulgaris. *Clue to diagnosis:* comedones.

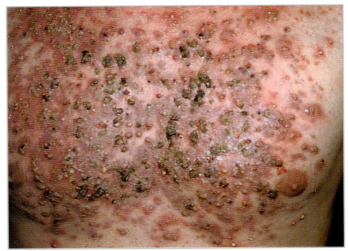

Figure 2.1.4 Acne vulgaris. *Clue to diagnosis:* cysts.

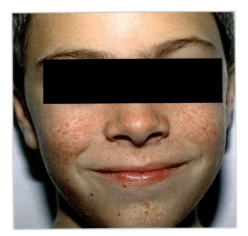

Figure 2.1.5 Adenoma sebaceum mimicking acne vulgaris.

2. ACNE ROSCEA VERSUS SYSTEMIC LUPUS ERYTHEMATOSUS

■ Features in common: malar redness

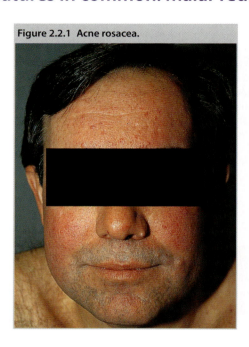

Figure 2.2.1 Acne rosacea.

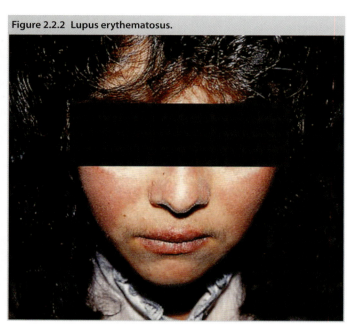

Figure 2.2.2 Lupus erythematosus.

■ Distinguishing features

	Acne rosacea	Systemic lupus erythematosus
Physical examination		
Morphology	Papules and pustules on erythematous base Rhinophyma in severe cases No discoid lesions seen	No papules or pustules No rhinophyma Occasionally discoid lesions present
Distribution	Face, chest, back	Central face, sun-exposed skin
History		
Symptoms	Patient asymptomatic; occasionally discomfort from papular-cystic lesions	Generalized malaise
Exacerbating factors	Sunlight, food, alcohol, heat, cold Also exacerbated by topical steroids	Occasionally drug-induced: hydralazine, procainamide
Associated findings	Conjunctivitis	Arthritis, pleurisy, renal insufficiency, anemia, central nervous system disorders, cardiac disorders
Epidemiology	Adults; predilection for men	Adults, much more common in women
Biopsy	No Perivascular and periappendiceal mixed inflammatory infiltrate Telangiectatic blood vessels	Occasionally Epidermal atrophy, hydropic changes, follicular plugging, superficial and deep lymphocytic infiltrate
Laboratory	None	Testing for antinuclear antibodies, anti-ds DNA, anti-Sm antibody, RO and LA antigens, and complement levels; complete blood count, platelet count, urinalysis
Outcome	Chronic	Chronic relapsing disease; in acute lupus erythematosus lesions heal without scarring

Differential diagnosis of macular facial rashes

Common causes
- Acne rosacea
- Contact dermatitis
- Photocontact dermatitis
- Phototoxic drug eruption
- Polymorphous light eruption
- Lupus erythematosus
- Seborrheic dermatitis
- Tinea faciei

Rarer causes
- Actinic reticuloid (chronic photosensitive dermatitis)
- Dermatomyositis
- Erysipelas
- Herpes zoster
- Keratosis pilaris atrophicans
- Leprosy
- Leishmaniasis
- Lupus pernio (sarcoidosis)
- Lymphoma
- Pemphigus foliaceus/erythematosus

Causes of facial flushing

- Rosacea
- Physiological/emotional
- Alcohol/drugs
- Foods: Chinese restaurant syndrome (reaction to monosodium glutamate)
- Carcinoid
- Mastocytosis
- Other rare tumors: medullary carcinoma thyroid, insulinoma, rare pancreatic
- POEMS syndrome (polyneuropathy, organomegaly, endocrinopathy, monoclonal gammopathy, skin changes)

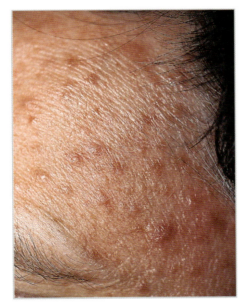

Figure 2.2.3 Rosacea. *Clue to diagnosis:* papules and pustules, but no comedones.

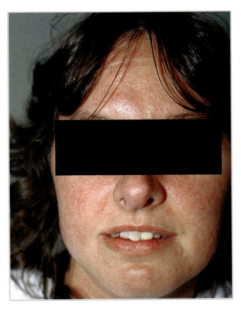

Figure 2.2.4 Lupus erythematosus: malar redness, no papules, no telangiectasias.

3. ACNE VULGARIS VERSUS PSEUDOFOLLICULITIS

■ Features in common: follicular based papules and pustules on the face

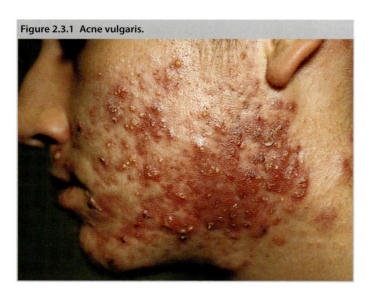

Figure 2.3.1 Acne vulgaris.

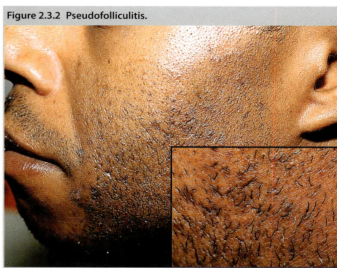

Figure 2.3.2 Pseudofolliculitis.

■ Distinguishing features

	Acne vulgaris	Pseudofolliculitis
Physical examination Morphology	Comedones present Nodular-cystic lesions may be present No ingrown hairs	No comedones No nodular-cystic lesions Ingrown hairs present
Distribution	Face, back, chest Neck rarely involved	Beard area and cheeks Neck area usually involved
History Symptoms	None	None
Exacerbating factors	Exacerbated by some cosmetics, chemicals, occlusion Drugs: see 'Differential diagnosis of acneiform eruption'	Exacerbated by shaving
Associated findings	Occasionally signs of androgen excess: hirsutism, oily skin Curly hairs (if present) coincidence	No androgen excess Majority of patients have curly hairs
Epidemiology	Primarily affects teenagers and young adults Genetic predisposition in many patients	Most common in black men Genetic predisposition may be present
Biopsy	No Follicular plugging with surrounding inflammation	No Hairs penetrating skin or hair shaft
Laboratory	None In case of suspected androgen excess: testosterone, free testosterone, dehydroepiandrosterone testing	None
Outcome	Chronic; end result of severe acne icepick-like scars	Chronic; may result in scars

4. SEBORRHEIC DERMATITIS VERSUS CONTACT DERMATITIS

■ Features in common: redness and scaling

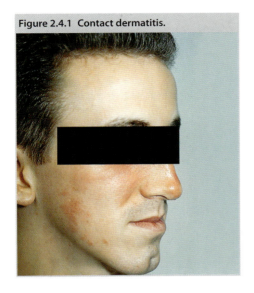

Figure 2.4.1 Contact dermatitis.

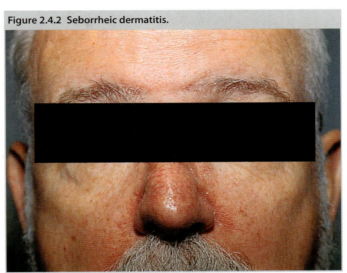

Figure 2.4.2 Seborrheic dermatitis.

■ Distinguishing features

	Seborrheic dermatitis	Contact dermatitis
Physical examination Morphology	Erythematous scaling patches Occasionally follicular papules No oozing or weeping No vesicles seen Yellow- to white-colored scale	Red patches with vesicles and erythematous plaques Oozing or weeping of serous fluid in established cases Vesicles may be present White-colored scale
Distribution	Involves areas with increased oil production (seborrhea): nasolabial areas, cheeks, eyebrows, scalp, axilla, anterior chest, groin	Can affect any cutaneous surface
History Symptoms	Asymptomatic or mildly pruritic	Usually very pruritic
Exacerbating factors	Infrequent washing, poor hygiene	Contact with irritant or allergen
Associated findings	Underlying diseases may be present such as human immunodeficiency virus infection, cardiac disease or Parkinson's disease	No associated disease
Epidemiology	Generally affects neonates, middle-aged, or older patients	Affects any age group
Biopsy	Epidermal spongiosis, parakeratotic mounds around follicular infundibuli	Epidermal spongiosis, parakeratotic mounds, superficial inflammatory infiltrate with few eosinophils
Laboratory	None	Patch testing
Outcome	Chronic; no scarring; good response to therapy	Self-limited once exposure to irritant or allergen halted

Differential diagnosis of red scaly seborrheic dermatitis-like eruptions

Common causes
- Contact dermatitis
- Lupus erythematosus
- Rosacea
- Photodermatitis
- Psoriasis (sebopsoriasis)
- Seborrheic dermatitis
- Tinea faciei

Rarer causes
- Histiocytosis X
- Leishmaniasis
- Leprosy
- Pellagra
- Pemphigus foliaceus/erythematosus
- Riboflavin, biotin, or pyridoxine deficiency
- Tuberculosis

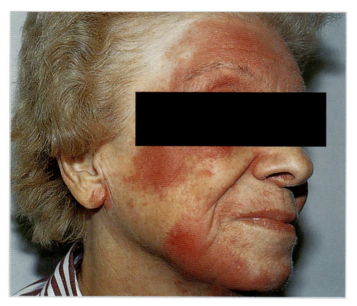

Figure 2.4.3 Contact dermatitis due to fragrance. *Clue to diagnosis:* well-circumscribed, geometric shape.

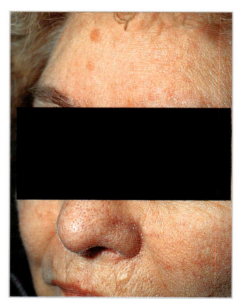

Figure 2.4.4 Seborrheic dermatitis: flaking of nasolabial folds.

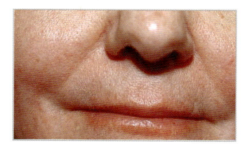

Figure 2.4.5 Contact dermatitis of the lips.

5. IMPETIGO CONTAGIOSA VERSUS HERPES SIMPLEX

Features in common: vesicles

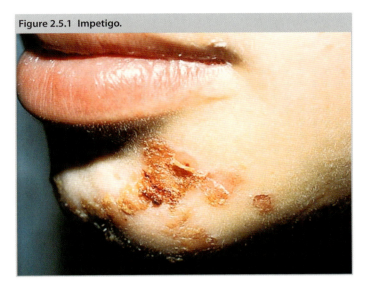

Figure 2.5.1 Impetigo.

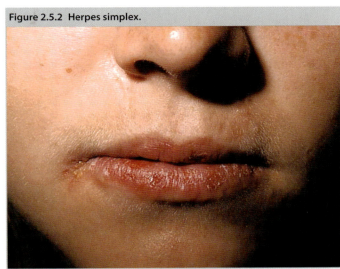

Figure 2.5.2 Herpes simplex.

Distinguishing features

	Impetigo contagiosa	Herpes simplex
Physical examination		
Morphology	Bullae may be present Blisters contain pus Blisters not grouped Blisters not umbilicated No scalloped borders Golden-orange-colored crust	No bullae No pus unless secondarily infected Blisters grouped Umbilicated blisters Scalloped borders Crust red-colored
Distribution	Any glabrous portion, frequently on face	Any skin surface, most frequently on lip
History		
Symptoms	No prodromal symptoms Not associated with fever	Prodromal tingling or burning sensation in most cases Primary lesions may be associated with fever and malaise
Exacerbating factors	Usually not recurrent Immunosuppression	May be recurrent Immunosuppression
Associated findings	None	Occasionally lymphadenopathy
Epidemiology	Most common in children	Common in children and adults
Biopsy	No Subcorneal pustule containing gram-positive organisms	No Ballooning necrosis of keratinocytes with multinucleated giant cells
Laboratory	Bacterial culture	Viral culture Tzanck preparation
Outcome	Excellent; heals without scarring	Good; no scarring, but may be recurrent

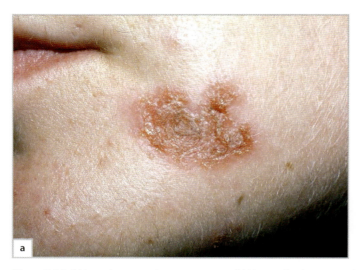 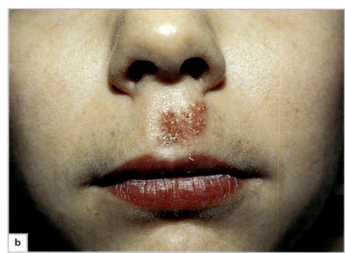

Figure 2.5.3 (a) Impetigo contagiosa: orange crust. (b) Herpes simplex: grouped vesicles.

6. POLYMORPHOUS LIGHT ERUPTION VERSUS LUPUS ERYTHEMATOSUS

Features in common: Red papules and plaques in sun-exposed skin, exacerbated by sunlight, polymorphous light eruption can clinically be confused with both discoid lupus erythematosus and systemic lupus erythematosus

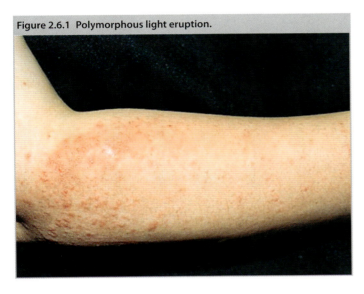

Figure 2.6.1 Polymorphous light eruption.

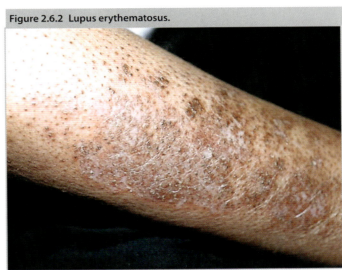

Figure 2.6.2 Lupus erythematosus.

Distinguishing features

	Polymorphous light eruption	Lupus erythematosus
Physical examination Morphology	Urticarial papules, vesicular eczematous plaques No atrophy, telangiectasias, or follicular plugging No pigmentary changes *Note:* Lesions of subacute lupus erythematosus indistinguishable from lesions of PMLE	Round, 'discoid' plaques Atrophy, follicular plugging telangiectasias present Hyper- and hypopigmentation frequently present
Distribution	Sun-exposed sites	Sun-exposed and also protected sites
History Symptoms	Eruption starts in spring Symptoms vary from burning to pruritus	Eruption may start any time of year Arthralgias, malaise if associated with systemic lupus erythematosus
Exacerbating factors	Sunlight	Sunlight Medications
Associated findings	None	Arthritis, hair loss, mouth ulcers, renal disease
Epidemiology	Children and young adults; more common in females	Young adults; more common in females
Biopsy	No Superficial and deep lymphocytic infiltrate with edema in papillary dermis	Occasionally Superficial and deep lymphocytic infiltrate Epidermal atrophy, follicular plugging, hydropic changes
Laboratory	Antinuclear antibody, SSA (Ro), SSB (LA) antigen tests negative; lesions sometimes reproduced by phototesting	Antinuclear antibody testing positive; frequently SSA (Ro) and SSB (La) antigen testing positive; low white blood cell and hemoglobin levels; platelets, urinalysis
Outcome	Chronic; nonscarring disease; tends to worsen with age	Chronic scarring disease

Differential diagnosis of photodistributed rashes

Common causes
- Lupus erythematosus
- Photocontact dermatitis
- Phototoxic drug eruption
- Phytophotodermatitis
- Polymorphous light eruption

Rarer causes
- Actinic reticuloid
- Actinic prurigo
- Dermatomyositis
- Hydroa vacciniforme
- Porphyria
- Photodistributed psoriasis
- Pellagra

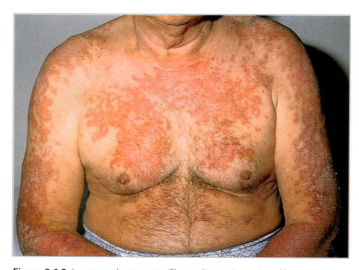

Figure 2.6.3 Lupus erythematosus. *Clue to diagnosis:* psoriasis-like photodistributed rash.

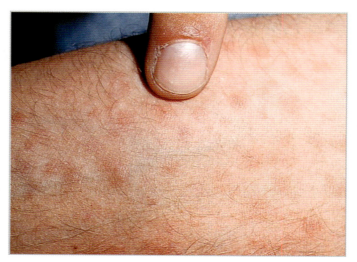

Figure 2.6.4 Polymorphous light eruption. *Clue to diagnosis:* urticarial-like papules.

7. SEBORRHEIC DERMATITIS VERSUS LUPUS ERYTHEMATOSUS

■ Features in common: red, scaly rash in malar distribution

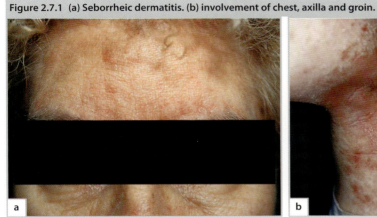

Figure 2.7.1 (a) Seborrheic dermatitis. (b) involvement of chest, axilla and groin.

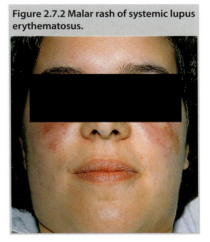

Figure 2.7.2 Malar rash of systemic lupus erythematosus.

■ Distinguishing features

	Seborrheic dermatitis	Lupus erythematosus
Physical examination Morphology	Persistent erythema	Acute cutaneous LE: transient erythema in malar area, minimal scaling
	Yellow- to white-colored, greasy- appearing scale	Chronic discoid LE: atrophy, telangiectasias, follicular plugging in round scaly plaques
	Telangiectasias due to sun damage	Telangiectasias in lesions
	Scaling and erythema most prominent in nasolabial fold	Nasolabial area usually spared
Distribution	Scalp, eyebrows, anterior chest, nasolabial area, occasionally axilla and groin	Sun-exposed sites and occasionally non-exposed sites
History Symptoms	Asymptomatic	If systemic disease: malaise, arthritis, pleurisy, fatigue
Exacerbating factors	Infrequent washing No medications	Sunlight Medications: procainamide, hydralazine
Associated findings	Parkinson's disease, human immunodeficiency virus infection, cardiac disease No associated physical findings	Arthritis, renal disease, anemia, pleurisy Diffuse or patchy hair loss Periungual telangiectasias Oral ulcers
Epidemiology	Older adults	Young adults, female predominance
Biopsy	No Superficial perivascular dermatitis with parakeratotic mounds around follicular orifices	Yes Superficial and deep perivascular and periappendiceal lymphocytic infiltrate Epidermal atrophy, telangiectasia, follicular plugging in DLE
Laboratory	None	Antinuclear antibody, anti-DS DNA, SS-A and SS-B antigen testing, complete blood count with differential; urinalysis
Outcome	Chronic; but nonscarring; good response to therapy	Chronic; may leave scars; fair response to therapy

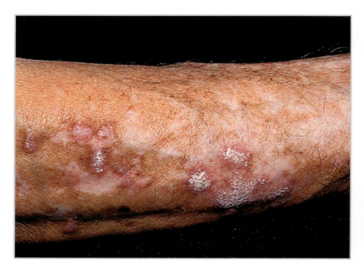

Figure 2.7.3 Cutaneous lupus erythematosus can also present with discoid 'round' scarring lesions.

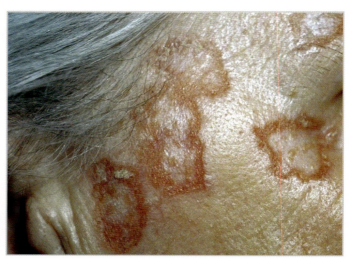

Figure 2.7.4 Cutaneous lupus erythematosus.

8. PERIORAL DERMATITIS VERSUS CONTACT DERMATITIS

Features in common: red, scaly patches and plaques on face

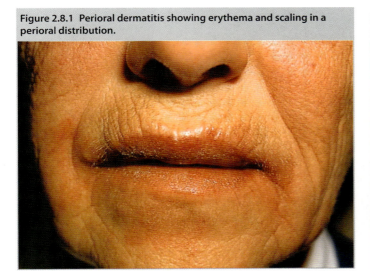

Figure 2.8.1 Perioral dermatitis showing erythema and scaling in a perioral distribution.

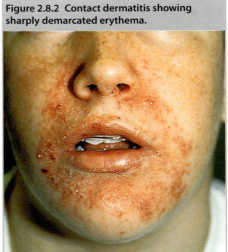

Figure 2.8.2 Contact dermatitis showing sharply demarcated erythema.

Distinguishing features

	Perioral dermatitis	Contact dermatitis
Physical examination		
Morphology	Erythema, scaling, and papules distributed around the mouth Pustules No geometric shape	Erythema, scaling, and vesicles in area of contact No pustules Eruption may have sharp borders or geometric shape
Distribution	Rim of normal skin surrounding mouth Perioral, rarely periocular	No area of sparing No particular distribution
History		
Symptoms	Little or no pruritus	Severe pruritus frequent
Exacerbating factors	Topical steroids	Fragrances and preservatives in cosmetics or toiletries are most common culprits
Associated findings	None	None
Epidemiology	Adult women	Any age or sex
Biopsy	No Spongiotic dermatitis with granulomatous folliculitis	No Spongiotic dermatitis
Laboratory	None	Patch testing
Outcome	Chronic Resolves over several months with therapy	Curable Rapid improvement over 1 to 2 weeks with therapy and avoidance of contactant

Possible causes of contact dermatitis of the face based on location

- Entire face: Cosmetics and topical pharmaceuticals
- Eyelids: Nail cosmetics, adhesives for artificial nails, eyedrops, mascara
- Nose: Eyeglasses, handkerchiefs, nasal medications
- Forehead: Hair care products
- Lips, perioral area: Lipstick, oral medications, foods
- Chin, beard area: Shaving products, chin straps

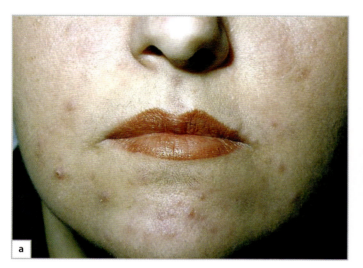 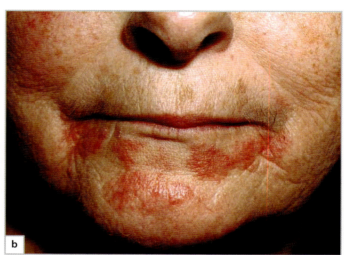

Figure 2.8.3 (a, b) Perioral dermatitis.

DISEASE DISCUSSION

Acne vulgaris

Definition and etiology
Acne is a follicular disease that is a result of blockage of pilosebaceous units by keratinous material and sebum. This forms a comedo, the primary lesion in acne. Subsequent inflammation results in papules, pustules, nodules, and cysts.

Clinical features
The blocked pore in acne becomes enlarged and produces a clinically visible comedo. If the opening of the pore is visible, the comedo clinically appears to be filled with black-colored debris known as a blackhead. If the pore opening is not visible, the comedo looks like a small white- to yellow-colored papule, the whitehead. The inflammatory response to colonization of the comedo by *Propionibacterium acnes* produces papular and pustular lesions. Rupture of the blocked pore produces nodular-cystic lesions. In an individual patient, the lesions may primarily be comedonal, papulopustular, cystic, or a combination of different types. The severity of acne can also be modulated by hormonal changes; hence, the onset during puberty. Other exacerbating factors include use of cosmetics such as hair pomade, occupational exposure to oils or occlusive chemicals, and use of medications like lithium and phenytoin (Dilantin) and epidermal growth factor, Mek and Braf inhibitors. Clinically, acne vulgaris is most commonly confused with acne rosacea. However, acne rosacea primarily affects middle-aged adults, and comedones are not present.

Treatment (Table 2.1)
Patients before seeing a physician have used some topical over the counter medications which usually contain salicylic acid, glycolic acids, or benzyl peroxide. The standard prescription treatment for acne is a combination of retinoids, antibiotics, and benzoyl peroxide. Topical retinoids help unclog the pores and prevent comedo formation; benzoyl peroxide has bacteriostatic and comedolytic activity; and antibiotics kill *Propionibacterium acnes*. Topical therapy with azelaic acid and sulfur preparations is also effective. Azelaic acid is class B unlike the other topical agents, and can be safely used in pregnant women. In severe nodular-cystic and scarring acne, oral therapy with a vitamin A derivative, *cis*-retinoic acid (Accutane), is very effective.

Acne rosacea

Definition and etiology
Rosacea, like acne, is a follicular disease of unknown origin. However, unlike acne, a vascular component is present, and comedones are not seen. The cause of rosacea is unclear, but most likely due to sun damage. Various potential etiologic factors include familial predisposition, psychogenic factors, sunlight, *Demodex* organisms, vasoactive peptides, and cell mediated and humoral immunity.

Clinical features
Acne rosacea is an asymptomatic but cosmetically bothersome disease of adults. Four clinical stages have been described in rosacea. In the first stage, intermittent flushing occurs. In the next stage, the erythema becomes persistent, and telangiectasias develop. In the third stage, papules and pustules develop. In the final stage (which rarely occurs), rhinophyma, which is enlargement of the nasal connective

Table 2.1 Treatment for acne vulgaris

Treatment	Precautions
Mild disease	
Tretinoin cream (0.025%, 0.05%, 0.1%)	Apply on dry skin and small amount or may be too irritation
Tretinoin gel (0.01%, 0.025%)	Apply on dry skin and small amount or may be too irritation
Adapalene cream (0.1%)	Apply at night-time since light may inactivate
Adapalene gel (0.1, 0.3%)	Do not pimple dab since trying to prevent new lesions
Moderate disease	
Use one of above and add Benzyl peroxide 2.5, 5 or 10% and/or Topical antibiotics Clindamycin 1% gel, lotion or solution bid Erythromycin 2% solution or gel	May be irritating: rare allergic reactions
Combination creams Epiduo (adapalene/benzoyl peroxide) Benzaclin/onexton (clindamycin/benzoyl peroxide) Ziana/Veltin (clindamycin/tretinoin) Benzamycin (benzyl peroxide/erythromycin)	Irritating, and may be very expensive
Severe disease	
Add oral antibiotics Minocycline 50–100 mg bid Doxycycline 20, 50–100 mg bid	Photosensitivity: can produce blue discoloration of gums and skin Rare lupus like syndrome with fevers, malaise, rash Photosensitivity Esophagitis Vaginal yeast infections
Other considerations for females	
Oral contraception	Risk of stroke, thrombus especially in smokers and older females
Spironolactone 25–50 mg bid	Avoid pregnancy
Chronic scarring or nodular acne	
Isotretinoin 0.5–1 mg/kg/day divided doses for 15–20 weeks	Class X: causes birth defects Xerosis, myalgias Rare pseudotumor cerebri Rare reports of depression and suicide Rare reports of coexistent or worsening of inflammatory bowel disease Check liver function tests and lipids, monthly pregnancy test
Miscellaneous treatments	
Azelaic acid 20% cream	Only treatment that is class B and can safely be used during pregnancy
Dapsone 5% gel	Alternative topical if allergic to others

tissue, develops, producing an enlarged, distorted nose. Clinically, because of the presence of papules, rosacea can be confused with acne. Acne rosacea is also commonly misdiagnosed as systemic lupus erythematosus because of the presence of erythema. The malar erythema in systemic lupus erythematosus is transient, and patients also suffer from systemic symptoms. Raynaud's phenomenon is commonly experienced. In discoid lupus erythematosus, atrophy, pigmentary changes, and follicular plugging occur.

Treatment (Table 2.2)

Treatment options for rosacea include oral doxycycline, topical metronidazole cream, retinoids, topical ivermectin, and sulfur preparations. For facial erythema brimonidine gel and oxymetzoline cream have recently been introduced. In patients with rhinophyma, use of the CO_2 laser or scalpel paring can be effective.

Contact dermatitis

Definition and etiology

Contact dermatitis is inflammation of the skin resulting from the interaction between the skin and chemicals. Contact dermatitis can be either an irritant type or an allergic type. Irritant contact dermatitis is a nonimmunologic reaction to a chemical that irritates the skin and causes inflammation. Conversely, allergic contact dermatitis is an individualized immunologic response to the chemical (i.e. the person who is allergic to the chemical will develop a rash when the chemical is absorbed through the skin, whereas another person who is not allergic to the chemical will not develop a rash upon contact). Irritant contact dermatitis is most frequently seen in the hands, whereas allergic contact dermatitis can occur in any part of the body in contact with the allergen.

Clinical features

In acute cases, erythema, scaling, vesicles, and swelling can be found. In patients with persistent disease, the erythema and scaling persist even though vesicles can no longer be found, and the skin becomes lichenified. The differential diagnosis includes acne rosacea, seborrheic dermatitis, perioral dermatitis, lupus erythematosus, pemphigus erythematosus, and tinea faciei. In pemphigus erythematosus, erosions may be found, and a biopsy for immunofluorescence demonstrates characteristic intercellular immunofluorescent staining pattern. Tinea faciei can be excluded by a negative potassium hydroxide (KOH) scraping or fungal culture. Since both irritant and allergic contact dermatitis can morphologically appear identical, patch testing remains the test of choice in confirming the diagnosis of allergic contact dermatitis. Contact dermatitis of the face can be a result of direct application of a pharmaceutical product, contact with a surface such as a pillow, or contact with airborne vapors, droplets, or dust particles. Rarely, contact dermatitis can also be transmitted from direct contact with other people ('consort' dermatitis). The allergen can also be transferred to the facial area from the hands. Eyelid dermatitis frequently occurs secondary to exposure to cosmetics in nail polish or adhesive resin used to glue on artificial nails.

Treatment (Table 2.3)

Contact dermatitis can be cured by avoidance of the appropriate allergen or irritant. Topical and oral steroids hasten the resolution of the rash.

Impetigo contagiosa

Definition and etiology

Impetigo contagiosa is a superficial blistering skin infection caused by either *Staphylococcus aureus* or *Streptococcus*.

Table 2.2 Treatment for rosacea

Treatment	Precautions
Universal	
Daily sunscreen	Patients notice the vasoconstrictive effect of steroids along with exacerbation when they stop taking them, so they may need hand-holding to wean them off such treatments
Avoid triggers	
Avoid topical steroids	
Topical therapies: mild disease	
Metronidazole 0.75% gel, lotion and cream or 1% cream and gel	Rarely irritating
Azelaic acid 15% gel bid	Occasional facial burning, stinging and itching
Sodium sulfacetamide-sulfur (a variety of combinations exist)	Some older formulations had unpleasant odor
Topical ivermectin (Soolantra Cream 1%) qd	Works best for papules and pustules. Mild irritation possible
Brimonidine 0.33% gel (Mirvaso) or 1% oxymetazoline hydrocholoride cream (Rhofade) qd	Works best for erythema. Theoretical risk of rebound redness
Systemic therapies: severe disease	
Antibiotics	
Doxycycline hyclate 20 mg bid	Higher doses may produce photosensitivity, esophagitis, and vaginal yeast infections
Tetracycline 250 mg qd	Higher doses may produce photosensitivity, esophagitis, and vaginal yeast infections
Miscellaneous therapies	
Pulsed dye therapy	Effective for erythema and telangiectasis
Surgery	Treatment of choice for rhinophyma
Isotretinoin	Treatment of last resort (see acne vulgaris)

Table 2.3 Treatment of allergic contact dermatitis

Treatment	Precautions
Universal	
Determine and avoid allergen	
Antihistamines for itching	
Oatmeal baths	
Mild-to-moderate disease	
Topical steroid such as clobetasol 0.05% cream bid	Avoid in intertriginous areas because of risk of atrophy Avoid on face since can produce steroid acne Glaucoma if applied on eyelids
Severe disease	
Systemic steroids for 2 weeks	Steroid side effects- hyperglycemia, insomnia, hypertension, fluid retention
Start at 40–60 mg prednisone a day for few days	Dermatitis may flare or recur if tapered too rapidly

Clinical features

Impetigo can occur on any cutaneous surface but frequently is seen in a perioral distribution, especially in children. Early on, a flaccid pus-filled blister may be present. Usually, since the blister occurs within the stratum corneum, it easily ruptures, and only erosions remain. The erosions are covered with an orange-colored crust. The major disease in the differential diagnosis is herpes simplex, especially since herpetic lesions can occasionally become secondarily infected. Unlike the lesions of herpes, the erosions and blisters in impetigo are large (centimeter-sized rather then millimeter-sized). The vesicles in herpes are also clustered and have scalloped borders with central umbilication. Patients with herpes infection also frequently have prodromal symptoms before lesions appear. In a primary infection, patients may also have a high fever with associated lymphadenopathy. In addition, herpes simplex may recur in the same site, whereas impetigo generally is not recurrent. In cases in which there is a diagnostic dilemma, a Tzanck preparation and culture should be performed.

Treatment (Table 2.4)

Impetigo can be treated either with topical mupirocin ointment or retapamulin ointment if localized. If the impetigo is generalized, a systemic antibiotic such as penicillin, dicloxacillin, erythromycin, or doxycycline in adults can be used. For generalized lesions the antibiotic choice is best modified or based on culture results and sensitivities.

Herpes labialis

Definition and etiology

Herpes labialis is a herpes simplex virus type 1 or (rarely) type 2 infection of the oral mucosa most commonly seen in children and young adults.

Clinical features

The eruption starts 2–10 days after subclinical exposure to herpes simplex virus. Usually, patients develop prodromal symptoms of burning, discomfort, or itching at the site of the impending eruption. In a primary episode, patients develop fever and malaise. The lesions start out as red macules on the vermilion border that rapidly become vesiculated and develop into widespread erosions. On closer inspection, the erosions are grouped and have scalloped borders characteristic of a herpesvirus infection. The lesions heal spontaneously in a few weeks.

The major diseases in the differential diagnosis are impetigo and contact dermatitis. Systemic and prodromal symptoms are rare in impetigo, the vesicles are not grouped, and scalloped borders are not seen. The golden-orange crust is also characteristic. However, clinicians should remember that herpetic lesions can become secondarily infected. In contact dermatitis, the vesicles are not grouped, bullae may be present, the rash is usually more widespread, and pruritus is very severe. In diagnostically difficult cases, the Tzanck smear should be performed; in herpes lesions, multinucleated giant cells are present. In older lesions, the Tzanck preparation results may be negative, and culture is more sensitive.

Treatment (Table 2.5)

Oral acyclovir, valacyclovir, or famciclovir, if started during the first 2 days of the infection, can limit the severity and duration of disease. Topical penciclovir cream, topical acyclovir cream, and acyclovir with hydrocortisone (Xerese) are also somewhat effective in reducing the severity of outbreaks.

Lupus erythematosus

Definition and etiology

Lupus erythematosus is an inflammatory autoimmune disease that affects the skin and extracutaneous tissue. It can be divided into relatively different homogeneous subsets. In one subset, discoid lupus erythematosus (DLE), the skin findings are the only manifestation. In subacute cutaneous lupus erythematosus, patients present with a photosensitive eruption that in approximately 50% of patients is associated with systemic disease. Systemic lupus erythematosus is a multiorgan disease. Patients can be classified into the appropriate subset based on a combination of clinical and laboratory data.

Clinical features

Lupus erythematosus occurs most frequently in young adult women. Classification of disease is independent of the morphology of the cutaneous eruption. For example, the skin lesions of discoid lupus

Table 2.4 Treatment of impetigo

Treatment	Precautions
Mild disease	
Mupirocin topical 2% cream or ointment tid x 7–14 days	Irritation
Retapamulin 1% ointment bid x 5 days	
Severe disease	
Oral antibiotics depending on culture and sensitivities	Systemic side effects possible
Consider cephalexin 500 mg bid, dicloxacillin 500 mg bid or, if methicillin resistant *Staphylococcus aureus* is a possibility, doxycycline 100 mg bid	

Table 2.5 Treatment of herpes labialis in immunocompetent patients

Treatment	Precautions
Avoid sun exposure/burn	
Topical sunscreens may help	
Mild disease	
Topicals	Less effective than systemic treatments
Acyclovir 5% cream or ointment 5 x daily for 4 days	
Penciclovir 1% cream q 2 hours while awake for 4 days	
Severe disease	
Acyclovir (200, 400, 800 mg pills) 400 mg tid for 5-10 days	Headache, nausea, diarrhea, vomiting, Rare psychosis, seizures, leukopenia, thrombocytopenia, Stevens–Johnson, TEN, etc.
Valacyclovir (500, 1000 mg pills) 2000 mg q12 x1 day	
Famciclovir (125, 250, 500 mg) 500 mg bid x 5–10 days or 1500 mg x 1	

erythematosus can be seen in patients with no systemic disease but can also be found in approximately 10% of patients with systemic disease.

The Systemic Lupus International Collaborating Clinics (SLICC) have established criteria for the diagnosis of systemic lupus erythematosus. In order to diagnose lupus erythematosus four criteria are needed at least one of which is clinical and one immunologic, or the patient must have lupus nephritis with circulating anti DS DNA antibodies. The clinical criteria are:
1. Acute cutaneous lupus:
    - Malar butterfly rash
    - Bullous lupus
    - Toxic epidermal necrolysis variant
    - Photosensitive rash
2. Chronic cutaneous lupus
    - Discoid rash
    - Verrucous hypertrophic lupus
    - Lupus panniculitis
    - Chilblain lupus
    - Discoid lupus/lichen planus overlap
    - Mucosal lupus
3. Oral ulcers
4. Nonscarring alopecia
5. Synovitis
6. Serositis
7. Renal disease
8. Neurologic disease
9. Hemolytic anemia
10. Leukopenia
11. Thrombocytopenia

The immunologic criteria are:
12. Positive ANA
13. Anti dsDNA antibody
14. Anti-SM
15. Antiphospholipid antibody positivity
16. Low complement.
17. Direct Coomb's test without hemolytic anemia

The classic butterfly-shaped malar rash is commonly known to be the cutaneous feature of systemic lupus erythematosus. Confluent erythematous macules overlying the cheeks form the wings of the butterfly, while erythema of the nose forms the body. The rash may be precipitated by sun exposure and lasts several hours to several days. The word 'discoid' is derived from the Greek word *discoīdēs*, meaning flat and circular. The cutaneous lesions of discoid lupus erythematosus are red, well-demarcated, scaly macules or papules that evolve into coin-shaped (discoid) plaques covered by an adherent scale, which is more prominent around dilated follicular orifices. By removing the scale, one can see keratotic spikes similar to carpet tacks. With time, the lesions expand, leaving atrophic telangiectatic scars in the center. Areas of hyper- and hypopigmentation also develop. The lesions of discoid lupus erythematosus most commonly occur on the face, scalp, ears, V area of neck, and arms. Unlike seborrheic dermatitis, the nasolabial area is usually spared. Scarring occurs in DLE.

In subacute cutaneous lupus erythematosus, patients present with a history of photosensitivity and antibodies against Ro (SS-A) and La (SS-B) antigens. Morphologically, the rash may appear to be either papulosquamous or annular polycyclic on sun-exposed skin. Unlike in discoid lupus erythematosus, the lesions heal without scarring, but postinflammatory hypopigmentation can be seen. The papulosquamous rash may clinically mimic psoriasis, but the lesions are less well-demarcated, have a papular component, and, unlike psoriasis, predominantly occur on sun-exposed skin. The annular polycyclic from of lupus can be confused with granuloma annulare, erythema multiforme, or erythema figuratum. The presence of slight scaling and photodistribution are helpful differentiating features.

Differential diagnosis

Although occasionally the rash may be persistent, most cases of chronic malar erythema in otherwise healthy patients are not due to lupus erythematosus. Persistent erythema of the face with overlying telangiectasias is most commonly seen in acne rosacea. The rash of dermatomyositis may also be confused with lupus erythematosus. In dermatomyositis, the erythema contains a violaceous hue, and periorbital erythema is a prominent feature. Gottron's papules, red papules and plaques overlying the knuckles, are seen in dermatomyositis. In cutaneous lupus, however, if skin lesions are present on the hands, they are more prominent between the joints.

Treatment (Table 2.6)

The treatment of lupus erythematosus is predicated on the extent of systemic involvement. For cutaneous lupus erythematosus, commonly used therapies include sun protection and avoidance, topical steroids, intralesional steroids, and oral antimalarials.

Perioral dermatitis

Definition and etiology

Perioral dermatitis is an idiopathic acneiform eczematous eruption characterized by a perioral distribution. The cause of perioral dermatitis is not known, but in one large series of 259 patients with the disease, 250 had been using topical corticosteroids. The topical steroids had been started for a variety of other rashes. The authors postulated that steroids may diminish the patients' tolerance to irritants in cosmetics or other contactants. Another hypothesis is that steroids may change the natural skin flora, thereby producing an acneiform eruption.

Clinical features

Perioral dermatitis is most commonly seen in adult women. A history of pruritus and cosmetic use can commonly be obtained. Papules, vesicles, and pustules on an erythematous base are seen surrounding the mouth. Some scaling resembling dermatitis is also commonly present. Rarely, perioral dermatitis can occur on the eyes, producing 'periocular dermatitis'. A characteristic clinical finding is a rim of uninvolved normal skin surrounding the vermilion border of the lips. Clinically, perioral dermatitis can be confused with contact dermatitis because of the presence of erythema and scaling or with an acneiform eruption such as acne vulgaris or acne rosacea if a papular or pustular component is prominent.

Treatment (Table 2.7)

Perioral dermatitis can be effectively treated with oral tetracycline or erythromycin. If patients have been taking potent topical steroids, a low-potency steroid preparation like 1% hydrocortisone may be used to prevent rebound upon stopping the high-potency steroid. Various topical creams or gels such as metronidazole gel, clindamycin, and sulfur preparations can also be used as adjunctive agents.

Polymorphous light eruption

Definition and etiology

Polymorphous light eruption is the most common idiopathic photodermatosis in the US and UK.

Table 2.6 Treatment of cutaneous lupus erythematosus

Treatment	Precautions
Universal	
Avoid heat sun and photosensitizing drugs Use sunscreen that blocks both UVA and UVB Wear sun protective clothing Cosmetics to cover/hide lesions	None
Mild disease	
Topical treatments Corticosteroids OTC hydrocortisone 1– 2% cream or Desonide 0.05% cream/ointment bid or Occasional pulse therapy	High potency steroids can produce skin atrophy and steroid induced rosacea on the face
Class I corticosteroids such as clobetasol cream/ointment 0.05% bid	
Tacrolimus (0.1% or 0.33%) ointment bid	Burning sensation
Severe disease	
Antimalarials Hydroxychloroquine 200 mg bid add Quinacrine 100 mg a day if no response or Chloroquine 150 mg PO q day	Response may take 2–3 months Eye toxicity may occur and patients need to have periodic ophthalmologic examination to evaluate for retinopathy
Acitretin 10–75 mg PO q day	Teratogen: monitor liver function tests and lipids for hypertriglyceridemia Hair loss also relatively common complaint
Azathioprine 25–100 mg q day	Functional testing for TPMP activity in order to ascertain how patients metabolize azathioprine Requires CBC monitoring along with LFT's and renal function
Methotrexate 10–25 mg q week	Requires monitoring of CBC and LFTs. Risk of hepatic cirrhosis
Thalidomide	Requires registration and monitoring for birth defects

Clinical features

As the word 'polymorphous' implies, the rash can assume a variety of different shapes; however, the appearance of the rash in a specific patient is relatively monomorphic. The disease starts in young adults, but in genetically predisposed individuals such as American Indians and the Scottish, the disease commonly starts in childhood. Females are more frequently affected than males. The eruption first appears in springtime and has a delayed onset of 24–48 hours after sun exposure.

With chronic sun exposure, hardening and improvement occur. The morphologic patterns include papulovesicles, eczematous lesions, edematous plaques, excoriated nodules, erythema multiforme-like lesions, and occasionally petechiae and hemorrhage. Pruritus is usually present, and lichenification due to chronic scratching can be seen.

Table 2.7 Treatment of perioral dermatitis

Treatment	Precautions
Universal	
Stop or taper any topical or systemic corticosteroid patient is taking	Expect flare with discontinuation of steroids
Mild/moderate disease	
Topical antibiotics	May be irritating
Metronidazole 0.75% bid	
Erythromycin 2% ointment bid	
Clindamycin 1% gel/lotion/solution bid	
Sulfacetamide 10% cream/wash bid	
Severe disease	
Systemic antibiotics	Risk of allergy, gastrointestinal upset, and photosensitivity
Tetracycline 250 mg to 500 mg bid	
Doxycycline 20 mg to 100 mg q day	
Consider patch testing if no resolution	

Differential diagnosis

Polymorphous light eruption can be distinguished from systemic lupus erythematosus by the lack of systemic symptoms, and it can be distinguished from discoid lupus erythematosus by the absence of atrophy, telangiectasias, and follicular plugging. In other diseases that can be confused with polymorphous light eruption (such as erythema multiforme, sarcoidosis, and tinea faciei), photosensitivity does not occur. In diagnostically challenging cases, a skin biopsy may be helpful. Finally, a photocontact or phototoxic eruption should always be excluded by taking a thorough history, including questions about topical or parenteral contact with a photosensitizing agent or by performing patch testing.

Treatment (Table 2.8)

Treatment consists of sun avoidance and broad-spectrum sunscreens. Topical steroids can be used during acute exacerbations. In severe cases, antimalarial therapy can be effective. Desensitization light therapy can also be used.

Pseudofolliculitis barbae

Definition and etiology

Pseudofolliculitis barbae is inflammation of the skin in the beard area of adult men caused by penetration of the skin by ingrown curved hair.

Clinical features

Pseudofolliculitis is a common problem in patients with curly hair and is seen most commonly in blacks. Physical examination reveals papules and pustules in the beard area. Closer examination will demonstrate curved and ingrown hairs. Scarring may form. The major diseases in the differential diagnosis are acne vulgaris and folliculitis. In pseudofolliculitis barbae, the eruption is localized to the beard area, and the rest of the face will not be involved (unlike in acne vulgaris). Comedones are not present. Infectious folliculitis most commonly involves the thigh and buttocks area. Culture of a pustule will be positive for *Staphylococcus aureus*.

Table 2.8 Treatment of polymorphous light eruption

Treatment	Precautions
Universal	
Sun avoidance	
Use sunscreen that blocks both UVA and UVB	
Mild disease	
Topical steroids such as Triamcinolone 0.1% bid	May produce steroid induced rosacea on face. Watch for steroid induced atrophy
Severe disease	
Short course of systemic prednisone	
Narrow band UV therapy	'Desensitization therapy', risk of burning
Antimalarials (hydroxychloroquine/Plaquenil 100 mg to 200 mg bid)	Needs monitoring for ocular toxicity/retinopathy
Occasionally other immunosuppressants such as azathioprine and cyclosporine	Third line therapy only as last resort. Needs close monitoring for toxicity

Table 2.9 Treatment of pseudofolliculitis barbae

Treatment	Precautions
Universal	
Consider growing beard, or not shaving as close	Not a reasonable option for many men
Mild disease	
Low-dose topical steroid after shaving	Watch for steroid induced acne
Topical retinoid daily	May be irritating
Topical clindamycin bid	May be irritating
Topical hydroquinone bid for hyperpigmentation	Risk of exacerbating hyperpigmentation and irritation
Severe disease	
Doxycycline 50 mg to 100 mg bid	Allergy, nausea, vomiting, esophagitis, photosensitivity
Consider topical epilating agents	May be irritating
Consider electrolysis or laser hair removal	May produce scarring

Treatment (Table 2.9)

The treatment of pseudofolliculitis is very difficult. Growing a beard will solve the problem, but this is not a desirable solution for everyone. Since shaving in itself can be irritating, shaving at nighttime instead of in the morning can give the skin some time to recover. Topical antibiotic and retinoid preparations offer some benefit. A low-potency hydrocortisone cream applied after shaving may also reduce some of the irritation.

■ Seborrheic dermatitis

Definition and etiology

Seborrheic dermatitis is a common form of dermatitis localized to areas with an increased number of sebaceous glands and increased sebum production such as the scalp, nasolabial folds, eyebrows, cheeks, anterior chest, axilla, and groin. The oil produced by the sebaceous glands facilitates the growth of Pityrosporum organisms, thereby producing inflammation and a dermatitis. In neonates, seborrheic dermatitis is called *cradle cap*, but it is most commonly seen in adults, with dandruff being its mildest manifestation. Severe seborrheic dermatitis is sometimes referred to as *tinea amiantacea*, but this term is confusing and is avoided here.

Clinical features

Seborrheic dermatitis is characterized by erythematous plaques covered with yellow, greasy scales. If seborrheic dermatitis involves the cheek, clinically it can be confused with systemic or discoid lupus or contact dermatitis. A seborrheic dermatitis-like rash can also occur in patients with riboflavin deficiency. The incidence of seborrheic dermatitis is increased in patients with human immunodeficiency virus infection, Parkinson's disease, dementia, or cardiac failure, as well as in alcoholics. Men are also more frequently affected than women.

Table 2.10 Treatment of seborrheic dermatitis

Treatment	Precautions
Universal	
Regular shampooing hair and washing face	Seborrheic dermatitis is a chronic disease with no cure
Consider selenium sulfide 1% or 2.5% and 1% zinc pyrithione containing shampoo or Nizoral shampoo 1% or 2% three times per week	
Mild disease	
Topical antifungal once or twice a day such as ketoconazole 1% cream	Combination of antifungal and cortisone may be more potent. High strength steroids may produce steroid acne
Topical cortisone such as 1% or 2.5% hydrocortisone q day or bid	
Topical calcineurin inhibitors	
Pimecrolimus 1% cream	Burning sensation
Severe disease	
Short course of systemic antifungal such as itraconazole	Follow for liver toxicity, drug interactions
Tacrolimus ointment 0.1% or 0.3% bid	Burning sensation

Treatment (Table 2.10)

Seborrheic dermatitis on the face usually responds well to low-potency topical steroids and imidazole creams such as ketoconazole. The scalp involvement can be treated with antidandruff shampoos containing ketoconazole, zinc oxide, and selenium sulfide. Benzoyl peroxide, zinc pyrithione, and selenium sulfide cleaners are also helpful.

Chapter 3 Oral mucosa

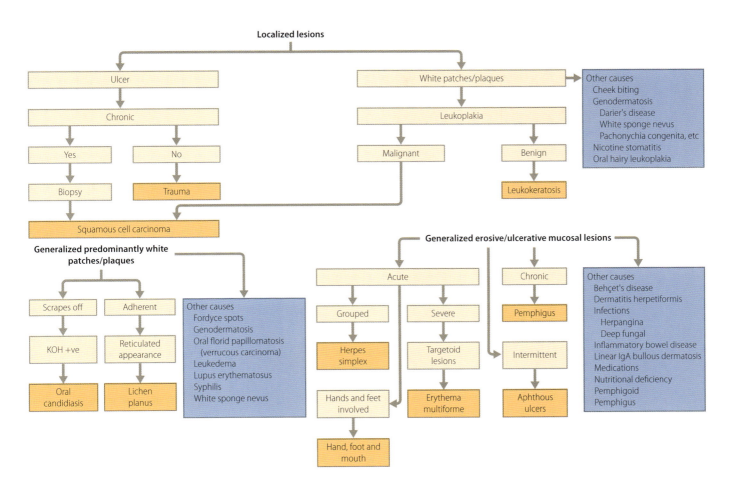

INTRODUCTION

Mucosal epithelium is different from the integument in that an outer keratinizing layer (stratum corneum) is not made in the absence of disease, adnexal structures are not present, and there is more rapid epithelialization. There is a limited repertoire of responses that mucosal epithelium can have to diseases. Therefore, oral diseases tend to look identical, and diagnoses made from clinical appearance and history may need to be supported by biopsy and blood test results. For example, white patches can be seen in entirely disparate diseases such as lichen planus, candidiasis, and squamous cell carcinoma. Oral lesions are especially important, since they can interfere with eating. In some diseases such as pemphigus, oral lesions may be the harbinger of a potentially fatal disease.

1. LICHEN PLANUS VERSUS ORAL CANDIDIASIS

Features in common: white mucosal lesions

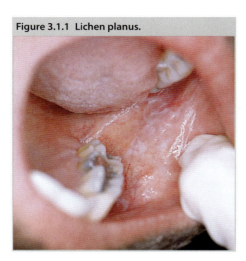

Figure 3.1.1 Lichen planus.

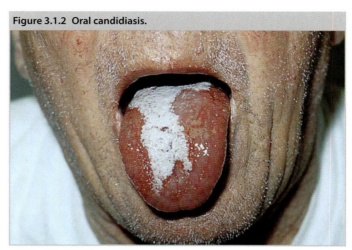

Figure 3.1.2 Oral candidiasis.

Distinguishing features

	Lichen planus	Oral candidiasis
Physical examination		
Morphology	White, reticulated plaque Ulcers commonly present White plaques do not rub off	White strands become confluent, forming plaques Ulcers rarely seen White plaques easily rub off
Distribution	Buccal mucosa, tongue, gingiva, palate, lips	Buccal mucosa, tongue, gingiva, palate, pharynx
History		
Symptoms	Asymptomatic or painful if ulcerated	Asymptomatic; occasionally burning mouth
Exacerbating factors	Iatrogenic: antimalarials, quinidine, β-blockers, diuretics, hypoglycemic agents Dental amalgams	Iatrogenic: steroids, antibiotics Immunosuppressant Dentures and implants
Associated findings	Violaceous papules and plaques on wrists, ankles, elsewhere in half of patients Nail dystrophy	Endocrine diseases: diabetes, thyroid, hypoparathyroidism Systemic diseases: lymphomas, autoimmune, immunodeficiencies (HIV)
Epidemiology	Adults	Any age
Biopsy	Yes Lichenoid infiltrate, irregular epidermal hyperplasia with sawtooth-like appearance, hypergranulosis	No Spores and pseudohyphae on surface of of epithelium (highlighted by periodic acid-Schiff stains)
Laboratory	None; KOH negative	Positive KOH
Outcome	Chronic course	Good response to therapy
HIV, human immunodeficiency virus; KOH, potassium hydroxide.		

Differential diagnosis of white oral plaques (leukoplakia)

Common causes
- Cheek biting (Morsicatio buccarum)
- Fordyce's spots
- Lichen planus
- Oral candidiasis
- Oral hairy leukoplakia
- Nicotine stomatitis
- Squamous cell carcinoma or dysplasia

Rarer causes
- White sponge nevus
- Oral florid papillomatosis
- Focal epithelial hyperplasia
- Leukoedema
- Mucous patch of syphilis
- White patches of genodermatosis: Darier's disease, pachyonychia congenita, dyskeratosis congenita

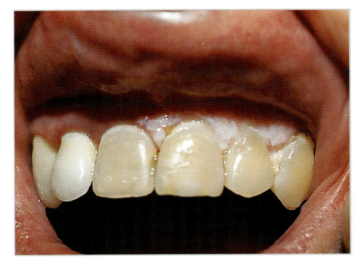

Figure 3.1.3 Lichen planus. *Clue to diagnosis:* reticulated white plaque on gingiva.

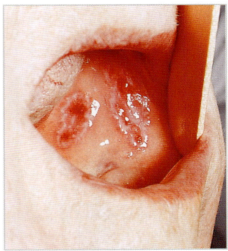

Figure 3.1.4 Lichen planus. *Clue to diagnosis:* ulcers in buccal mucosa with surrounding white reticulated plaques.

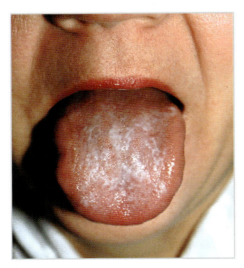

Figure 3.1.5 Lichen planus

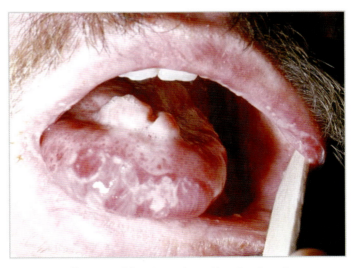

Figure 3.1.6 Chronic candidiasis in a patient with graft vs. host disease.

2. APTHOUS ULCERS VERSUS PEMPHIGUS VULGARIS

Features in common: oral ulcer

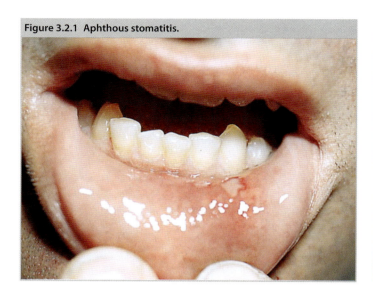

Figure 3.2.1 Aphthous stomatitis.

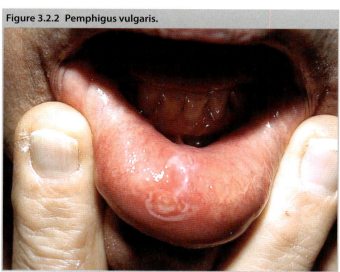

Figure 3.2.2 Pemphigus vulgaris.

Distinguishing features

	Aphthous ulcers	Pemphigus vulgaris
Physical examination		
Morphology	Minor aphthae: 4–8 mm round or oval lesions, yellow center and erythematous rim Major aphthae: similar appearance but large 1–3 cm ulcers Herpetiform: grouped small 1-mm erosions that coalesce into large ulcers	Large (often several centimeters in size) in coalescent ulcers and erosions Vesicles not grouped
Distribution	Buccal mucosa and occasionally tongue, soft palate, oropharynx	Buccal mucosa, tongue, palate, gingiva, occasionally oropharynx
History		
Symptoms	Intermittent oral sores Four stages: premonitory, preulcerative, ulcerative, healing Premonitory stage: asymptomatic or paresthesia and burning sensation Preulcerative and ulcerative stage: pain	Chronic oral sores Severe pain and discomfort
Exacerbating factors	Stress, nutritional deficiencies, food allergy, infections, trauma	Occasionally drug-induced: penicillamine, penicillin, captopril, phenobarbital
Associated findings	Ulcers of genital mucosa occasionally (if uveitis consider Behçet's disease)	Erosions in glabrous skin Positive Nikolsky's sign
Epidemiology	Common Can occur at any age, but most prevalent in young adults	Rare Primarily affects middle-aged adults
Biopsy	No Nonspecific ulceration	Yes Epidermal acantholysis, eosinophilic infiltrate, tombstoning of the basal epithelial layer
Laboratory	Occasionally vitamin B12, folic acid, iron deficiency	Positive indirect and direct immunofluorescence results
Outcome	Chronic relapsing course	Mortality of 60–90% prior to glucocorticoid treatment Chronic disease

Differential diagnosis of oral ulcers

- Aphthous stomatitis
- Autoimmune blistering
  - Cicatricial pemphigoid
  - Dermatitis herpetiformis
  - Linear IgA bullous dermatosis
  - Pemphigus vulgaris
- Behçet's syndrome
- Cytotoxic drugs (e.g. methotrexate, 6-mercaptopurine)
- Epidermolysis bullosa
- Infections
  - Herpetic gingivostomatitis
  - Candidiasis
  - Herpangina
  - Hand-foot-and-mouth disease
  - Deep fungal infections
- Lichen planus
- Neoplasia carcinoma
- Nutritional deficiency
  - Noma
- Trauma
- Ulcerative colitis
- Vasculitis
  - Wegener's granulomatosis

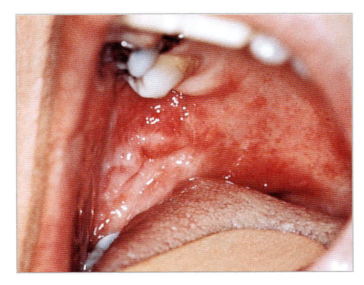

Figure 3.2.3 Pemphigus vulgaris. *Clue to diagnosis:* chronic unremitting oral ulcers.

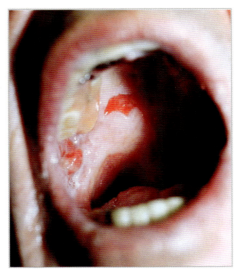

Figure 3.2.4 Pemphigus vulgaris.

3. LICHEN PLANUS VERSUS LEUKOPLAKIA

■ Features in common: white mucosal lesions

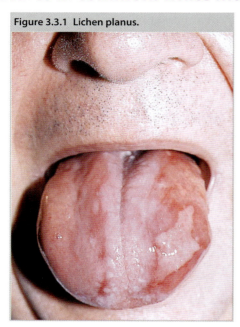

Figure 3.3.1 Lichen planus.

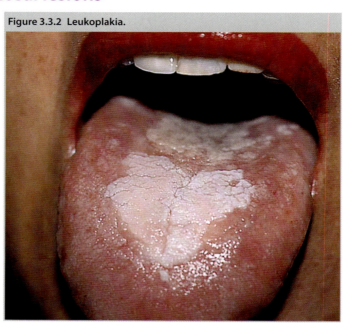

Figure 3.3.2 Leukoplakia.

■ Distinguishing features

	Lichen planus	Leukoplakia
Physical examination Morphology	White reticulated plaque Erosions/ulcers commonly present	Localized white patch/plaque Lesions may be small or large Ulcers only after long-standing duration or trauma Lesions become leathery and thick with time Erythematous speckled or warty appearance in premalignant lesions
Distribution	Buccal mucosa, tongue, gingiva, palate, lips	Buccal mucosa, retrocommissural mucosa, alveolar ridge, tongue, hard palate, rarely sublingual area and gingiva
History Symptoms	Not related to tobacco products Asymptomatic or painful if ulcerated	Smokers or tobacco chewers Asymptomatic
Exacerbating factors	Iatrogenic: antimalarials, quinidine, β-blockers, diuretics, hypoglycemic agents Dental amalgams	None
Associated findings	Violaceous papules and plaques on wrists, ankles, elsewhere in half of patients Nail dystrophy	Squamous cell carcinoma Occasionally poor dental hygiene
Epidemiology	Men and women	Predominantly men
Biopsy	Occasionally Lichenoid infiltrate, sawtoothing of epithelium, hypergranulosis	Yes Epithelial acanthosis with varying amounts of dysplasia
Laboratory	None	Occasionally candida overgrowth found on potassium hydroxide test
Outcome	Chronic disease	May regress upon stopping tobacco use or may develop into squamous cell carcinoma

Differential diagnosis of white oral plaques (leukoplakia)

Common causes
- Cheek biting (morsicatio buccarum)
- Fordyce's spots
- Lichen planus
- Oral candidiasis
- Oral hairy leukoplakia
- Nicotine stomatitis
- Squamous cell carcinoma or dysplasia

Rarer causes
- White sponge nevus
- Oral florid papillomatosis
- Focal epithelial hyperplasia
- Leukoedema
- Mucous patch of syphilis
- White patches of genodermatosis:
- Darier's disease, pachyonychia congenita, dyskeratosis congenita

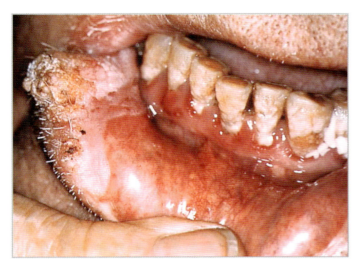

Figure 3.3.3 Squamous cell carcinoma arising within a plaque of leukoplakia. Clue to diagnosis: crusted nodule and erythema within an area of leukoplakia.

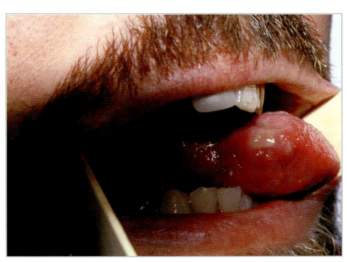

Figure 3.3.4 Squamous cell carcinoma of the tongue arising in leukoplakia.

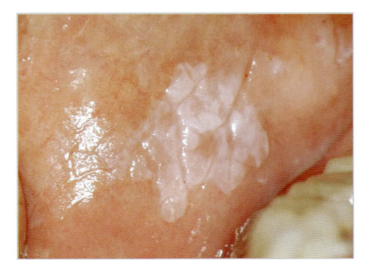

Figure 3.3.5 Leukoplakia.

4. HERPES STOMATITIS VERSUS ERYTHEMA MULTIFORME

■ Features in common: oral erosions and vesicles

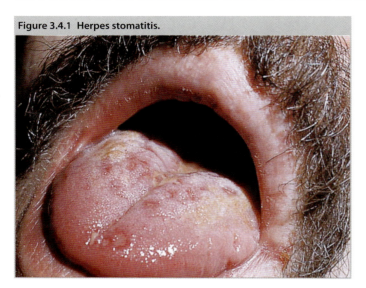

Figure 3.4.1 Herpes stomatitis.

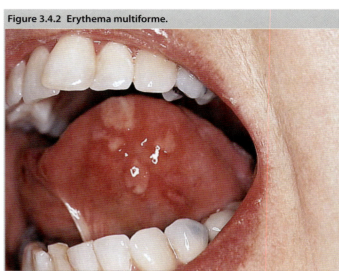

Figure 3.4.2 Erythema multiforme.

■ Distinguishing features

	Herpetic gingivostomatitis	Erythema multiforme
Physical examination Morphology	Generalized mucosal grouped vesicles and erosions Scalloped border may be present	Generalized erosions and ulcers with pseudomembrane formation No scalloped border
Distribution	Entire oral mucosa in primary infection Other mucosal surfaces not involved No target lesions Localized lymphadenopathy	Entire oral mucosa Involvement of other mucosal surface common (eyes, nose) Targetoid lesions on skin Generalized lymphadenopathy
History Symptoms	History of exposure to herpes virus 2 – 10 days previously (in some cases) Fevers, malaise commonly present Cannot eat or drink Pain and discomfort	Occasional prodromal upper respiratory tract infection Ingestion of new medication Fever rarely, presents more commonly with prodrome, malaise Cannot eat or drink Pain and discomfort
Exacerbating factors	Immunosuppression	None
Associated findings	None	Over 50 reported associations including the following: Infections: *Mycoplasma pneumoniae*, herpes simplex Most common medications: nonsteroidal anti-inflammatory agents, antibiotics, barbiturates Rarely associated with neoplasm or connective tissue disease
Epidemiology	Primarily involves children	Primarily involves young adults aged 20–40 years
Biopsy	No Ballooning necrosis of epidermis Multinucleated giant cells within epidermal vesicles	Occasionally Necrotic keratinocytes with areas of epidermal necrosis, interface lymphocytic dermatitis
Laboratory	Positive culture for herpes simplex Tzanck preparation: multinucleated giant cells	Chest X-ray if pulmonary symptoms Tzanck test and culture negative unless secondary to herpes infection
Outcome	Good Resolves over 1–2 weeks No scarring	Usually good Resolves over 4–6 weeks May have residual scarring Eye involvement may lead to blindness Occasionally fatal due to secondary sepsis

Differential diagnosis of erosive oral disease

- Aphthous stomatitis
- Autoimmune blistering
  - Cicatricial pemphigoid
  - Dermatitis herpetiformis
  - Linear IgA bullous dermatosis
  - Pemphigus vulgaris
- Behçet's syndrome
- Cytotoxic drugs (e.g. methotrexate, 6-mercaptopurine)
- Epidermolysis bullosa
- Infections
  - Herpetic gingivostomatitis
  - Candidiasis
  - Herpangina
  - Hand-foot-and-mouth disease
  - Deep fungal infections
- Lichen planus
- Neoplasia carcinoma
- Nutritional deficiency
  - Noma
- Trauma
- Ulcerative colitis
- Vasculitis
  - Wegener's granulomatosis

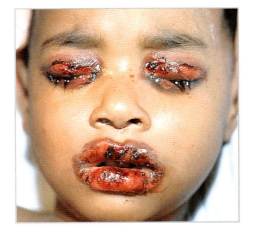

Figure 3.4.3 Erythema multiforme. *Clue to diagnosis:* involvement of other mucosal skin.

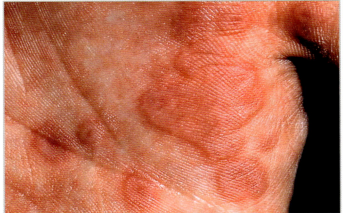

Figure 3.4.4 Erythema multiforme. *Clue to diagnosis:* targetoid lesions on palms.

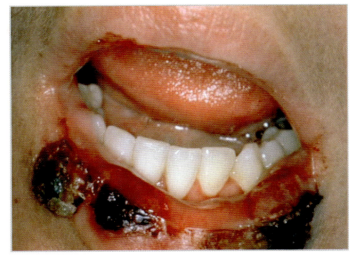

Figure 3.4.5 Herpes infection in a patient with AIDS.

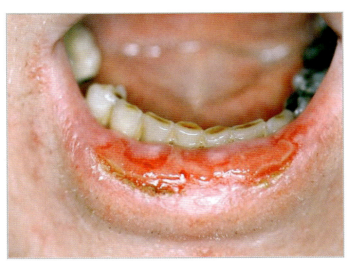

Figure 3.4.6 Herpes labialis. Resolving herpes labialis. Note scalloped borders.

5. LOCALIZED LESIONS

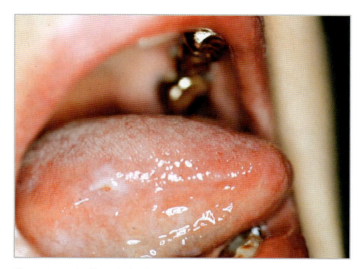

Figure 3.5.1 Oral hairy leukoplakia.

6. GENERALIZED PREDOMINANTLY WHITE PATCHES/PLAQUES

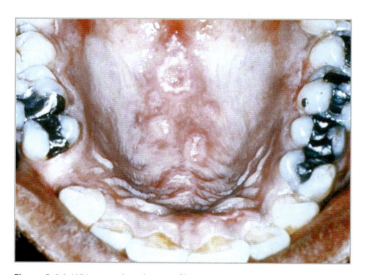

Figure 3.6.1 White atrophic plaques of lupus erythematosus.

7. GENERALIZED EROSIVE/ULCERATIVE MUCOSAL LESIONS

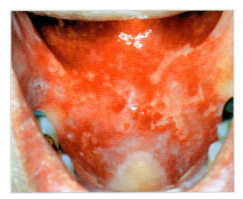

Figure 3.7.1 Cicatricial pemphigoid.

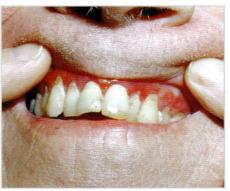

Figure 3.7.2 Desquamative gingivitis secondary to cicatricial pemphigoid. Other causes of desquamative gingivitis includes lichen planus and pemphigus.

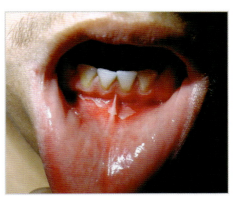

Figure 3.7.3 Hand-foot-and-mouth disease.

8. OTHER EXAMPLES

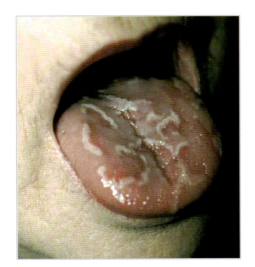

Figure 3.8.1 Geographic tongue.

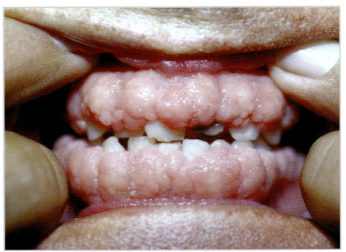

Figure 3.8.2 Gingival hyperplasia secondary to Dilantin. Other drugs that can produce gingival hyperplasia include cyclosporine and calcium channel blockers.

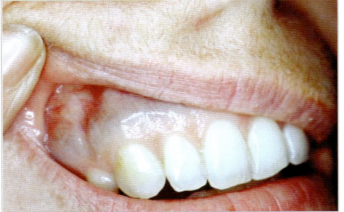

Figure 3.8.3 Mucosa hyperpigmentation secondary to minocycline.

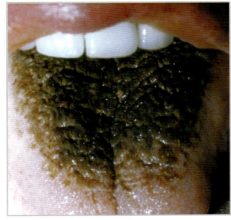

Figure 3.8.4 Black hairy tongue (lingua nigra).

DISEASE DISCUSSION

Apthous stomatitis

Definition and etiology
Recurrent aphthous stomatitis, commonly called a canker sore, is an ulcerative disease of the oral mucosa of unknown cause.

Clinical features
Aphthous ulcers are the most common ulcerative disease of the oral mucosa. Twenty percent of the general population may suffer from aphthous ulcerations at some time in their lives.

Patients with aphthous ulcers commonly experience a tingling or burning sensation at the site of the initial lesions. The ulcers are most commonly seen on the buccal mucosa but can also involve the lips, tongue, soft palate, and oropharynx. Morphologically, aphthous ulcers can be classified as minor, major, or herpetiform lesions. Minor aphthae, the most common form, are characterized by small ulcers a few millimeters in size covered with a yellow scab and surrounded by erythema. The lesions usually heal without scarring in 7–10 days, but recurrences are common. Major aphthous ulcers (Sutton's disease) have a similar appearance to minor aphthae; however, they are a few centimeters in size and persist up to one month. Scarring can also occur. In patients with the herpetiform variant, small, grouped popular vesicles that coalesce into a larger plaque are present. Herpes culture is negative.

The differential diagnosis includes other ulcerating diseases such as herpes simplex stomatitis and pemphigus vulgaris. Herpes gingival stomatitis usually involves children. Skin involvement is not seen, and the lesions have a characteristic grouped appearance. The herpetiform variant of aphthous ulcers can be distinguished only by means of culture or skin biopsy; however, herpes gingivostomatitis, unlike herpes labialis, is usually not a recurrent disease. Autoimmune blistering diseases such as pemphigus vulgaris and cicatricial pemphigoid usually are chronic, not recurrent. In both pemphigus vulgaris and cicatricial pemphigoid, skin involvement can occur. In cicatricial pemphigoid, conjunctival, nasal, or pharyngeal involvement occurs in a majority of patients. Other causes of oral ulcers (such as medications, a nutritional deficiency state, or inflammatory bowel disease) can usually be excluded based upon the history.

Treatment (Table 3.1)
Since the ulcers in aphthous stomatitis are usually self limited, treatment is usually only palliative. Hot, spicy, and acidic foods should be avoided. Topical anesthetics can provide temporary relief from the pain but also numb the taste buds resulting in tasteless dining. Topical steroids are also frequently prescribed. For severe cases systemic treatment is necessary.

Oral candidiasis

Definition and etiology
Oral candidiasis, also known as oral thrush or acute pseudomembranous candidiasis, is infection of the oropharyngeal cavity with *Candida albicans*, a yeast.

Clinical features
Oral candidiasis can be seen in any age group. Candidiasis starts as small, white, droplike macules and papules on the buccal mucosa, tongue, gingiva, palate, and pharynx. The lesions have been described

Table 3.1 Treatment of aphthous stomatitis

Treatment	Precautions
Mild/moderate disease	
Fluocinonide gel 0.05%, triamcinolone in benzocaine 20% paste (Orabase) qid	Secondary *Candida* infection (thrush)
Dyclonine hydrochloride solution 1% prn	Loss of taste
Lidocaine jelly 2% prn	Loss of taste
Severe disease	
Intralesional triamcinolone 10 g/mL	
Prednisone: start at 40–60 mg/day and taper	Avoid long term – hyperglycemia, insomnia, hypertension, fluid retention, infection, osteoporosis
Colchicine 0.6 mg daily or bid	Gastrointestinal – nausea, vomiting, diarrhea, myelosuppression
Pentoxifylline 400 mg tid	Renal or hepatic impairment

as resembling milk curds or cottage cheese. With time and in severe cases, large plaques with pseudomembranes, erosions, or ulcers may develop. The base and surrounding mucosa are often erythematous.

Other diseases with white plaques include morsicatio buccarum (cheek biting), lichen planus, leukoplakia, leukoedema, oral florid papillomatosis, white sponge nevus, and squamous cell carcinoma. Unlike in the other diseases, the white plaques in candidiasis usually are easily rubbed off. In morsicatio buccarum, white plaques are produced owing to chronic cheek biting of the buccal mucosa, and white patches are oriented parallel to the gum line. Leukoedema is an idiopathic, asymptomatic swelling of the oral mucosa and lips. The diffuse white discoloration of the mucosa disappears upon stretching the skin. White sponge nevus is an autosomal dominant disease in which white patches are found mainly on the buccal mucosa. In oral florid papillomatosis, a cancerous condition of the oral cavity caused by a papillomavirus infection, localized white papillomatous cauliflower-like vegetations are seen on the buccal mucosa. In lichen planus (discussed in greater detail later in this chapter), the white plaques are arranged in a reticular and lacelike pattern. Finally, in both leukoplakia and squamous cell carcinoma, localized white plaques are found. The plaques may ulcerate or may have a vegetative appearance.

Oral candidiasis is commonly seen in newborns and infants when the mucosa becomes colonized by yeast from the mother's birth canal. In children and adults, oral candidiasis is commonly secondary to underlying systemic disease or is iatrogenically produced. Some common systemic diseases associated with candidiasis include endocrine disorders (diabetes, hypoparathyroidism, hypothyroidism), immune deficiencies (human immunodeficiency virus infection, acquired immunodeficiency syndrome), nutritional deficiencies, and malignancies. Iatrogenic factors include broad-spectrum antibiotics, corticosteroid therapy, immunosuppressive agents, cytotoxic agents, dentures, and other prostheses.

Treatment (Table 3.2)
The first caveat of treatment is to identify and, when possible, eliminate any predisposing factors. The next step is to eliminate the causative organisms by using either topical or systemic therapy. Topically, a 2- to

Table 3.2 Treatment of oral candidiasis

Treatment	Precautions
Mild/moderate disease	
Nystatin suspension 500,000 units qid swish and swallow	None
Clotrimazole troches 10 mg qid	None
Severe disease	
Fluconazole 200 mg daily	Hepatic or renal impairment

3-week course of nystatin suspension or clotrimazole troches is effective. For more severe, recurrent, or chronic cases, oral ketoconazole or fluconazole may be used.

Erythema multiforme

Definition and etiology

Erythema multiforme is an inflammatory reactive skin disease secondary to a wide variety of triggers. Common causes include medications and infections, such as *Mycoplasma pneumoniae* or herpes simplex. The possible triggers include the following:

- Infections: viral, bacterial, mycobacterial, fungal (especially coccidioidomycosis and histoplasmosis), protozoal
- Medications: sulfonamides, penicillins, nonsteroidal anti-inflammatory agents, barbiturates, phenytoin (Dilantin), hydralazine, penicillamine, tetracycline, allopurinol
- Neoplasms (especially lymphoma)
- Connective tissue diseases
- Physical agents: radiation therapy
- Foods
- Contactants: bromofluorine, fire sponge, toxicodendron
- Topical agents
- Miscellaneous: pregnancy, sarcoidosis, inflammatory bowel disease

Clinical features

Erythema multiforme commonly involves both mucosal and glabrous skin. Generalized erosions with formation of pseudomembrane and crust are seen in the mouth. Sometimes the mucosal involvement can precede the skin findings, which typically include symmetric urticarial macules and papules. Rarely, mucosal involvement is the only manifestation of erythema multiforme. Within the first few days, some of the lesions develop concentric color changes owing to necrosis. This produces the characteristic 'target' or 'iris' lesion. Blisters may also develop. The lesions appear first on extremities and then extend to the trunk. Patients complain of pain from the mucosal involvement, along with mild malaise or itching. In the severe form, known as *erythema multiforme* major, fevers, arthralgia, severe malaise, and even death due to secondary infection can occur. Erythema multiforme major is defined by mucous membrane involvement (oral, nasal, or eye), as well as severe and widespread skin involvement. The relationship between erythema multiforme and toxic epidermal necrolysis (TEN), a disease with widespread tissue desquamation, continues to be debated. In TEN, target lesions are not present. If skin involvement is present, erythema multiforme can be easily diagnosed. If only mucosal involvement is present, the differential diagnosis includes herpetic gingivostomatitis or other erosive diseases like aphthous ulcers.

Table 3.3 Treatment of oral erythema multiforme

Treatment	Precautions
Universal	
Remove/treat precipitating factor – drug, infection Supportive care	
Mild/moderate disease	
Fluocinonide gel 0.05%, Triamcinolone in benzocaine 20% paste (Orabase) qid	Secondary *Candida* infection (thrush)
Dyclonine hydrochloride solution 1% prn	Loss of taste
Lidocaine jelly 2% prn	Loss of taste
Severe disease	
Prednisone 40–60 mg daily tapered over 2–3 weeks	Hyperglycemia, hypertension, insomnia, mood change, weight gain, infection, osteoporosis
Intravenous immunoglobulin	Controversial, expensive, risk of an allergic reaction and rare cases of anaphylaxis in IgA deficiency

Treatment (Table 3.3)

Erythema multiforme usually resolves spontaneously with supportive care if the precipitating factor is eliminated. Some physicians advocate the use of systemic steroids in the first few days of disease involvement, but the efficacy of steroids has been controversial. Prolonged steroid use is not advised because signs of underlying infection may be missed. Ophthalmologic consultation should be obtained if eye involvement is suspected to prevent synechiae development or scarring. Topical dressings may help lesions to heal. In severe cases, patients should be treated in a burn unit, and electrolyte and fluid balance must be closely monitored.

Herpetic gingivostomatitis

Definition and etiology

Acute herpetic gingivostomatitis is a primary herpes simplex virus infection of the oral mucosa most commonly seen in children and young adults. It occurs in only a small number of patients with first-time exposure to herpes simplex.

Clinical features

The eruption starts 2–10 days after exposure to herpes simplex virus. Many patients are unaware of their source of exposure. Patients develop fever, malaise, and painful erosive stomatitis and pharyngitis. Lesions frequently start in the interdental gingival papillae and spread to involve the entire mucosal surface. The lesions start out as red macules that rapidly become vesiculated and develop into widespread erosions. Intact blisters are rarely found because moisture and maceration in the mouth cause vesicles to rupture. On closer inspection, the erosions are grouped and have scalloped borders characteristic of a herpesvirus infection. The lesions heal spontaneously within a few weeks. The major disease in the differential diagnosis is aphthous stomatitis, which usually is recurrent, unlike herpes gingivostomatitis. Other common blistering diseases in the differential diagnosis are discussed in the section on aphthous stomatitis. A Tzanck preparation or biopsy can help confirm the diagnosis by revealing multinucleated giant cells. A culture or immunofluorescent tests for herpes can also quickly confirm the diagnosis

Table 3.4 Treatment of herpetic gingivostomatitis

Treatment	Precautions
First episode – primary	
Condoms may help prevent spread with oral sex	
Valacyclovir 1000 mg bid for 7 days	Headache, nausea, diarrhea, vomiting. Rarely psychosis, seizures, leukopenia, thrombocytopenia, Stevens–Johnson, toxic epidermal necrolysis
Acyclovir 400 mg tid for 7 days	Same as valacyclovir
Famciclovir 250 mg tid for 7 days	Same as valacyclovir
Recurrent	
Valacyclovir 2000 mg bid for 1 day	As above
Acyclovir 800 mg tid for 2 days	As above
Famciclovir 1 g bid for 1 day	As above
Topicals – acyclovir ointment 5%, Penciclovir cream 1%, docosanol cream 10% use 5–6 times daily until healed	Irritation
Chronic suppressive	
Valacyclovir 1000 mg daily	As above
Acyclovir 400 mg bid	As above
Famciclovir 250 mg bid	As above

Treatment (Table 3.4)

Oral acyclovir, valacyclovir, or famciclovir, if started during the first 2 days of the infection, can limit the severity and duration of disease. Viscous lidocaine can be used for pain and discomfort.

Leukoplakia

Definition and etiology

Leukoplakia is a descriptive term, not a disease entity. Leukoplakia is defined as a persistent white patch of the oral mucosa that can be either idiopathic or produced by external irritants. The most common etiologic factor is tobacco smoking or use of chewing tobacco.

Clinical features

The clinical features depend on both the severity of disease and its duration. The lesions start out as small white patches resembling candle wax and with time can become thick, leathery plaques. The lesions usually are sharply demarcated and involve the buccal mucosa. Other sites of involvement include the alveolar ridge, tongue, lips, gingiva, and palate. Squamous cell carcinoma can develop in foci of leukoplakia. Lesions of leukoplakia that are evolving into squamous cell carcinomas frequently have a red color and are called erythroplakia.

The differential diagnosis includes other white patches and plaques of the oral mucosa, such as lichen planus and candidiasis. Areas of leukoplakia can frequently become secondarily infected with candidiasis; however, unlike in candidiasis, the white plaques are adherent and do not scrape off. In lichen planus, the lesions usually have a reticulated appearance, and glabrous skin may be involved. Other rarer entities in the differential diagnosis include the mucous patch of syphilis, white sponge nevus, leukoedema, cheek biting (morsicatio buccarum), and oral florid papillomatosis. A biopsy should be performed in all cases of suspected leukoplakia to confirm the diagnosis and to rule out underlying squamous cell carcinoma.

Table 3.5 Treatment of leukoplakia

Treatment	Precautions
Universal	
Remove irritant – tobacco, physical trauma, etc.	
Moderate/severe disease	
Cryotherapy	Scar
Laser	Scar
Surgery	Scar

Treatment (Table 3.5)

In many cases, the lesions can resolve spontaneously if the stimulus (such as smoking) is removed. Good dental hygiene can also help. In persistent lesions, topical retinoids and surgery have been used.

Lichen planus

Definition and etiology

Lichen planus is an idiopathic inflammatory dermatitis that may involve both glabrous skin and mucosa. The cause of lichen planus is not known, but certain drugs such as methyldopa, ß-blockers, thiazide diuretics, gold, penicillamine, and nonsteroidal anti-inflammatory agents can produce an oral eruption indistinguishable from classic idiopathic lichen planus. Lichen planus-like eruptions have also been related to use of gold in dental restorations. Associations between oral lichen planus and hepatitis C infection have been reported, and rare reports suggest that lichenoid lesions indistinguishable from lichen planus may be seen as a paraneoplastic phenomenon. These findings need to be confirmed.

Clinical features

Lichen planus most commonly occurs between the ages of 30 and 60 years and affects both sexes equally. The buccal mucosa is the most frequently involved intraoral site, but lichen planus can also involve the tongue, lips, palate, and gingiva. Approximately 15% to 25% of patients with oral lichen planus do not have skin lesions. Conversely, mucous membranes are affected in approximately half of patients with skin lesions.

If the characteristic white reticulated pattern is present, the diagnosis of oral lichen planus can be made clinically. In other cases, a biopsy is necessary to exclude entities such as candidiasis, contact stomatitis, leukoplakia, leukoedema, white sponge nevus, and oral florid papillomatosis. (See discussion of candidiasis.)

Treatment (Table 3.6)

Treatment of oral lichen planus is usually unsatisfactory. Any suspected causative drug should be eliminated. Drug-induced lichen planus may take a few months to subside after discontinuation of the offending drug. In rare cases, removal of gold or amalgam dental restorations may also be helpful, especially in patients proven by patch testing to be sensitive to mercuric compounds or gold. Irritants like tobacco and alcohol should be avoided. Topical steroid gels, pastes, or

Table 3.6 Treatment of oral lichen planus

Treatment	Precautions
Mild/moderate disease	
Fluocinonide gel 0.05%, triamcinolone in benzocaine 20% paste (Orabase) qid	Secondary candida infection (thrush)
Tretinoin gel 0.025% bid	Irritation
Cyclosporine solution: 5 mL of a 100 mg/mL swish and spit qid	Do not swallow
Severe disease	
Prednisone 40–60 mg daily tapered over 2–3 weeks	Hyperglycemia, hypertension, insomnia, mood change, weight gain, infection, osteoporosis. Avoid chronic administration
Immunosuppressants	Numerous

sprays are applied to lesions 3–4 times daily. Other therapies include topical cyclosporine, and topical or systemic retinoids.

Pemphigus vulgaris

Definition and etiology

Pemphigus vulgaris is an intraepidermal autoimmune blistering disease. Blisters can be found both in the oral cavity and on glabrous skin.

Clinical features

Pemphigus vulgaris is rare, occurring in approximately 1 of 100,000 persons. It can occur at any age but most commonly affects middle-aged adults. A genetic predisposition in people of Jewish heritage is present. Pemphigus affects both glabrous and mucosal skin but starts in the oral mucosa in approximately 50–70% of patients. The most common intraoral site of involvement is the buccal mucosa, but the palate, pharynx, larynx, and gingiva can also be involved. Physical examination reveals generalized ulcers and erosions that may be several centimeters in diameter and that can be extended with peripheral pressure (Nikolsky's sign). In cases with involvement of glabrous skin, intact blisters are less commonly found, since they easily rupture and leave superficial erosions.

The major disease in the differential diagnosis of oral pemphigus vulgaris is aphthous stomatitis. The ulcers and erosions in aphthous stomatitis are usually intermittent and of short duration (1–3 weeks), unlike those of pemphigus vulgaris, which are persistent. The lesions of pemphigus are usually symmetric; if asymmetric ulcers are found, malignancy or trauma should be suspected. Other rarer causes of generalized ulcers, such as medications (e.g. methotrexate, bismuth, chlorpromazine, phenytoin), nutritional deficiency, inflammatory bowel disease, infections (such as herpes), or deep fungi, should also be considered.

The differential diagnosis of pemphigus vulgaris includes other forms of pemphigus such as pemphigus foliaceus, pemphigus erythematosus, pemphigus vegetans, endemic pemphigus (fogo selvagem), and paraneoplastic pemphigus. In pemphigus foliaceus and pemphigus erythematosus, the blister is more superficial on biopsy specimens. The mucosal surface is rarely involved. Malar involvement resembling lupus erythematosus is seen in pemphigus erythematosus. Pemphigus vegetans is a variant of pemphigus vulgaris in which blisters occur predominantly in intertriginous folds. Lesions develop a vegetating appearance. Paraneoplastic pemphigus is a variant of pemphigus associated with internal malignancies, usually lymphomas, in which severe mucosal ulcerations occur along with an erythema multiforme-like skin eruption. Fogo selvagem is a form of pemphigus endemic to parts of Brazil and is thought to be secondary to an infectious agent yet to be identified.

Although the diagnosis of pemphigus vulgaris can be suspected on clinical grounds, it should always be confirmed with biopsy and immunofluorescent studies. Biopsy reveals a blister with intraepidermal acantholysis (disruption of the normal attachments between keratinocytes). Indirect immunofluorescent studies show circulating autoantibodies directed against epidermal adhesion molecules in approximately 90% of patients. Samples for direct immunofluorescent studies should be taken from perilesional inflamed skin. Intercellular staining for IgG and C3 will occur in approximately 90% of biopsy specimens. Lesional skin or long-standing lesions have many secondary changes that obscure the characteristic immunofluorescent findings.

Treatment (Table 3.7)

The treatment of choice for pemphigus vulgaris is oral prednisone. Immunosuppressive agents such as mycophenolate mofetil, azathioprine, cyclophosphamide, and methotrexate are frequently used as either primary agents or steroid-sparing agents. Other therapies include topical steroids, cyclosporine, dapsone, parenteral gold, rituximab, and plasmapheresis.

Table 3.7 Treatment of oral pemphigus vulgaris

Treatment	Precautions
Mild/moderate disease	
Fluocinonide gel 0.05%, triamcinolone in benzocaine 20% paste (Orabase) qid	Secondary *Candida* infection (thrush)
Severe disease	
Prednisone 40–60 mg daily tapered as warranted by clinical response	Hyperglycemia, hypertension, insomnia, mood change, weight gain, infection, osteoporosis
Immunosuppressants	Numerous
Rituximab 1000 mg infusion × 2 separated by 2 weeks	Severe infusion and mucocutaneous reactions, reactivation of hepatis B virus, progressive multifocal leukoencephalopathy
Dapsone 50–300 mg daily	Hematologic – hemolysis, dyscrasias, methemoglobinemia, G6PD deficiency, rare neuropathy

Chapter 4 Hands and feet

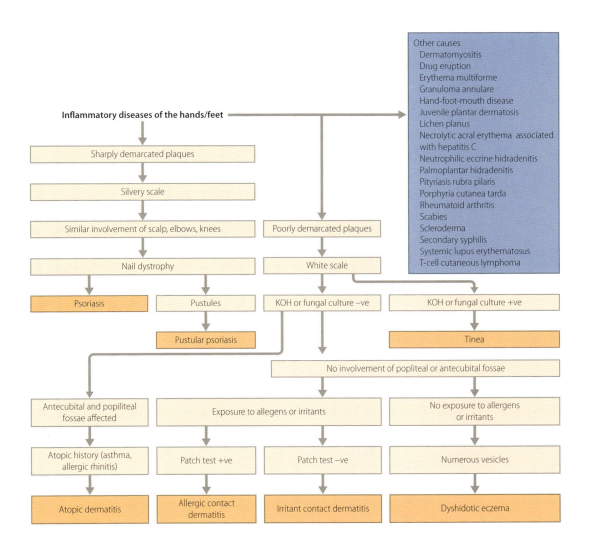

INTRODUCTION

Eruptions of the hands and feet are common and frequently are disabling. Inflamed fissured, blistered, and weeping hands or feet make the activities of daily life and work difficult, if not impossible. It is therefore very important to arrive at an accurate diagnosis on which treatment can be based. With the proper diagnosis and treatment, inflammatory diseases of the hand or foot usually markedly improve or clear completely.

The physical examination is often similar and non-distinguishing when examining the hands or feet alone. The complete skin examination sometimes reveals involvement elsewhere, which will secure the diagnosis. For example, psoriasis of the hands or feet may be associated with typical involvement of the elbows, knees, and scalp. Hand and foot eruptions almost always have associated scaling, and a potassium hydroxide (KOH) preparation or fungal culture should be accomplished to rule out a very treatable disease (e.g., tinea pedis or tinea manuum). For eczematous eruptions of the hands and feet, contact dermatitis, atopic dermatitis, and nonspecific or dyshidrotic eczema need to be considered. For any individual with a hand or foot eruption, one should ultimately ask the question, could this be contact dermatitis? Patch testing with appropriate allergens is the most important diagnostic test to rule out allergic contact dermatitis. For these individuals, removal or avoidance of the allergen or irritant is curative.

1. ALLERGIC CONTACT DERMATITIS VERSUS IRRITANT CONTACT DERMATITIS

Features in common: inflamed patches and plaques

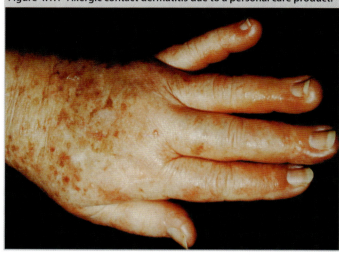

Figure 4.1.1 Allergic contact dermatitis due to a personal care product.

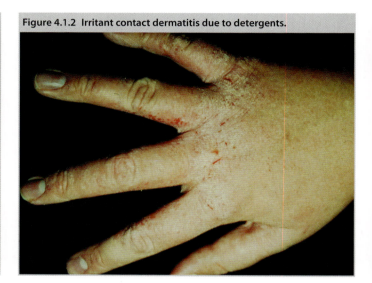

Figure 4.1.2 Irritant contact dermatitis due to detergents.

Distinguishing features

	Allergic contact dermatitis	Irritant contact dermatitis
Physical examination Morphology	Intertriginous areas often uninvolved	Intertriginous areas often involved
History Symptoms	Burning not prominent Pruritus	Burning prominent Pruritus
Exacerbating factors	Exposure to allergen	Exposure to irritant
Associated findings	None	None
Epidemiology	25% of contact dermatitis	75% of contact dermatitis
Biopsy	No	No
Laboratory	Patch test positive	Patch test not done
Outcome	Curable	Curable

Differential diagnosis of inflamed patches and plaques

- Psoriasis
- Tinea
- Atopic dermatitis
- Dyshidrotic eczema
- Reactive arthritis/keratoderma blennorrhagicum
- Pityriasis rubra pilaris
- Lichen planus
- T-cell cutaneous lymphoma (mycosis fungoides)
- Id reaction

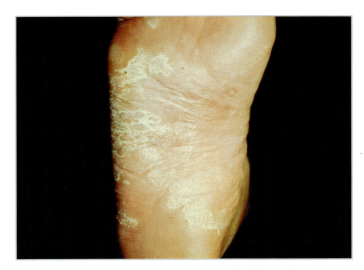

Figure 4.1.3 Allergic contact dermatitis due to insole of shoes. *Clue to diagnosis:* involvement corresponds to area of contact.

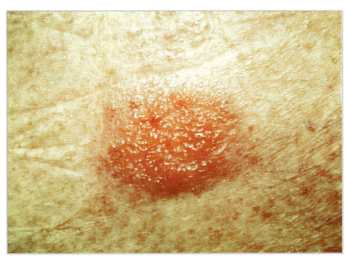

Figure 4.1.4 Allergic contact dermatitis. *Clue to diagnosis:* positive patch test.

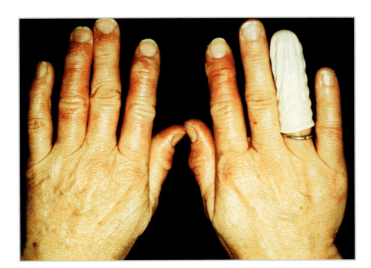

Figure 4.1.5 Allergic contact dermatitis due to finger cot.

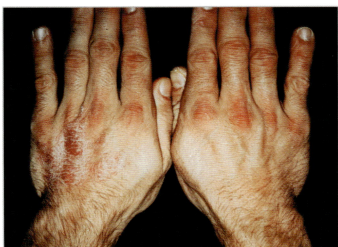

Figure 4.1.6 Irritant contact dermatitis due to glove worn on left hand. *Clue to diagnosis:* negative patch tests.

2. DYSHIDROTIC VERSUS CONTACT DERMATITIS

■ Features in common: inflamed patches and plaques

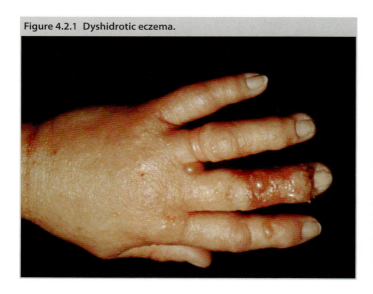

Figure 4.2.1 Dyshidrotic eczema.

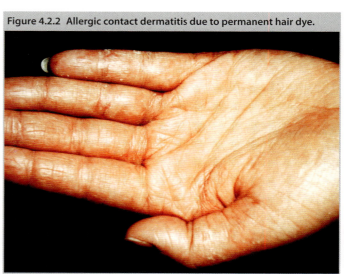

Figure 4.2.2 Allergic contact dermatitis due to permanent hair dye.

■ Distinguishing features

	Dyshidrotic eczema	Contact dermatitis
Physical examination		
Morphology	Prominent vesicles and bullae Hyperhidrosis frequently present	Less prominent vesicles and bullae No hyperhidrosis
Distribution	Dorsum of hands and feet uninvolved Sides of digits involved	Dorsum of hands and feet involved Sides of digits spared
History		
Symptoms	Marked pruritus and burning	Moderate pruritus and burning
Exacerbating factors	Stress	No stress
Associated findings	None	None
Epidemiology	Adults Not occupational	Children and adults May be occupational illness
Biopsy	No	No
Laboratory	None	Patch test
Outcome	Chronic with acute flare-ups	Clears

Causes of contact dermatitis of the hands/feet

Allergic
- Medicaments: benzocaine, neomycin, bacitracin
- Preservatives: barrier and moisturizing creams,
- Work materials (e.g. metal-working fluids)
- Rubber compounds: gloves, shoes
- Epoxy resins: paints, glues
- Metals: tools, cement
- Fragrances: personal care products

Irritant
- Soaps and detergents
- Solvents
- Acids
- Alkalies
- Wet work

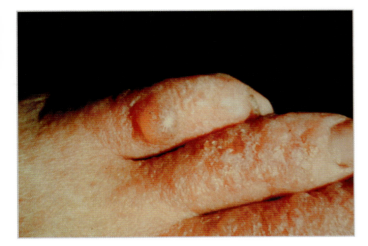

Figure 4.2.3 Dyshidrotic eczema. *Clue to diagnosis:* numerous vesicles and bullae on digits.

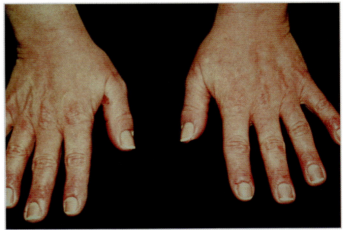

Figure 4.2.4 Allergic contact dermatitis. *Clue to diagnosis:* involvement where there is contact with nail polish.

3. PSORIASIS VERSUS ATOPIC DERMATITIS

Features in common: scaling patches and plaques

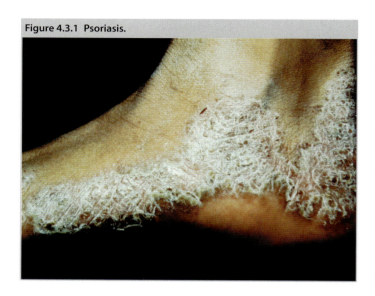

Figure 4.3.1 Psoriasis.

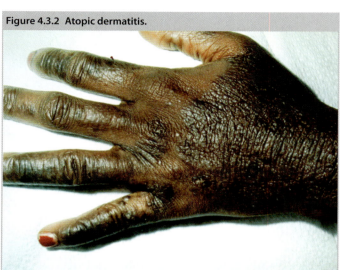

Figure 4.3.2 Atopic dermatitis.

Distinguishing features

		Psoriasis	Atopic dermatitis
Physical examination			
Morphology		Well demarcated Silvery scaling No lichenification Pustules	Ill marginated White scaling Lichenification No pustules
Distribution		Scalp, elbows, knees, nails	Antecubital and popliteal fossae
History			
Symptoms		Mild to moderate pruritus	Marked pruritus
Exacerbating factors		Sunlight improves Skin trauma Strep throat Not heat or sweating Not clothes	Sunlight not helpful Not skin trauma Not strep throat Sweating, heat Clothes, particularly wool
Associated findings		Arthritis Metabolic syndrome No allergic respiratory disease No secondary infection	No arthritis Allergic respiratory disease: asthma and rhinitis Frequent secondary infection with *Staphylococcus aureus*
Epidemiology		Predominantly adults	Predominantly children
Biopsy		No	No
Laboratory		None	None
Outcome		Chronic No remission	Chronic Most children 'outgrow' their eczema

Differential diagnosis of scaling patches

- Contact dermatitis
- Tinea
- Dyshidrotic eczema
- T-cell cutaneous lymphoma (mycosis fungoides)
- Lupus erythematosus
- Lichen planus

Differential diagnosis of pustular hand dermatoses

- Psoriasis
- Acrodermatitis
- Infected dermatitis
- Tinea
- Reactive arthritis/keratoderma blennorrhagicum
- Drug eruption

Major criteria for diagnosis of atopic dermatitis

- Pruritus
- Morphology and distribution:
  - Infants: excoriated juicy papules and patches on extensor extremities and face
  - Infants, children, adults: excoriated, lichenified patches and plaques on flexor extremities (antecubital and popliteal fossae) and face
- Chronic relapsing course
- Atopic disease (asthma, hay fever, eczema) in family or self

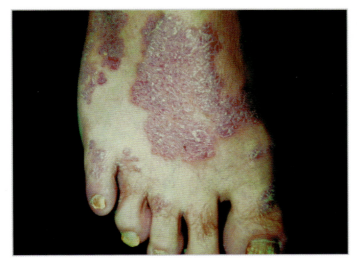

Figure 4.3.3 Psoriasis. *Clue to diagnosis:* well-demarcated plaques; note nail dystrophy.

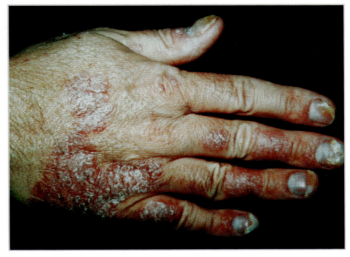

Figure 4.3.4 Psoriasis. *Clue to diagnosis:* well-demarcated plaques; note nail dystrophy.

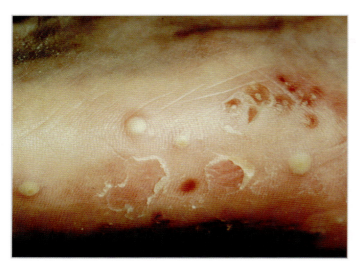

Figure 4.3.5 Pustular psoriasis.

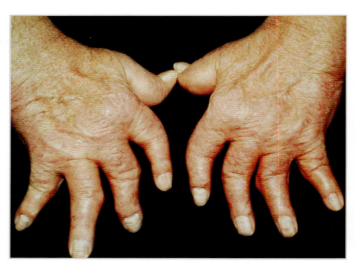

Figure 4.3.6 Psoriatic arthritis.

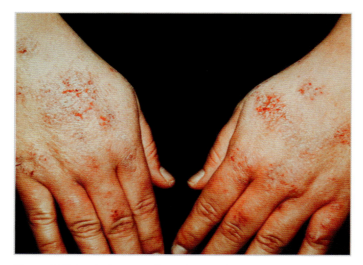

Figure 4.3.7 Atopic dermatitis. *Clue to diagnosis:* ill-marginated patches and plaques.

4. TINEA VERSUS CONTACT DERMATITIS

Features in common: scaling patches and plaques

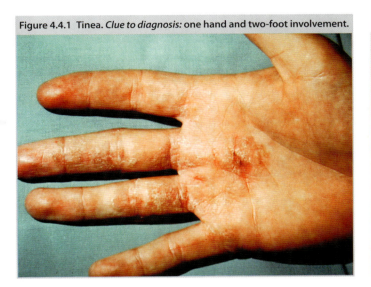

Figure 4.4.1 Tinea. *Clue to diagnosis:* one hand and two-foot involvement.

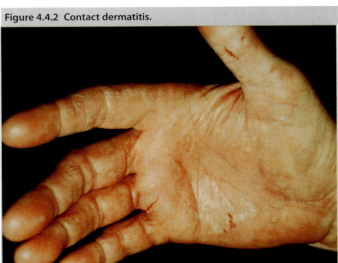

Figure 4.4.2 Contact dermatitis.

Distinguishing features

	Tinea	Contact dermatitis
Physical examination Morphology	Feet: interdigital maceration, diffuse plantar scaling, vesiculopustular eruptions One hand affected Nails dystrophic, thick	Feet: no maceration, lichenified plaques, no pustules Two hands affected Nails not affected
Distribution	Usually both feet; when hand involvement, one hand and two feet	Dermatitis where contact with allergen or irritant
History Symptoms Exacerbating factors	Asymptomatic or pruritus No allergen or irritant	Moderate pruritus and burning Allergen or irritant
Associated findings	Tinea elsewhere, especially nails No dermatitis	No tinea Dermatitis elsewhere
Epidemiology	Not occupational	May be an occupational illness
Biopsy	No	No
Laboratory	Potassium hydroxide test or culture	Patch test
Outcome	Clears	Clears

Differential diagnosis of scaling patches of the hands and feet

- Psoriasis
- Atopic dermatitis
- Dyshidrotic eczema
- Cellulitis
- Xerosis

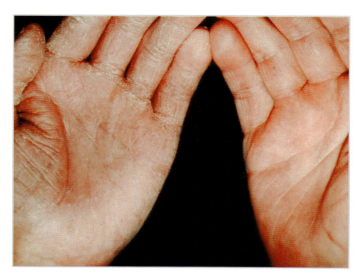

Figure 4.4.3 Tinea manuum. *Clue to diagnosis:* only one hand infected.

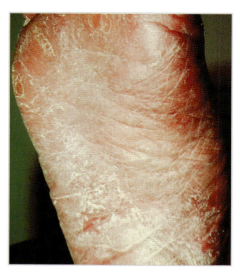

Figure 4.4.4 Tinea pedis. *Clue to diagnosis:* diffuse plantar scaling in 'moccasin' distribution.

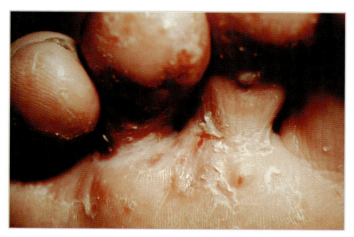

Figure 4.4.5 Tinea pedis with interdigital involvement.

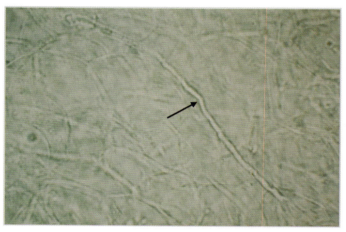

Figure 4.4.6 Tinea pedis and manuum. *Clue to diagnosis:* positive potassium hydroxide test result. Arrow shows fungal hyphae.

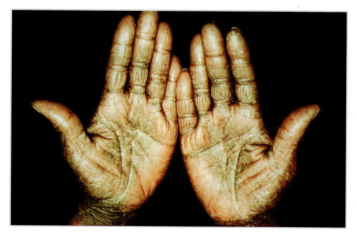

Figure 4.4.7 Contact dermatitis. *Clue to diagnosis:* involvement where there is contact with hand cream.

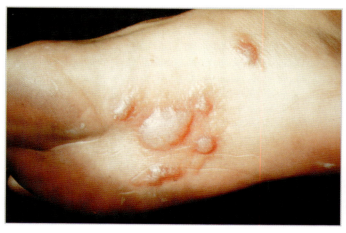

Figure 4.4.8 Contact dermatitis. *Clue to diagnosis:* involvement with contact with poison ivy.

DISEASE DISCUSSION

Atopic dermatitis

Definition and etiology
Atopic dermatitis is a chronic, markedly pruritic, eczematous eruption which is thought to be caused by skin barrier and immune dysfunction. It is usually associated with a personal or family history of atopy (e.g. asthma, allergic rhinoconjunctivitis, or atopic dermatitis).

Clinical features
Atopic dermatitis is predominantly a childhood disease, with up to 17% of children affected. It usually manifests before 5 years of age. For adults, hand dermatitis may be the most common presentation of atopic dermatitis. It is, however, unusual for adults to develop atopic dermatitis without a history of childhood eczema. Allergic respiratory disease is found in the majority of patients or in their family members. Characteristically, pruritus is the most prominent and distressing symptom in patients with atopic dermatitis. For many, pruritus precedes the eruption and is so severe that it disrupts sleep and other activities of daily life. Atopic dermatitis is a chronic disease punctuated by acute and severe flare-ups.

The examination reveals ill-marginated, lichenified, erythematous scaling patches and plaques that affect the dorsum and the palmar surface of the hands and feet. This may be the only manifestation of atopic dermatitis in adults. Usually, however, there are eczematous patches and plaques scattered elsewhere, particularly affecting the antecubital and popliteal fossae. Generalized dry skin is often found.

The differential diagnosis of atopic hand-and-foot dermatitis includes any eczematous-appearing eruption. This includes contact dermatitis, dyshidrotic eczema, psoriasis, superficial fungal infection, scabies, and rare disorders such as pityriasis rubra pilaris. A skin biopsy is usually not necessary to differentiate among these conditions (with the exception of pityriasis rubra pilaris). If done, the skin biopsy reveals the characteristics of any eczematous eruption. Acute and subacute dermatitis shows epidermal spongiosis and chronic dermatitis shows hyperkeratosis with acanthosis of the epidermis.

Treatment (Table 4.1)
Since atopic hand-and-foot dermatitis is a chronic condition, the goal of treatment should be symptomatic relief of itching and control of inflammation. This is accomplished with antihistamines, potent topical steroids, ultraviolet light, and short bursts of systemic steroids. Compresses or soaks with tar or oatmeal emulsions are soothing and help with oozing, if present. Most important, protection of the hands and avoidance of irritants are necessary to ameliorate the inflammatory process. For those whose occupation requires exposure to irritating chemicals, wearing gloves may be helpful. However, a change in jobs may be necessary. The frequent use of moisturizers for dry and lichenified dermatitis of the hands and feet is also quite helpful.

Contact dermatitis

Definition and etiology
Contact dermatitis is an inflammatory reaction to an exogenous chemical, irritant, or allergen that comes in contact with the skin. Irritant contact dermatitis is precipitated by a substance that has direct toxic properties, whereas allergic contact dermatitis is triggered by a delayed-type hypersensitivity reaction. Irritating chemicals include acids, alkalies, solvents, and detergents. There are numerous allergens, including plants (poison ivy and oak), metals (nickel), rubber chemicals, personal care products (cosmetic) ingredients (fragrances, preservatives), and topical medicines (neomycin and bacitracin).

Clinical features
Contact dermatitis of the hands is responsible for a significant proportion of occupational skin diseases. More commonly, the cause is irritant contact dermatitis due to cumulative exposure to wet work, solvents, and detergents, as seen in hairdressers, housewives, nurses, and machinists. These weaker irritants require multiple applications over a period of days before the irritant contact dermatitis appears. For

Table 4.1 Treatment of dermatitis

Treatment	Precautions
Universal	
Avoid irritants and allergens	None
Moisturizers	
Mild cleansing agents such as Dove or Aveeno	
Mild disease	
Hydrocortisone cream/ointment 1% bid	Rarely causes allergic contact dermatitis
Pimecrolimus cream 1% bid	Burning sensation
Moderate disease	
Triamcinolone cream/ointment 0.1% bid	Atrophy with chronic application; especially intertriginous areas
	Steroid acne of face
	Glaucoma and cataracts if apply on eyelids
Tacrolimus ointment 0.1% bid	Burning sensation
Cetirazine 10 mg bid, Diphenhydramine 25–50 mg qid	Sedation
Gabapentin 100–300 mg qid	
Oatmeal or tar baths	None
Bleach baths for skin infections: 1/4 cup in half full bathtub	
Severe disease	
Clobetasol cream/ointment 0.5% bid	Atrophy with chronic application; especially intertriginous areas
	Steroid acne of face
	Glaucoma and cataracts if apply on eyelids
Prednisone 40–60 mg daily tapered over 2–3 weeks	Hyperglycemia, hypertension, insomnia, mood change, weight gain, infection, osteoporosis
Mycophenolate mofetil 1000–1500 mg bid	Nausea, diarrhea, bone marrow suppression, infection
	Birth defects
Ultraviolet light: nUVB	Burning, skin cancer
Antipuritics and baths as for moderate	

strong irritants, symptoms develop within minutes to hours, and the diagnosis is readily apparent. For allergens, because of the delayed-type hypersensitivity reaction, onset occurs after one day to several days. This makes identification of the allergen more difficult, and it often goes unrecognized. This is particularly true in the case of daily contact with allergens such as rubber chemicals found in gloves or shoes, personal care products, and medicines applied to the hands and feet.

Contact dermatitis varies from acute to chronic, which results in varying appearances. Acute contact dermatitis has marked epidermal edema, or spongiosis, which causes papules, vesicles, bullae, and secondary changes such as oozing and crusting. The hallmark of chronic contact dermatitis is lichenification or thickening of the epidermis associated with scaling and fissuring. The distribution of the dermatitis corresponds with the areas of contact. Streaks, geometric outlines, and sharp margins typically occur, particularly elsewhere on the body (e.g. where there has been application of the contactant or brushing of the leaf or stem of posion ivy or oak). For gloves, both the palmar and the dorsal surface may be involved. Since the stratum corneum is much thinner on the dorsum of the hands and allows penetration of the allergen more easily, however, the dorsum is more commonly affected. For the feet, the distribution depends on what portion of the shoe is causing the contact dermatitis. For example, the insole of the shoe causes diffuse dermatitis on the soles of the feet.

On physical examination, contact dermatitis of the hands and feet can be acute, subacute, or chronic, depending on the strength of the contactant and the nature of exposure. Strong irritants and allergens cause acute contact dermatitis, manifested by a vesicular bullous eruption. Weaker irritants and allergens to which there has been repeated exposure cause chronic lichenified contact dermatitis. Contact dermatitis elsewhere may occur owing to transmission of the irritant or allergen via the hands by touching other areas of the body, such as the face.

Since the morphology of different dermatitic eruptions is identical, dyshidrotic (nonspecific) eczema and atopic dermatitis should be considered. Other eczematous appearing dermatoses that should be ruled out include superficial fungal infection, psoriasis, and cellulitis. The diagnosis of irritant contact dermatitis is one of exclusion. There is no standard testing for irritation. For allergic contact dermatitis, the allergen can be identified by patch testing.

Treatment (Table 4.1)

The management of contact dermatitis should emphasize prevention by complete avoidance of the offending irritants or allergens. This may require a change in occupation or lifestyle. Protective clothing such as gloves may be helpful. Substitution of less toxic materials may be accomplished. The principal treatment is topical steroids of medium to potent strength applied twice a day. For those individuals with severe or widespread contact dermatitis, a short course of systemic steroids is indicated. General majors such as astringent soaks or compresses, applied 15 minutes twice a day are used to reduce weeping. Colloidal oatmeal or tar emulsion baths or compresses reduce inflammation and itching. Antihistamines can be taken for itching.

■ Dyshidrotic eczema

Definition and etiology

Dyshidrotic eczema, also known as pompholyx, is characteristically a vesicular eruption of the hands and feet of unknown cause.

Clinical features

The characteristic appearance of dyshidrotic eczema is deep-seated vesicles that resemble the pearls in tapioca pudding and involve the palms, soles, and sides of the digits. The vesicles usually occur bilaterally and symmetrically. Vesicles may coalesce, forming bullae or, when slow in resolving, may be replaced by the chronic eczematous changes of erythema, scaling, and lichenification. This disease often has a waxing and waning course with sudden flare-ups of vesicles characterized by marked pruritus and burning. Patients often have associated hyperhidrosis.

The differential diagnosis includes other eczematous eruptions such as contact and atopic dermatitis, psoriasis, tinea, mycosis fungoides, lupus erythematosus, and lichen planus. Although a biopsy is usually not necessary, results reveal spongiosis typical of dermatitis.

Treatment (Table 4.1)

Treatment of dyshidrotic eczema is similar to that of other eczematous eruptions, with steroids being the mainstay. For symptomatic relief, soaks or compresses with astringents as well as oral antihistamines are helpful.

■ Psoriasis

Definition and etiology

Psoriasis is an inflammatory disease characterized by increased epidermal proliferation. The cause of psoriasis is unknown, but abnormal epidermal kinetics as well as the activation of the immune system within the skin must be taken into account.

Clinical features

Approximately one-third of patients have a family history positive for psoriasis. This is a relatively common skin disease affecting about 2–5% of the population in the United States. The most common age of onset is in the third decade, but it can present at any time. The major precipitating or aggravating factors include streptococcal pharyngitis, trauma to the skin, emotional stress, use of drugs such as β-blocking agents and lithium, and human immunodeficiency virus infection.

The examination of the hands and feet reveals sharply demarcated, erythematous, silvery, scaling plaques. Pustules within these plaques are found in pustular psoriasis. Dystrophic nail changes (pits, onycholysis, brown discoloration, and thickened nail plate) often occur. Typical involvement elsewhere includes the extensor surfaces of the elbows and knees and the scalp.

The differential diagnosis of hand-and-foot psoriasis includes contact dermatitis, tinea, dyshidrotic eczema, atopic dermatitis, T-cell cutaneous lymphoma (mycosis fungoides), lupus erythematosus, and lichen planus. Usually, a skin biopsy is not necessary, but if one is done, findings reveal characteristic hyperkeratosis, parakeratosis, acanthotic epidermis, inflammatory infiltrate in the dermis, and neutrophils migrating into the epidermis, forming microabscesses.

Treatment (Table 4.2)

Treatment modalities include topical preparations containing steroids, tars, anthralin, and calcipotriol. When the disease is severe, ultraviolet light, methotrexate, acetretin, cyclosporine, and biologic agents are used.

Table 4.2 Treatment of psoriais

Treatment	Precautions
Mild disease	
Moisturizers	None
Tars, anthralin	Stain, irritation
Hydrocortisone cream/ointment 1% bid	Rarely causes allergic contact dermatitis
Pimecrolimus cream 1% bid	Burning sensation
Moderate disease	
Ultra violet light: nUVB 2–3 times/week	Burning, skin cancer
Triamcinolone cream/ointment 0.1% bid	Atrophy with chronic application; especially intertriginous areas
	Steroid acne of face
	Glaucoma and cataracts if apply on eyelids
Tacrolimus ointment 0.1% bid	Burning sensation
Calcipotriene cream/ointment	Irritation. Overuse can cause hypercalcemia
Apremilast 30 mg bid	Weight loss, depression
Severe disease	
Clobetasol cream/ointment 0.5%	Atrophy with chronic application; especially intertriginous areas
	Steroid acne of face
	Glaucoma and cataracts if apply on eyelids
Ultraviolet light: nUVB, PUVA 2–3 times/week	Burning, skin cancer
Acitretin 25 mg daily	Dry skin, hair loss, elevated serum lipids and liver functions, birth defects
Methotrexate 10–20 mg once a week	Bone marrow suppression, liver toxicity/cirrhosis, nausea/diarrhea
Biologics (etanercept, adalimumab, infliximab, ustekinumab, secukinumab, etc.)	Infection, possible increase in lymphoma, injection site reactions

Table 4.3 Treament of tinea manum/pedis

Treatment	Precautions
Universal	
Periodic antifungals to prevent recurrence	
For feet, reduce sweating/moisture	
Mild/moderate disease	
Clotrimazole 1%, miconazole 2%, or terbinafine 1% cream daily or bid	None
Severe disease	
Terbinafine 250 mg/day for 4–8 weeks	Rare hepatic toxicity
Fluconazole 200 mg/day for 4–8 weeks	Rare hepatic toxicity
Griseofulvin 500 mg/day for 4–8 weeks	Rare hepatic toxicity

Tinea manuum and pedis

Definition and etiology

Tinea manuum and tinea pedis are superficial fungal infections of the hands and feet, respectively, caused by dermatophytes, usually *Trichophyton rubrum*, *Trichophyton mentagrophytes*, or *Epidermophyton floccosum*.

Clinical features

Tinea manuum is relatively uncommon, whereas tinea pedis affects approximately 4% of the general population. Spread of tinea pedis occurs easily in settings such as locker rooms, where high spore counts and bare feet are found. Hot, humid climates; sweating; and occlusive shoes encourage fungal infections. Tinea manuum typically affects one hand and is associated with bilateral tinea pedis in what is called 'one hand, two feet' syndrome. The reason for involvement of only one hand is unknown. The palmar surface is usually affected by mild, diffuse, white scaling. Tinea pedis can appear as interdigital maceration, diffuse plantar scaling, or a vesiculopustular eruption. Often, onychomycosis is associated with tinea manuum and pedis.

The differential diagnosis of tinea manuum and pedis includes atopic and dyshidrotic eczema, psoriasis, xerosis, and occasionally cellulitis. Although usually an infection of adults, tinea should be considered in the differential diagnosis of children with an eczematous eruption of the feet. A KOH preparation or fungal culture confirms the diagnosis.

Treatment (Table 4.3)

Topical therapy for tinea manuum and pedis is usually effective in controlling or clearing the eruption. When the disease is associated with onychomycosis, oral antifungal agents are required to clear the nails. The most effective agent is probably terbinafine (Lamisil), but also very effective are the azoles, such as ketoconazole, miconazole, or clotrimazole. Measures to reduce recurrence of tinea pedis include using topical antiperspirants to reduce sweating, wearing nonocclusive shoes, changing socks frequently, and not going barefoot in public areas such as locker rooms.

Chapter 5: Nails

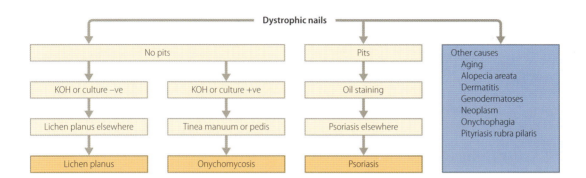

INTRODUCTION

In addition to having significant cosmetic value, the nail protects the distal end of the fingers and toes from trauma and is used for fine grasping and scratching. The nail unit is not a static horny appendage but a dynamic growing structure consisting of matrix, bed, folds, hyponychium, and plate. These components of the nail unit are affected by a number of diseases, which ultimately can alter the appearance of the nail plate and cause nail dystrophy. The dystrophic physical appearance of the nail cannot be used reliably to make a diagnosis. For the three diseases discussed in this chapter – onychomycosis, psoriasis, and lichen planus – other entities in the differential diagnosis include aging, trauma, and secondary changes due to dermatitis. A history, skin examination, and appropriate laboratory tests are required to arrive at a definite diagnosis. This is particularly important with respect to onychomycosis, since it is treatable with systemic antifungals.

1. ONYCHOMYCOSIS VERSUS PSORIASIS

■ Features in common: dystrophic nails

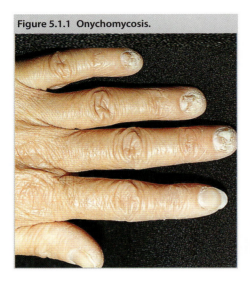

Figure 5.1.1 Onychomycosis.

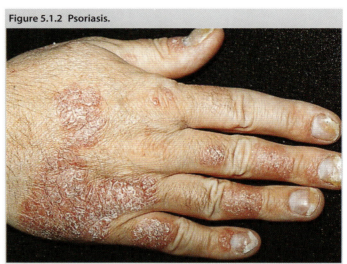

Figure 5.1.2 Psoriasis.

■ Distinguishing features

	Onychomycosis	Psoriasis
Physical examination		
Morphology	No pits No oil spots	Pits Oil spots
Distribution	No elbow, knee involvement	Elbow, knee involved
History		
Symptoms	Asymptomatic or some discomfort	Asymptomatic or some discomfort
Exacerbating factors	Not stress Sweating	Stress Not sweating
Associated findings	Tinea manuum and pedis No arthritis	No tinea manuum or pedis Arthritis
Epidemiology	Common	Common
Biopsy	No	No
Laboratory	KOH or culture positive	KOH or culture negative
Outcome	Cure	Chronic

KOH, potassium hydroxide

Differential diagnosis of dystrophic nails

- Aging
- Trauma
- Dermatitis
- Lichen planus

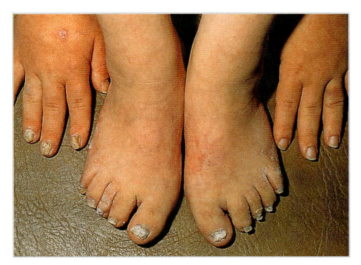

Figure 5.1.3 Onychomycosis. *Clue to diagnosis:* one hand, two foot involvement.

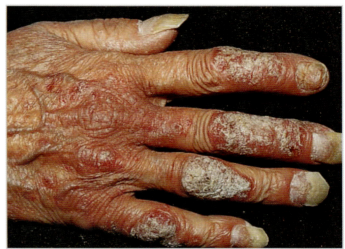

Figure 5.1.4 Psoriasis. *Clue to diagnosis:* associated psoriasis of fingers.

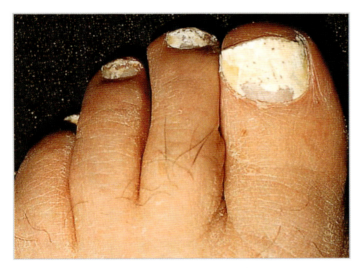

Figure 5.1.5 Onychomycosis with superficial white infection.

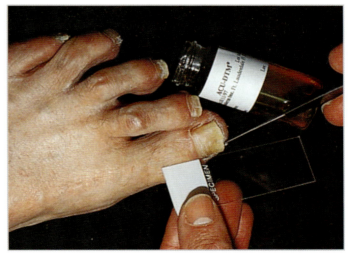

Figure 5.1.6 Onychomycosis. Confirm diagnosis with potassium hydroxide test and culture.

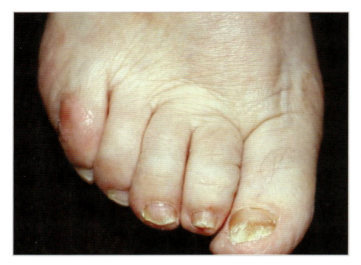

Figure 5.1.7 Onychomycosis.

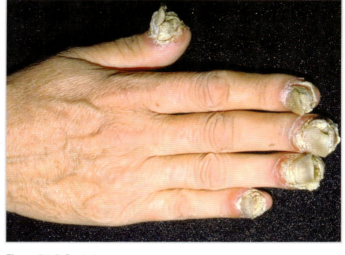

Figure 5.1.8 Psoriasis.

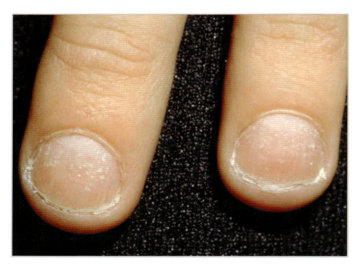

Figure 5.1.9 Psoriasis: note pits.

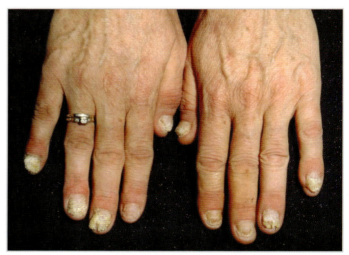

Figure 5.1.10 Psoriasis.

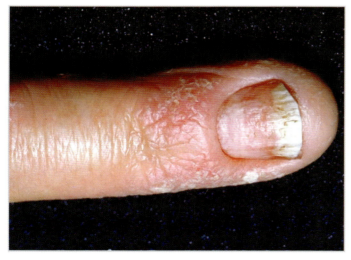

Figure 5.1.11 Psoriasis: note nail separation and yellow discoloration.

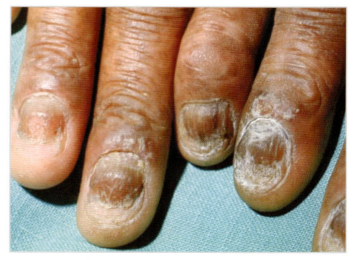

Figure 5.1.12 Psoriasis.

2. PSORIASIS VERSUS LICHEN PLANUS

Features in common: dystrophic nails

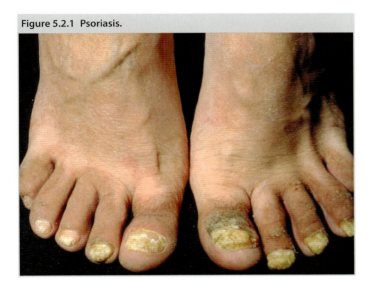

Figure 5.2.1 Psoriasis.

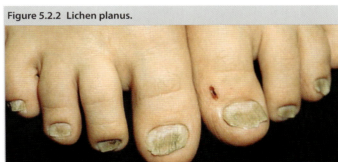

Figure 5.2.2 Lichen planus.

Distinguishing features

	Psoriasis	Lichen planus
Physical examination		
Morphology	Pits No pterygium	No pits Pterygium
Distribution	Elbows, knees involved Mouth uninvolved	No elbow, knee involvement Mouth may be involved
History		
Symptoms	Asymptomatic or some discomfort	Asymptomatic or some discomfort
Exacerbating factors	Physical or emotional stress or illness	None
Associated findings	Arthritis	No arthritis
Epidemiology	Common	Uncommon
Biopsy	No	No
Laboratory	No	No
Outcome	Chronic	Chronic

Differential diagnosis of dystrophic nails

- Aging
- Trauma
- Dermatitis
- Lichen planus

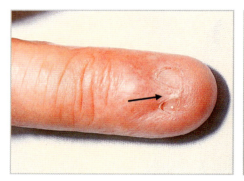

Figure 5.2.3 Lichen planus. *Clue to diagnosis:* pterygium formation (arrow).

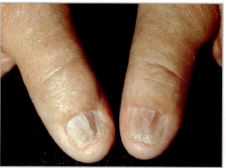

Figure 5.2.4 Lichen planus.

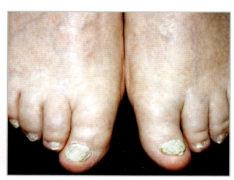

Figure 5.2.5 Lichen planus.

3. DYSTROPHIC NAILS

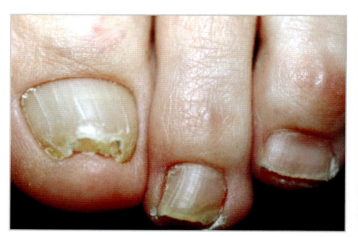

Figure 5.3.1 Trauma.

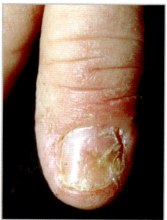

Figure 5.3.2 Allergic contact dermatitis from artificial nails.

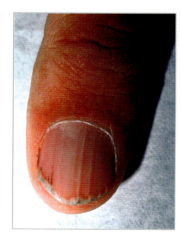

Figure 5.3.3 Darier's disease.

Dystrophic nails

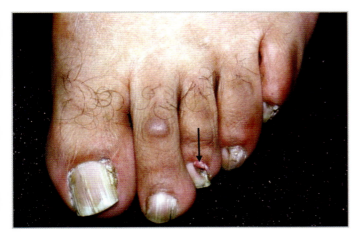

Figure 5.3.4 Tuberous sclerosis: note the fibromas (arrow).

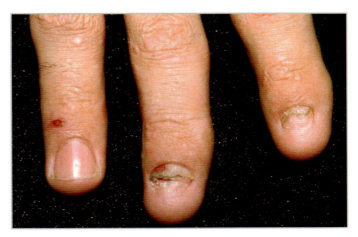

Figure 5.3.5 Epidermolysis bullosa: dominant dystrophic.

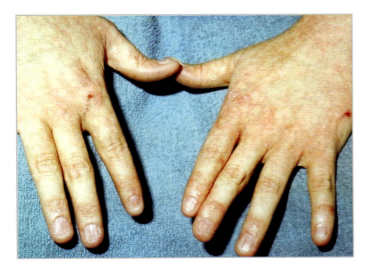

Figure 5.3.6 Dyskeratosis congenita.

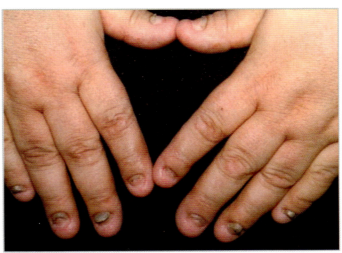

Figure 5.3.7 Pachyonychia congeniata.

4. OTHER EXAMPLES

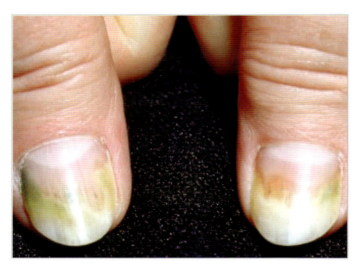

Figure 5.4.1 Pseudomonas infection.

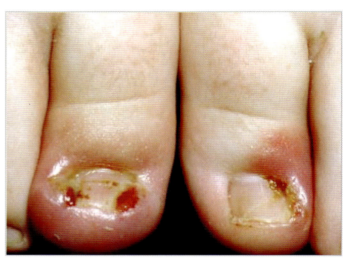

Figure 5.4.2 Ingrown toenails.

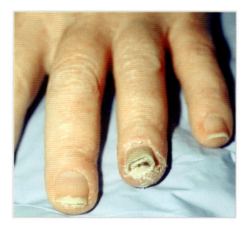

Figure 5.4.3 Scabies.

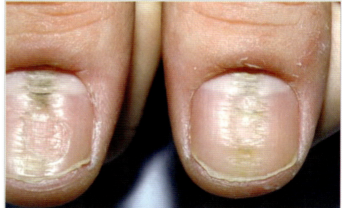

Figure 5.4.4 Nail tic.

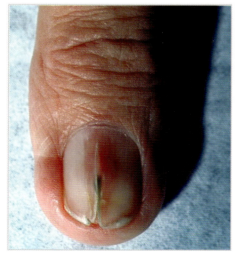

Figure 5.4.5 Median canal of Heller.

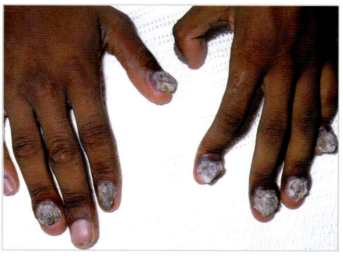

Figure 5.4.6 Mucocutaneous candidiasis.

DISEASE DISCUSSION

Lichen planus

Definition and etiology
Lichen planus is an idiopathic inflammatory process affecting the nails, hair, skin, and mucous membranes.

Clinical features
Lichen planus is a relatively uncommon disorder, usually of adults. The skin is most commonly affected by pruritic papules, and the mucous membranes develop asymptomatic white patches or painful erosions. A minority of cases (approximately 10%) have nail involvement. Rarely, lichen planus involves only the nails without associated skin or mucous membrane findings.

The nail affected by lichen planus has a variety of appearances. Most commonly, the nail plate is thickened or thinned and is separated from the nail bed (onycholysis). Occasionally, scarring occurs with formation of a characteristic pterygium.

The differential diagnosis of lichen planus of the nails includes psoriasis, onychomycosis, aging, trauma, and dermatitis. Some entities in the differential diagnosis include genodermatoses, alopecia areata, onychophagia, and 20-nail dystrophy, which is a nail disorder primarily seen in children that is thought to be a variant of lichen planus only affecting the nails. Associated lichen planus found elsewhere, particularly on the wrists, ankles, and mucous membranes of the mouth, confirms the diagnosis. A negative potassium hydroxide (KOH) test result or fungal culture will rule out onychomycosis.

Treatment (Table 5.1)
There is no good treatment for lichen planus affecting the nails. Topical steroids are usually ineffective but may be tried.

Onychomycosis

Definition and etiology
Onychomycosis, also termed tinea unguium, is a superficial fungal infection of the nail caused by the dermatophytes *Trichophyton rubrum* and *Trichophyton mentagrophytes*.

Clinical features
Onychomycosis is almost always associated with tinea pedis or manuum. Infection of the toenails is more common than infection of the fingernails. It is uncommon for all 10 toenails to be involved at the same time or to the same degree. There are three patterns of nail involvement: proximal, distal, and white superficial.

The examination of an onychomycotic nail reveals white, yellow, or brown discoloration. In the distal type, which is the most common, the plate is usually thickened with distal subungual debris, and it may be crumbling. Occasionally, the dermatophyte infects only the top surface of the nail plate, causing a white, crumbling superficial onychomycosis. Rarely, the thickening and debris occur in the proximal nail plate. Usually, both feet are affected. On occasion, a typical presentation will be the so-called 'one hand, two feet' syndrome, in which the nails of one hand and both feet are infected in association with tinea manuum and pedis.

The differential diagnosis of onychomycosis includes psoriasis, lichen planus, and other causes of dystrophic nails such as aging, trauma, and dermatitis. Onychomycosis cannot be diagnosed reliably by physical examination alone; a KOH Test, nail clipping for pathology, or a fungal culture *must* be done to confirm the diagnosis.

Treatment (Table 5.2)
Treatment must be with an oral antifungal. We prefer terbinafine (Lamisil) given continuously for 6 weeks for fingernails and 12 weeks for toenails is usually effective. Alternatively, itraconazole (Sporanox) or fluconazole (Diflucan) can be given in pulse doses. Topical antifungal agents work poorly and are not usually recommended for treatment. However, they may work to prevent recurrence once oral treatment has cleared the nails, especially for tinea pedis as a source of fungus for the nail. Preventative measures to reduce recurrence include applying topical agents to reduce sweating, wearing nonocclusive shoes, changing damp socks frequently, and not going barefoot in public areas such as locker rooms.

Psoriasis

Definition and etiology
Psoriasis is an inflammatory disease characterized by increased epidermal proliferation. The cause of psoriasis is unknown, but abnormal epidermal kinetics as well as the activation of the immune system within the skin must be taken into account.

Clinical features
Approximately one-third of patients have a family history positive for psoriasis. This is a relatively common skin disease affecting about

Table 5.1 Treatment of nail lichen planus

Treatment	Precautions
Universal: poor outcomes	Do not miss tinea
Clobetasol cream/ointment 0.5% bid	Atrophy
Intralesional triamcinolone (Kenalog) 10 mg/mL to nail matrix	Painful

Table 5.2 Treatment of onychomycosis

Treatment	Precautions
Universal: treat tinea pedis periodically to prevent recurrence	
Terbinafine 62.5 mg for weight <20 kg, 125 mg for weight 20–40 kg, 250 mg >40 kg daily For fingernails: 6 weeks For toenails: 12 weeks	Rare hepatic toxicity
Itraconazole: For toenails: 200 mg daily for 12 weeks For fingernails: 200 mg bid for 1 week, repeat once after 3 weeks	Hepatic toxicity, drug interactions

2% of the population in the United States. The most common age of onset is in the third decade, but it can present at any time. The major precipitating or aggravating factors include streptococcal pharyngitis, trauma to the skin, emotional stress, and use of drugs such as ß-blocking agents and lithium.

The examination of the psoriatic nail typically reveals pitting, yellow oil staining, thickening, and separation of the nail plate from the nail bed (onycholysis). All or just a few nails may be involved. It is uncommon for psoriasis to affect only the nails without associated cutaneous disease.

The differential diagnosis of psoriatic nails includes other causes of dystrophic nails such as onychomycosis, lichen planus, aging, and dystrophy secondary to eczema or another inflammatory process of the nail fold. Typical psoriatic involvement elsewhere, such as the extensor surface of the elbows and knees and the scalp, confirms the diagnosis. Biopsy of the nail is rarely done.

Table 5.3 Treatment of nail psoriasis

Treatment	Precautions
Universal: poor outcomes unless systemic therapy	Do not miss tinea
Clobetasol cream/ointment 0.5% bid	Atrophy
Intralesional triamcinolone (Kenalog) 10 mg/mL to nail matrix	Painful

Treatment (Table 5.3)

Psoriasis of the nail is chronic, with a waxing and waning course. Treatment is difficult and rarely effective. Systemic medications used to control psoriasis elsewhere often help the nail involvement. However, nail involvement alone does not warrant use of these potentially toxic drugs.

Chapter 6 Legs

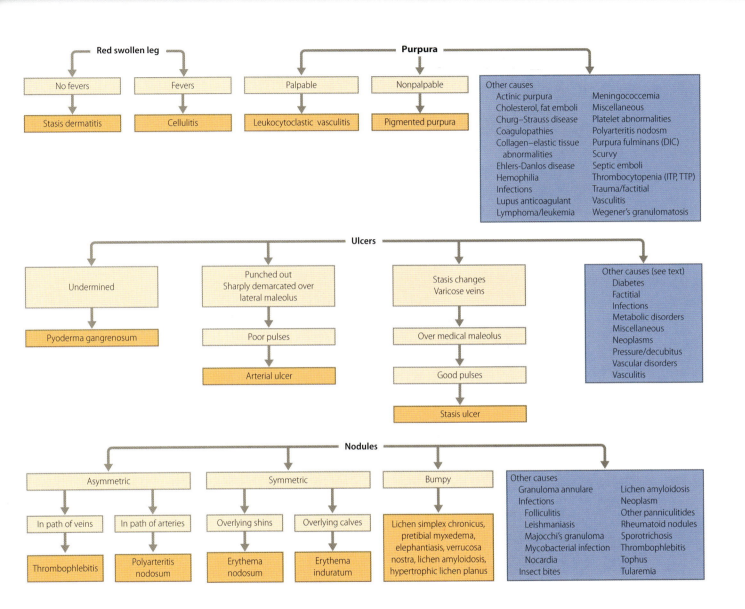

INTRODUCTION

Circulatory diseases most often present on the legs. Gravity, distance from the heart, increased venous pressure, and the lower temperature of the limbs compared with core body temperature all compromise the function of blood vessels in the legs and predispose them to the development of lesions. Gravity and increased venous pressure affect the venous circulation and lead to venous insufficiency. Over time, valves become incompetent, and varicosities develop. Eventually, venous incompetence results in extravasation of blood into the skin, producing stasis dermatitis, fibrosis, and ulceration. Emboli may lodge in arteries because they end in capillary beds without adequate collateral circulation. Venous insufficiency and resultant stasis dermatitis need to be differentiated from arterial disease or pyoderma gangrenosum because the treatments for these disorders are different. In patients with vasculitis, circulating immune complexes lodge in small vessels in dependent sites, producing palpable purpura. Nonpalpable purpura due to capillaritis (i.e. pigmented purpura) is also most commonly found on the legs. Panniculitis frequently presents on the shins and calves. Other rashes with a predilection for the shins include necrobiosis lipoidica diabeticorum and pretibial myxedema. Each of these disorders shares an affinity for the legs and is associated with certain clues that allow for accurate differentiation among them. This chapter outlines helpful clues in their differential diagnosis.

1. ERYTHEMA NODOSUM VERSUS ERYTHEMA INDURATUM

■ Features in common: red nodules and plaques on lower extremities

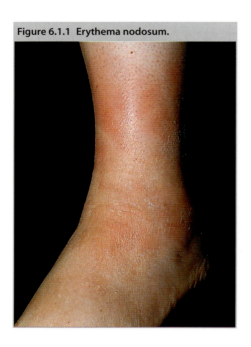

Figure 6.1.1 Erythema nodosum.

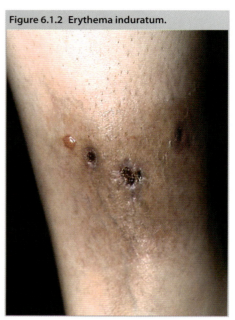

Figure 6.1.2 Erythema induratum.

■ Distinguishing features

	Erythema nodosum	Erythema induratum
Physical examination		
Morphology	Lesions do not ulcerate Resolving lesions: purpuric bruise-like nodules	Lesions frequently ulcerate Ulcers have ragged violaceous margin No purpuric lesions
Distribution	Pretibial area, rarely elsewhere	Predilection for calves Occasionally shins and thighs
History		
Symptoms	Pain	Pain
Exacerbating factors	Prolonged standing, limb dependencies	None
Associated findings	Medications: oral contraceptives Infections: streptococcal infections, deep fungal infections, Immunologic diseases: sarcoidosis, Behçet's disease Inflammatory bowel disease	No medications Infections: tuberculosis No immunologic disease No bowel disease
Epidemiology	More in common in women Common	More in common in women Rare
Biopsy	Occasionally Septal panniculitis with mixed inflammatory infiltrate	Yes Lobular panniculitis with histiocytes and caseation necrosis, vasculitis of medium- sized venules and occasionally arteries
Laboratory	Anti-streptolysin O titer, chest X-ray	Purified protein derivative, chest X-ray
Outcome	Self-limited, resolves over several weeks	Chronic

Differential diagnosis of leg nodules

Common causes
- Erythema nodosum
- Furunculosis
- Thrombophlebitis
- Insect bites
- Infections: Majocchi's granuloma

Rarer causes
- Granuloma annulare
- Gouty tophus
- Infections: leishmaniasis, mycobacterial infection, Nocardia, parasitic infection, sporotrichosis, tularemia
- Rheumatoid nodule
- Erythema induratum
- Polyarteritis nodosa
- Malignant neoplasms: lymphoma, metastases
- Benign neoplasms: lipoma, adnexal tumors

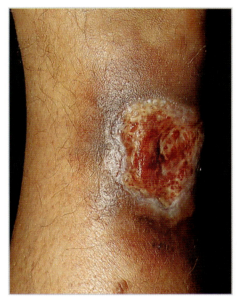

Figure 6.1.3 Erythema induratum. *Clue to diagnosis*: location over the calves and ulceration.

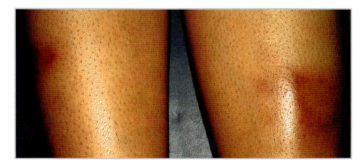

Figure 6.1.4 Erythema nodosum. *Clue to diagnosis*: a lesion with a bruise like appearance (erythema contusiformis).

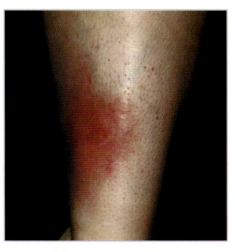

Figure 6.1.5 Erythema nodosum.

2. LEUKOCYTOCLASTIC VASCULITIS VERSUS PIGMENTED PURPURA

Features in common: purpura on lower legs

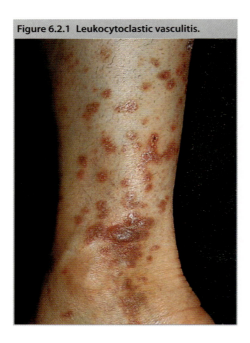

Figure 6.2.1 Leukocytoclastic vasculitis.

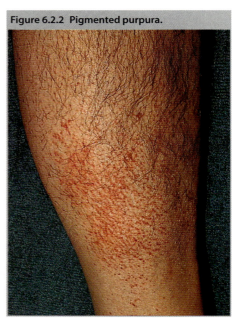

Figure 6.2.2 Pigmented purpura.

Distinguishing features

	Leukocytoclastic vasculitis	Pigmented purpura
Physical examination Morphology	Urticarial lesions Lesions palpable No cayenne-pepper-like macules	No urticarial lesions Lesions not palpable Orange-brown cayenne-pepper-like macules
Distribution	Occasionally ulcers and vesicles Lower legs and dependent areas	No ulcers or vesicles Lower legs
History Symptoms	Fever, malaise, pain, burning, itching	Asymptomatic or mild itching
Exacerbating or causative factors	Drugs Infections Collagen vascular diseases Malignancies Miscellaneous: paraproteinemia, cryoglobulinemia	Occasionally drugs
Associated findings	Occasionally extracutaneous vasculitis: kidney, central nervous system, gastrointestinal tract, lung, joints, heart	No systemic vasculitis
Epidemiology	Uncommon No sex predominance	Uncommon Slight male predominance
Biopsy	Yes Fibrinoid necrosis of blood vessels, neutrophilic infiltrate, leukocytoclasis, endothelial swelling, extravasated erythrocytes	No Superficial lymphocytic infiltrate, extravasated erythrocytes, hemosiderin
Laboratory	Anti-streptolysin O titer, erythrocyte sedimentation rate, complete blood count with differential, cryoglobulins, serum protein electrophoresis, antinuclear anti- body, hepatitis screen in suggestive clinical history, chest X-ray	None
Outcome	Acute or chronic depending on associated disease or cause	Chronic

Differential diagnosis of purpura

- Connective tissue abnormality
  - Actinic purpura
  - Scurvy
  - Ehlers–Danlos syndrome
- Vascular abnormality
- Vasculitis – usually palpable
  - Henoch–Schönlein purpura
  - Leukocytoclastic (allergic) disease
  - Finkelstein's disease
  - Granulomatosis with polyangitis
  - Polyarteritis nodosa
  - Thrombophlebitis
- Pigmented purpura
- Hematologic abnormality
  - Thrombocytopenia
  - Idiopathic thrombocytopenic purpura
  - Thrombotic thrombocytopenia
  - Coagulopathies (hemophilia)
  - Purpura fulminans (disseminated intravascular coagulation)
  - Leukemia
- Infections
  - Meningococcemia
  - Rocky Mountain spotted fever
  - Endocarditis
  - Acute hemorrhagic fever
- Miscellaneous
  - Amyloidosis
  - Cholesterol/fat emboli
  - Drug-induced (corticosteroid) disorder
  - Dysproteinemia
  - Trauma/bites
  - Panniculitis
  - Wiskott–Aldrich syndrome
  - Langerhans cell granulomatosis
  - Increased intravascular pressure: coughing, Valsalva's maneuver

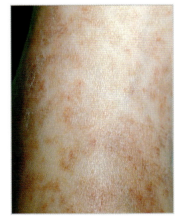

Figure 6.2.3 Pigmented purpura. *Clue to diagnosis*: cayenne-pepper like appearance.

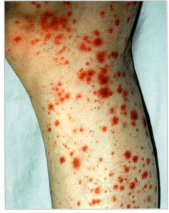

Figure 6.2.4 Leukocytoclastic vasculitis: palpable purpura.

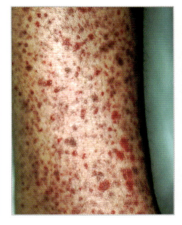

Figure 6.2.5 Leukocytoclastic vasculitis: palpable purpura.

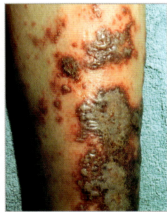

Figure 6.2.6 Leukocytoclastic vasculitis with incipient ulceration.

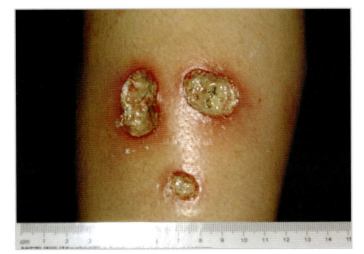

Figure 6.2.7 Punched-out ulcers due to leukocytoclastic vasculitis in patient with rheumatoid arthritis.

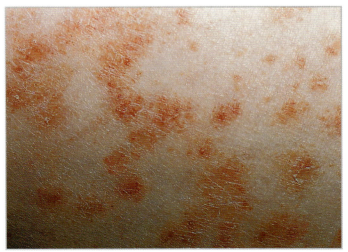

Figure 6.2.8 Pigmented purpura.

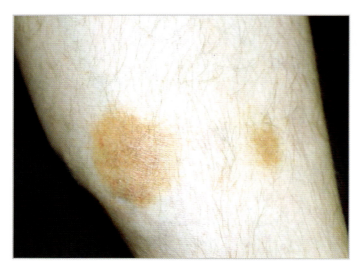

Figure 6.2.9 Lichen aureus variant of pigmented purpura. *Clue to diagnosis:* gold colored with petechiae.

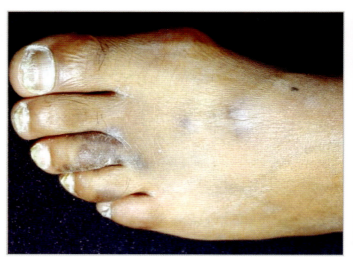

Figure 6.2.10 Cholesterol emboli. Embolic phenomena can be mistaken for vasculitis but usually lesions are fewer, asymmetric, and more nodular and infarctive.

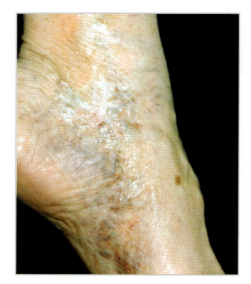

Figure 6.2.11 Livedoid vasculitis. Although livedoid vasculitis is labeled as a vasculitis the primary etiology is a hypercoagulative state with secondary vasculitis. *Clue to diagnosis:* white atrophic scar.

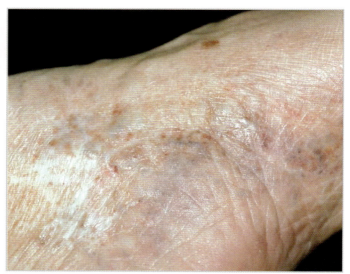

Figure 6.2.12 Livedoid vasculitis.

3. ERYTHEMA NODOSUM VERSUS POLYARTERITIS NODOSA

Features in common: red nodules on lower extremities

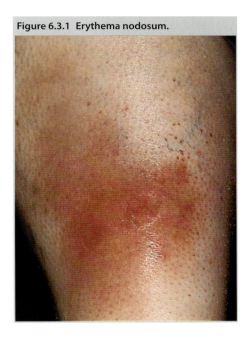

Figure 6.3.1 Erythema nodosum.

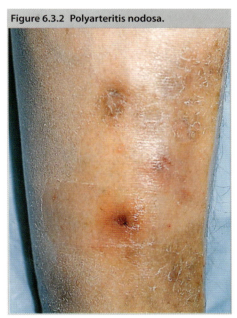

Figure 6.3.2 Polyarteritis nodosa.

Distinguishing features

	Erythema nodosum	Polyarteritis nodosa
Physical examination		
Morphology	No ulcers Lesions do not follow arteries No livedo pattern	Ulcers (occasionally) Lesions follow course of arteries Livedo pattern occasionally present
Distribution	Pretibial area, rarely elsewhere	Variable, most common on lower legs
History		
Symptoms	Pain No suppuration No fever or malaise No central nervous system symptoms	Pain Suppuration Fever, malaise Central nervous system symptoms
Exacerbating factors	Prolonged standing, limb dependencies	Prolonged standing, limb dependency
Associated findings	Medications: oral contraceptives Infections: streptococcal infection, deep fungal infections, Yersinia, Campylobacter Malignancies Immunologic diseases: sarcoidosis, Behçet's disease	No medications Infections: hepatitis B infection No malignancies No immunologic disease
Epidemiology	Uncommon Young female predominance	Rare
Biopsy	No Septal panniculitis with mixed inflammatory infiltrate	Yes Vasculitis of medium-sized arteries
Laboratory	Anti-streptolysin O titer, chest x-ray	Hepatitis B screen Childhood variant: ASO positive Angiography Erythrocyte sedimentation rate
Outcome	Self-limited, resolves over several weeks	Variable with significant morbidity and mortality; patients with only cutaneous manifestations have a good prognosis

Causes of erythema nodosum

- Medications
  - Oral contraceptives
  - Bromides
  - Sulfonamides
- Inflammatory bowel disease
  - Ulcerative colitis, Crohn's disease
- Infections
  - Bacterial: *Streptococcus*, *Yersinia*, enterocolitis, *Mycoplasma pneumoniae*, leptospirosis,
  - Tularemia, cat-scratch disease
  - Fungal: coccidioidomycosis, blastomycosis, histoplasmosis, dermatophytosis
  - Viruses: hepatitis
- Malignancies
  - Lymphoma
  - Rarely solid tumors
- Autoimmune diseases
  - Sarcoidosis
  - Behçet's disease
- Miscellaneous
  - Postradiation therapy
- Idiopathic factors

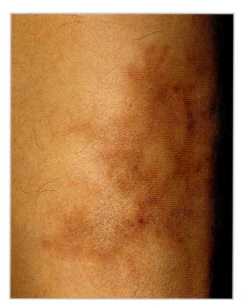

Figure 6.3.3 Polyarteritis nodosa. Clue to diagnosis: poikilodermatous skin with underlying nodules.

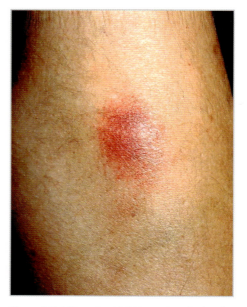

Figure 6.3.4 Thrombophlebitis: can be mistaken for polyarteritis nodosa but the nodules are localized to veins.

4. PYODERMA GANGRENOSUM VERSUS STASIS ULCER

■ Features in common: undermined ulcers on lower extremities

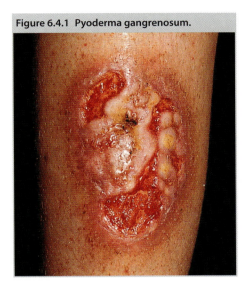

Figure 6.4.1 Pyoderma gangrenosum.

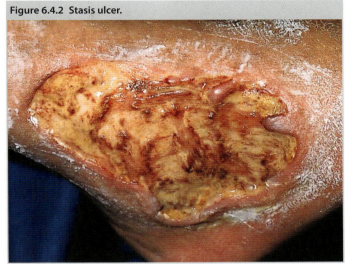

Figure 6.4.2 Stasis ulcer.

■ Distinguishing features

	Pyoderma gangrenosum	Stasis ulcer
Physical examination		
Morphology	No dermatitis Ulcer with undermined purple edge No venous insufficiency No papillomatosis	Surrounding dermatitis No undermined edge Venous insufficiency: varix Chronic lesions: papillomatosis, elephantiasis
Distribution	71% multiple lesions: lower legs > thighs > buttocks > chest	Lower legs: most commonly overlying medial malleolus
History		
Symptoms	Severe pain not helped by leg elevation	Dull pain that improves with leg elevation
Exacerbating factors	Active bowel disease	Standing
Associated findings	Ulcerative colitis Crohn's disease Rheumatoid arthritis Idiopathic Leukemia	Deep vein phlebitis
Epidemiology	Variable age, equal in men and women	Elderly; multiparous women
Biopsy	Yes	No
	Dermal abscess that early on is follicular centered, lymphocytic vasculitis in periphery	Dermal edema, fibrosis, hemosiderin deposition and spongiosis
Laboratory	Rheumatoid factor, erythrocyte sedimentation rate, serum protein electrophoresis	Ultrasound
Outcome	Chronic course, lesions heal with cribriform scarring	Chronic; stasis papillomatosis (elephantiasis verrucosum nostras)

Differential diagnosis of ulcers

- Infections
  - Abscess
  - Anthrax
  - Amebiasis
  - Ecthyma gangrenosum
  - Deep fungal: histoplasmosis, chromoblastomycosis, cryptococcosis, mycetoma
  - Fournier's gangrene
  - Mycobacterial infection
  - Sexually transmitted disease: syphilis, chancroid
- Metabolic disorders
  - Diabetes
  - Necrobiosis lipoidica diabeticorum
  - Prolidase deficiency
- Miscellaneous
  - Bites (human, pet, and insect, especially brown recluse spider)
- Miscellaneous (continued)
  - Pyoderma gangrenosum
  - Neuropathic disorders
  - Pressure/decubitus ulcers
  - Factitial disorders
  - Erythema induratum or other panniculitis
  - Sickle cell anemia
- Neoplasms
  - Lymphoma
  - Squamous cell carcinoma
  - Basal cell carcinoma
  - Other
- Vascular disorders
  - Stasis ulcer (atrophie blanche)
  - Arterial ulcer
  - Vasculitis
  - Calciphylaxis

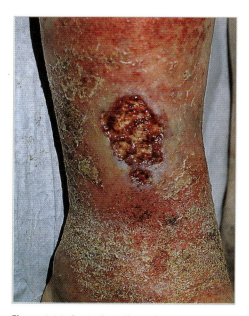

Figure 6.4.3 Stasis ulcer. *Clue to diagnosis:* eczematous skin surrounding ulcer.

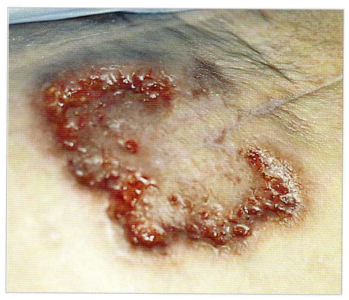

Figure 6.4.4 Pyoderma gangrenosum. *Clue to diagnosis:* undermined ulcer healing with a cribriform scar.

Pyoderma gangrenosum versus stasis ulcer

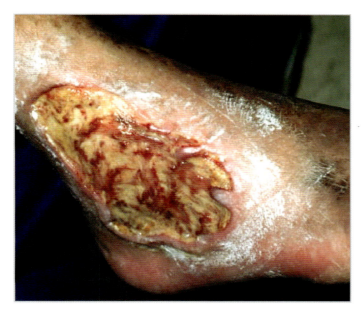

Figure 6.4.5 Pyoderma gangrenosum. *Clue to diagnosis:* violaceous rim of skin surrounding the ulcer.

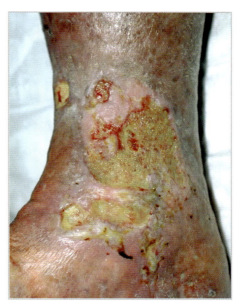

Figure 6.4.6 Stasis dermatitis.

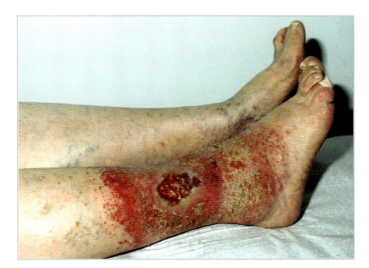

Figure 6.4.7 Stasis dermatitis.

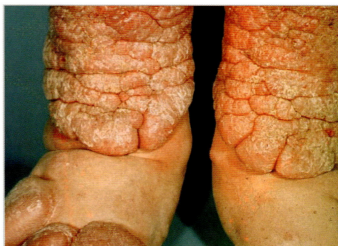

Figure 6.4.8 Elephantiasis verrucosa nostra. Chronic stasis can result in thick leathery and warty plaques.

5. STASIS ULCER VERSUS ARTERIAL ULCER

Features in common: ulcers on lower extremities

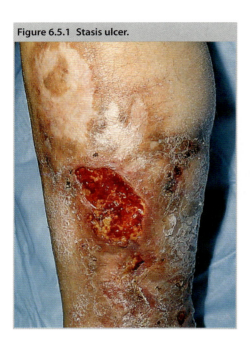

Figure 6.5.1 Stasis ulcer.

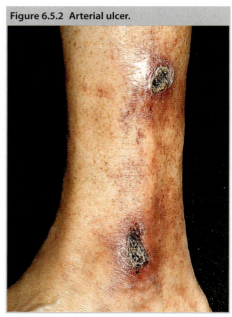

Figure 6.5.2 Arterial ulcer.

Distinguishing features

		Stasis ulcer	Arterial ulcer
Physical examination	Morphology	Skin erythematous Good capillary refill Prominent varix Pitting edema No hair loss Surrounding dermatitis Elephantiasis may develop	Skin pale, cyanotic Poor capillary refill No prominent varix No pitting edema Hair loss occasionally present No surrounding dermatitis No elephantiasis
	Distribution	Lower legs: most commonly overlying medial malleolus	Most common over lateral malleolus
History	Symptoms	Dull pain that improves with leg elevation No claudication	Severe pain worsens with leg elevation Claudication
	Exacerbating factors	Deep vein phlebitis	Hypertension, renal disease, arteriosclerosis, smoking
Associated findings		Venous insufficiency Good pulses No murmur Extremities cold Lipodermatosclerosis	Arterial insufficiency Poor pulses Vascular murmur Extremities warm No lipodermatosclerosis
Epidemiology		Elderly; multiparous women	Elderly men
Biopsy		No Dermal edema, fibrosis, lobular proliferation of blood vessels, hemosiderin deposition, epidermal acanthosis and spongiosis	No Thickened blood vessels
Laboratory		Photoplethysmography Venous hypertension on ultrasound occasionally	Arteriogram, Doppler ultrasound
Outcome		Chronic Elephantiasis	Chronic Untreated: gangrene

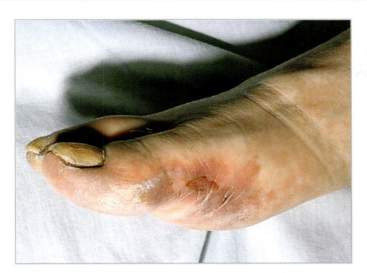

Figure 6.5.3 Healing arterial ulcer. *Clue to diagnosis:* cyanotic skin due to peripheral vascular disease.

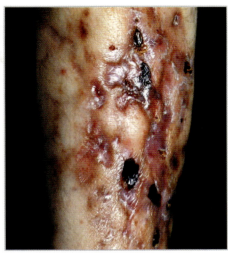

Figure 6.5.4 Factitial ulcer due to injection of drugs. *Clue to diagnosis:* linearity of ulcers with geographic borders.

6. PRETIBIAL MYXEDEMA VERSUS STASIS DERMATITIS

Features in common: red plaques on lower extremities

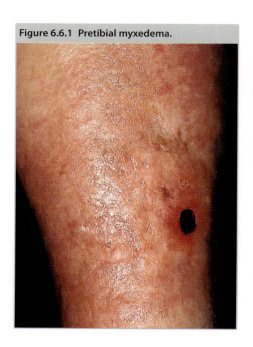

Figure 6.6.1 Pretibial myxedema.

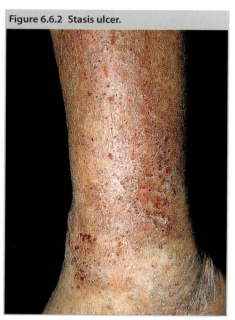

Figure 6.6.2 Stasis ulcer.

Distinguishing features

	Pretibial myxedema	Stasis dermatitis
Physical examination	Primarily dermal changes No scales	Primarily epidermal changes Scales present
Morphology	Nonpitting edema Does not ulcerate Chronic lesions: waxy thickened skin with woody feel and peau d'orange	Pitting edema May ulcerate Chronic lesions: papillomatosis, elephantiasis
Distribution	Shins	Lower legs
History Symptoms Exacerbating factors	Asymptomatic Hyperthyroidism	Dull pain that improves with leg elevation Deep vein phlebitis
Associated findings	Exophthalmos, thyroid disease	Thrombophlebitis
Epidemiology	Adult women	Elderly; multiparous women
Biopsy	Yes Epidermal acanthosis and papillomatosis in old lesions, dermal mucin, frequently grenz zone of uninvolved collagen in superficial papillary dermis	No Dermal edema, fibrosis, lobular proliferation of blood vessels, hemosiderin and mucin deposition, epidermal acanthosis and spongiosis
Laboratory	Thyroid receptor antibodies, thyroid-stimulating hormone, long-acting thyroid-stimulating hormone	Venous hypertension, ultrasound
Outcome	Chronic and persistent, poor response to therapy	Chronic, stasis papillomatosis

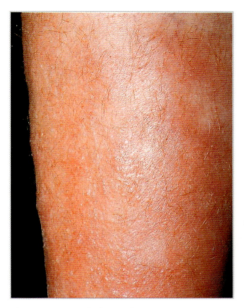

Figure 6.6.3 Pretibial myxedema.

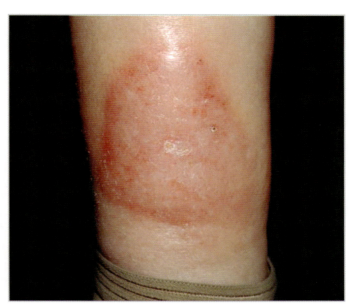

Figure 6.6.4 Pretibial myxedema.

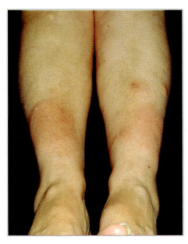

Figure 6.6.5 Pretibial myxedema.

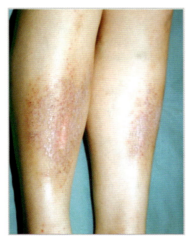

Figure 6.6.6 Lichen planus: can mimic pretibial myxedema. *Clue to diagnosis:* purple pruritic polygonal papules.

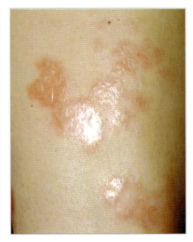

Figure 6.6.7 Necrobiosis lipoidica. Unlike pretibial myxedema or stasis dermatitis the lesions are usually atrophic, may ulcerate, and have characteristic orange yellow color.

7. STASIS DERMATITIS VERSUS CELLULITIS

Features in common: swollen red extremity

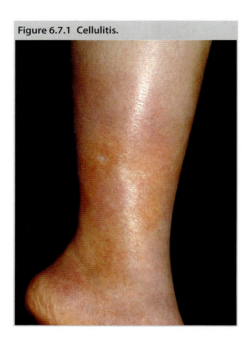

Figure 6.7.1 Cellulitis.

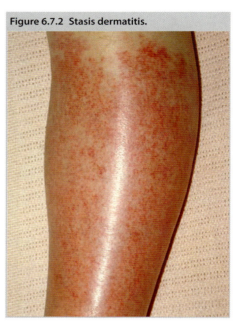

Figure 6.7.2 Stasis dermatitis.

Distinguishing features

	Stasis dermatitis	Cellulitis
Physical examination Morphology Distribution	Pitting edema Varicose veins May ulcerate	Acute redness and edema Area of redness rapidly enlarging
History Symptoms Exacerbating factors	No fevers, dull pain	High fevers Malaise
Associated findings	Thrombophlebitis	Occasional tinea pedis Intertrigo between toes, Leg ulcer, wound, or preceding dermatitis
Epidemiology	Elderly	Prior leg surgery, prior cellulitis or dermatitis
Biopsy	No Dermal edema, fibrosis, lobular proliferation of blood vessels, hemosiderin and mucin deposition, epidermal acanthosis and spongiosis	No Dermal edema with sparse neutrophilic infiltrate. Bacteria usually not visible
Laboratory	Venous hypertension, ultrasound	Increased WBC
Outcome	Occasional ulceration, chronic thick papillomatous skin (elephantiasis)	Good

DISEASE DISCUSSION

Arterial ulcer

Definition and etiology
Arterial ulcers occur secondary to necrosis of skin and soft tissue owing to insufficient arterial circulation.

Clinical features
The ulcers occur commonly in adult men who smoke. Coexisting atherosclerotic coronary artery disease is frequently present. Examination reveals poor pulses; pale, cold extremities; and poor capillary refill. Occasionally, vascular murmurs can be heard in the inguinal area over the femoral artery. The ulcers commonly are very painful at rest and frequently made worse with leg elevation. The ulcers are sharply punched out and commonly occur overlying the lateral malleolus. Loss of hair on the toes and the dorsum of the foot may occur. The toenails may become thick and dystrophic. The end result of chronic untreated arterial insufficiency is dry gangrene with loss of toes or part of the extremity.

The major disease in the differential diagnosis is stasis ulcer. Stasis ulcers most commonly occur in the medial malleolus and do not have a punched-out appearance. The surrounding skin is erythematous, not pale, and dermatitis is frequently present. The skin may also be indurated owing to inflammation in the fat (i.e. lipodermatosclerosis, hypodermitis sclerodermiformis). Varicose veins and a history of thrombophlebitis are common features. Stasis ulcers are painful; however, unlike with arterial ulcers, the pain can be relieved by leg elevation. In severe cases, pitting edema and chronic thickening of the skin producing elephantiasis verrucosum nostras occur. Other diseases in the differential diagnosis include pyoderma gangrenosum, factitial, infectious, vasculitic, diabetic, pressure, and malignant ulcers. The ulcers of pyoderma gangrenosum have an undermined violaceous border and heal with a characteristic cribriform scar. Diabetic ulcers most commonly occur on the plantar surface of the foot as a result of neuropathy and trauma due to walking in poorly fitting shoes. The lesions of necrobiosis lipoidica diabeticorum can also ulcerate, but the surrounding atrophic yellow-colored plaques should not be confused with other entities. Ulcers due to vasculitis, such as arterial ulcers, are sharply punched out, and palpable purpura is usually present. Pressure ulcers occur at sites of pressure on the skin (such as over the heel) owing to chronic immobility. Pressure ulcers occur in comatose patients as well as in those with neuropathy or central nervous system disease, since these patients cannot feel the pain caused by the chronic pressure. Malignant ulcers have a rough irregular base and, frequently, heaped-up borders; however, since squamous cell carcinoma can also develop in chronic stasis ulcer, malignancy should be considered in any nonhealing ulcer and must be excluded by biopsy. Infectious ulcers usually occur secondary to trauma and have purulent drainage.

Treatment (Table 6.1)
The crux of the treatment is to improve the arterial circulation. Patients should stop smoking. Diabetes, hypertension, hypercholesterolemia should also be controlled. Aspirin and dipyridamole (Persantine) may be helpful. Severe cases require vascular surgery.

Table 6.1 Treatment of arterial ulcer

Treatment	Precautions
Universal	
Treat risk factors for arteriosclerosis such as smoking, diabetes, hypertension, hypercholesterolemia, obesity, and hypothyroidism	
Debride necrotic tissue	
Treat secondary infection Exercise increases blood flow	
Mild disease	
Antiplatelet therapy	Pentoxifylline has not been shown to be beneficial
	Aspirin and dipyridamole together may be more effective
Wound care/dressings	
Severe disease	
Surgery if possible	
Hyperbaric oxygen	

Cellulitis

Definition and etiology
Cellulitis is an acute infection of the skin and soft tissue characterized by rapidly spreading red edematous patch associated with fever and malaise. The most common bacteria causing cellulitis are *Streptococcus pyogenes* and *Staphylococcus aureus*.

Clinical features
Patients present with acute onset of a warm, swollen red tender patch, with rapidly spreading margins. Patients universally have fevers often associated with malaise. The leg is the most common location of cellulitis, but cellulitis can occur anywhere on the body. Cellulitis on the face is frequently referred to as erysipelas. Erysipelas usually has more well defined borders than cellulitis located elsewhere. Predisposing factors for cellulitis includes diabetes, tinea pedis, and trauma. Morphologically the lesions present as red confluent macule/patch, but occasionally blisters can occur, and ulcers form. Clinically there can also be overlapping features between cellulitis and deeper infection necrotizing fasciitis.

The differential includes stasis dermatitis, contact dermatitis, and insect bite reaction. In none of these entities do fevers occur, and the absence of fevers and malaise can be used as evidence against the diagnosis. Patients with allergic contact dermatitis frequently complain of severe itching. In patients with stasis dermatitis signs of venous insufficiency such as varicose veins and petechiae are usually present. Of note is that patients with stasis dermatitis.

Treatment (Table 6.2)

Table 6.2 Treatment of cellulitis

Treatment	Precautions
Universal	
Look for predisposing factor such as tinea pedis	
Mild disease	
Oral antibiotics such as cephalexin 500 mg bid or doxycycline 100 mg bid	Allergic reaction, rash, photosensitivity with doxycycline
Severe disease	
IV antibiotics	Numerous

Erythema nodosum

Definition and etiology
Erythema nodosum is panniculitis characterized by tender, red nodules and plaques on the pretibial surface. Erythema nodosum can be caused by a variety of different entities. The most common causes include oral contraceptives, streptococcal infections, sarcoidosis, inflammatory bowel disease, and gastrointestinal infections due to *Salmonella, Campylobacter,* or *Yersinia*.

Clinical features
Females are more commonly affected than males. Most cases occur in young adults. Patients present with sudden onset of tender, red nodules overlying the extensor surface of the legs. The lesions may last 3 to 6 weeks; lesions older than 2 weeks become purpuric, resembling an old bruise. Rarely, the upper extremities or other cutaneous surfaces can be involved. Arthralgia may be present.

The major clinical diseases in the differential diagnosis are erythema induratum, other panniculitides, polyarteritis nodosa, insect bites, cellulitis, Majocchi's granuloma, and thrombophlebitis. Unlike erythema nodosum, erythema induratum involves the calves and frequently ulcerates. The lesions of erythema nodosum never ulcerate. The lesions of thrombophlebitis predominantly affect the sides of the legs, are hard and firm, and are attached to a vein. Venous insufficiency is usually apparent. Early on, the acute lesions of erythema nodosum can resemble cellulitis, but cellulitis is usually unilateral. In addition, nodules are not present in cellulitis, and patients are febrile. Majocchi's granuloma is a fungal infection involving hair follicles and is usually asymmetric and slightly scaly. These patients have been exposed to a source of tinea. Insect bites may also present with dermal nodules, on closer inspection, however, a central punctum can be found, and the lesions are not symmetric. Other panniculitides such as lupus pernio can also be confused with erythema nodosum. Helpful distinguishing features in the case of lupus pernio are the association with exposure to cold and the location of the lesions predominantly over distal extremities. Patients with polyarteritis usually have systemic manifestations of disease such as fever or renal insufficiency. The lesions most commonly follow the course of blood vessels and are frequently found in the popliteal fossa. Sometimes, however, an excisional biopsy is needed to exclude these other diseases.

Treatment (Table 6.3)
Patients with erythema nodosum should be evaluated for an underlying cause. The routine work-up is a throat culture, measurement of anti-streptolysin O antibody or streptozyme levels to exclude a streptococcal infection, and chest X-ray to exclude sarcoidosis or other pulmonary infection. A gastroenterology work-up should also be performed if there are gastrointestinal symptoms. Once the underlying cause is eliminated, the lesions will spontaneously improve. To hasten the resolution, systemic steroids, topical steroids, nonsteroidal anti-inflammatory agents, dapsone, and potassium iodide (SSKI) can be helpful. Patients should also elevate their legs and avoid prolonged standing or physical activity.

Erythema induratum

Definition and etiology
Erythema induratum is a form of chronic recurrent panniculitis. In Europe, it is frequently secondary to tuberculosis. In the United States, the association between erythema induratum and tuberculosis is rare.

Table 6.3 Treatment of erythema nodosum

Treatment	Precautions
Universal	
Look for and treat underlying cause	
Leg elevation and rest	
Mild disease	
Non-steroidal anti-inflammatory agents	Avoid in patients with renal disease. Higher risk of myocardial infarction. May cause or exacerbate gastritis/esophagitis
Short course prednisone	Avoid in diabetic patients. May predispose to aseptic femoral necrosis. Long term induction of osteoporosis
Potassium iodide 300 mg tid and titrate up as needed	Very unpleasant taste. Gastrointestinal upset, may cause hypothyroidism
Severe disease	
Colchicine 1 mg bid	Diarrhea, gastrointestinal upset, bone marrow suppression
Immunosuppressants such as cyclosporine	Numerous
Infliximab	Risk for infection and malignancy
Thalidomide	May produce neuropathy, teratogen

More commonly, erythema induratum is believed to be an idiopathic vasculitis and is often termed *nodular vasculitis*.

Clinical features
Females are affected more commonly than males. Erythema induratum presents with erythematous, tender, subcutaneous nodules with a predilection for the calf area. Ulceration is common, and the lesions heal with scarring. In cases associated with tuberculosis, there is a strongly positive result with purified protein derivative testing. The major disease in the differential diagnosis is erythema nodosum. Erythema nodosum predominantly affects the shins, not the calves, and the lesions do not ulcerate or heal with scarring, as in erythema induratum. As in erythema nodosum, the differential diagnosis would also include other panniculitides, infections, polyarteritis nodosa, and thrombophlebitis. Although the disease may be clinically suspected, the diagnosis of erythema induratum requires pathologic examination. Histologic analysis demonstrates lobular panniculitis with caseation necrosis and with vasculitis of a medium-sized blood vessel.

Treatment (Table 6.4)
Cases associated with tuberculosis can be successfully treated with triple anti-tuberculid therapy. The idiopathic form can be treated with topical, intralesional, or systemic steroids, dapsone, and SSKI.

Leukocytoclastic vasculitis

Definition and etiology
Leukocytoclastic vasculitis (necrotizing vasculitis, hypersensitivity vasculitis) represents an inflammatory destructive process of postcapillary venules due to deposition of immune complexes. The stimuli for immune complex formation are protean, including collagen vascular diseases, infections, medications, cryoglobulins, paraprotein, and malignancies.

Table 6.4 Treatment of erythema induratum

Treatment	Precautions
Universal	
Test for tuberculosis with PPD or QuantiFERON-TB	If positive treat for tuberculosis
Mild disease	
Nonsteroidal antiinflammatory agents	Avoid in patients with renal disease Higher risk of myocardial infarction May cause or exacerbate gastritis/esophagitis
Severe disease	
Mycophenolate mofetil	Pregnancy category D. Screen for prior hepatitis B and C Increased risk of infection Monitor CBC
Oral prednisone	Avoid in diabetic patients May cause aseptic femoral necrosis Long term use may result in osteoporosis

Table 6.5 Treatment of leukocytoclastic vasculitis

Treatment	Precautions
Universal	
Look for underlying cause and treat	
Leg elevation and rest	
Mild disease	
Non-steroidal anti-inflammatory agents	Avoid in patients with renal disease Higher risk of myocardial infarction May cause or exacerbate gastritis/esophagitis
Severe disease	
Oral prednisone	Avoid in diabetic patients May cause aseptic femoral necrosis Long term use may result in osteoporosis
Colchicine	Diarrhea, gastrointestinal upset, bone marrow suppression
Azathioprine	Baseline TPMP genotyping in order to ascertain patients can metabolize azathioprine Requires CBC monitoring along with LFTs and renal function
Methotrexate	Monitor CBC and liver functions Can cause cirrhosis of liver
Dapsone	Monitor CBC Risk of hemolytic anemia

Clinical features

During the first few hours, urticarial papules develop in dependent sites, such as the lower legs and buttocks. The lesions rapidly develop into the classic palpable purpuric macules and papules. In severe cases, necrosis, ulcers, livedo reticularis, and even vesicles occur. Commonly associated symptoms include fever and arthralgias. Rarely, glomerulonephritis and gastrointestinal symptoms such as nausea, vomiting, diarrhea, and pain can occur. The pigmented purpuras can be distinguished from leukocytoclastic vasculitis by their lack of palpable lesions and lack of systemic symptoms. In questionable cases, biopsy can be helpful. The differential diagnosis could also include other types of vasculitis. The lesions of Henoch-Schönlein purpura (HSP) are identical to those of leukocytoclastic vasculitis. HSP is most commonly seen in children, and abdominal pain and renal involvement occur more frequently than in leukocytoclastic vasculitis. The definitive diagnosis of HSP can be made only if direct immunofluorescent studies demonstrate IgA immunoreactants in blood vessels. In Wegener's granulomatosis (granulomatosis and polyarteritis), palpable purpura can also be found along with ulcers, papules, and plaques. If respiratory tract symptoms occur along with renal involvement, Wegener's granulomatosis should be suspected. In polyarteritis nodosa, nodules are found along the course of arteries. Erythema elevatum diutinum is a chronic variant of leukocytoclastic vasculitis in which nodules are found overlying hand, elbow, and knee joints.

Treatment (Table 6.5)

In all cases of leukocytoclastic vasculitis, an underlying cause should be sought, eliminated, and treated. Treatments include nonsteroidal anti-inflammatory agents, dapsone, and brief courses of systemic steroids.

Pigmented purpura

Definition and etiology

Pigmented purpura is a benign, usually idiopathic, capillaritis that can appear in several different overlapping clinical patterns. Rarely, a pigmented purpuric eruption can be attributed to a medication.

Clinical features

The pigmented purpuras are characterized by nonpalpable purpura, most commonly on the lower extremities. The purpura is associated with yellow-to-red petechiae and eczematous plaques. If petechiae predominate, this is called *Schamberg's disease*. Sometimes the lesions have an annular distribution, then the eponym *Majocchi's disease* (purpura annularis telangiectodes) applies. Other variants includes Gougerot–Blum syndrome (pigmented purpuric lichenoid dermatitis), in which small red papules can be found, and lichen aureus, in which the lesions have a golden rust-colored hue. Histologically, all the different subtypes have similar findings a superficial perivascular lymphocytic infiltrate, extravasated erythrocytes, and hemosiderin deposition. An overlying dermatitis can be found in Majocchi's disease, and the inflammation is denser and more lichenoid in Gougerot–Blum syndrome and lichen aureus variant.

The major diseases in the differential diagnosis are stasis dermatitis, leukocytoclastic vasculitis, and petechiae secondary to thrombocytopenia. The lesions of pigmented purpura are nonpalpable, unlike the lesions of leukocytoclastic vasculitis. Systemic involvement and an early urticarial phase are also not present. Although in stasis dermatitis, petechiae and yellow plaques can also be found, signs of venous insufficiency such as edema and varicose veins are prominent features. Petechiae secondary to thrombocytopenia are usually widespread and involve the mucous membranes, and epistaxis and internal bleeding can be present. Patients with purpuric variant of mycosis fungoides have generalized skin patches, not localized to the lower extremity.

Treatment (Table 6.6)

Since the pigmented purpuras are only of cosmetic concern, no treatment is necessary; however, topical steroids can be beneficial in severe cases.

Pyoderma gangrenosum
Definition and etiology

Pyoderma gangrenosum is a clinically distinct, painful skin ulcer related to a variety of systemic diseases. The most commonly associated systemic diseases are inflammatory bowel disease and rheumatoid arthritis. Other rarer associations include leukemia, myeloma, and paraproteinemia.

Table 6.6 Treatment of pigmented purpura

Treatment	Precautions
Universal	
Discontinue any possible associated medications	
Mild disease	
No treatment may be necessary since may spontaneously resolve	
Topical corticosteroids	Monitor for skin atrophy
Rutoside 50 mg × 2 qd and ascorbic acid 1000 mg qd	None
Severe disease	
Narrow band UVB	Risk of burning

Clinical features

The first lesions usually develop in a site of trauma, most commonly in the lower legs, but can be found in any cutaneous surface. Pyoderma gangrenosum starts out as a follicular-based papulovesicle or pustule that over a few days becomes necrotic, enlarged, and ulcerated. Upon presentation, large ulcers with a violaceous undermined border are present. The ulcers characteristically are very painful and heal with a cribriform scar. The characteristic clinical course and appearance allow easy differentiation from other causes of ulcers discussed previously. A biopsy is occasionally helpful to rule out other causes of ulcers, such as infections or malignancies. The histologic findings in pyoderma gangrenosum are not diagnostic; however, early lesions may show a follicular-centered abscess. The base of the ulcer in pyoderma gangrenosum shows an abscess, but a biopsy specimen taken from the edge of the ulcer will show lymphocytic vasculitis.

Treatment (Table 6.7)

Underlying systemic diseases should be sought and appropriately treated. The most commonly used treatment is high-dose oral prednisone. Cyclosporine is also highly effective in refractory cases. Other therapies include intralesional steroid injection, IVIG, cyclophosphamide, chlorambucil, thalidomide, dapsone, minocycline, occlusive dressings, topical cromolyn, and hyperbaric oxygen.

■ Polyarteritis nodosa

Definition and etiology

Polyarteritis nodosa is vasculitis of medium-sized arteries. The commonly affected organs include skin, kidneys, central nervous system, peripheral nervous system, lungs, heart, and gastrointestinal tract. A rare variant primarily affecting the skin, joints, and peripheral nervous system can also occur. The cause is unclear, but some cases have been associated with hepatitis B infection.

■ Clinical features

Patients are usually sick and suffer from multiple systemic complaints. The most common findings are fever, weight loss, arthritis, mononeuritis multiplex, cutaneous disorders, renal involvement, gastrointestinal symptoms, asthma, hypertension, and cardiac failure. Cutaneous findings include erythematous nodules that follow the course of the superficial arteries. The nodules are most prominent in the popliteal fossa, anterior lower leg, and dorsum of the foot. Severe involvement can lead to ulcer formation, necrosis, and gangrene. Purpuric lesions

Table 6.7 Treatment of pyoderma gangrenosum

Treatment	Precautions
Universal	
Treat any underlying systemic disease	
Pain killers as necessary	
Wound care	
Mild disease	
Topical corticosteroids	Atrophy, steroid induced acne
Intralesional steroid injection	Atrophy
Topical tacrolimus	Report of renal insufficiency due to topical use in pyoderma gangrenosum
Minocycline 100 mg bid	Case reports may be helpful Monitor for hyperpigmentation, rare lupus-like syndrome
Severe disease	
Systemic corticosteroids/prednisone	Avoid in diabetic patients May cause aseptic femoral necrosis Long term use may result in osteoporosis
Cyclosporine	Monitor renal function, blood pressure, along with increased risk of infection
Infliximab or other TNF inhibitors	Test for tuberculosis and monitor for infection
IVIG	Risk of allergic reaction Rare cases of anaphylaxis in IgA deficient patients Risk of viral infection Rare cases of thrombotic events such as stroke
Other immunosuppressants	

due to extravasated erythrocytes can also frequently be found along with livedo reticularis. The major diseases in the differential diagnosis are thrombophlebitis and panniculitides such as erythema nodosum. The lesions of thrombophlebitis follow the course of veins, not arteries, and varicose veins are usually present. Systemic symptoms are also lacking. The lesions of erythema nodosum are unrelated to vasculature pattern and predominantly occur overlying the shins. Livedo reticularis, ulcers, and necrosis do not occur in erythema nodosum. Purpura only occurs in old resolving lesions.

Treatment (Table 6.8)

The therapy for polyarteritis nodosa is high-dose systemic steroids. Immunosuppressive agents such as cyclophosphamide and cyclosporine can also be used.

■ Pretibial myxedema

Definition and etiology

Pretibial myxedema is the deposition of mucin in the pretibial area in patients with Graves' disease.

Clinical features

Early on, patients develop symmetric bilateral erythema overlying the shins. With time, the lesions become indurated, firm, nonpitting plaques. The follicular orifices become prominent, and localized hypertrichosis may be present. The associated clinical findings due to Graves' disease includes exophthalmos, thyroid acropachy, and a

Disease discussion

Table 6.8 Treatment of polyarteritis nodosa

Treatment	Precautions
Universal	
Look for underlying hepatitis B or streptococcal infection	
Work up for systemic involvement	Consider angiogram if renal abnormalities or CNS findings
Serum study for ANCA	
Mild disease	
Topical or intralesional corticosteroid	Atrophy
Oral prednisone	Diabetes, hypertension, insomnia, weight gain, osteoporosis, aseptic femoral necrosis
TNF inhibitor	Risk of infection and malignancy
Severe disease	
Intravenous corticosteroids	Diabetes, hypertension, insomnia, weight gain, osteoporosis, aseptic femoral necrosis
IVIG	Risk of allergic reaction Rare cases of anaphylaxis in IgA deficient patients Risk of viral infection Rare cases of thrombotic events such as stroke
Cyclosporine	Monitor renal function, blood pressure, along with increased risk of infection
Cyclophosphamide	Monitor for myelosuppression Increased risk infection secondary malignancies Hemorrhagic cystitis

diffuse goiter. Laboratory examination reveals circulating antibody against thyroid-stimulating hormone receptor in the majority of patients. Pretibial myxedema needs to be differentiated from stasis dermatitis. In stasis dermatitis, pitting edema, pigmentary changes due to dermal melanin and hemosiderin deposition, and eczematous scaly plaques are present. Although upon biopsy of the lesions, mucin can be found in both stasis dermatitis and pretibial myxedema, in pretibial myxedema a grenz zone of normal-appearing collagen is present in the superficial papillary dermis.

Treatment (Table 6.9)

There is no adequate treatment for pretibial myxedema. Topical and intralesional steroids have been of limited benefit.

Stasis dermatitis and ulcer

Definition and etiology

Stasis dermatitis is an eczematous rash on lower extremities associated with venous insufficiency. Stasis dermatitis can ulcerate over time if left untreated.

Clinical features

Stasis dermatitis starts on the lower legs. Pitting edema is frequently present along with prominent varicose veins. The legs often are bright red edematous and can be mistaken for cellulitis. Unlike cellulitis often eczematous changes such as scale and serous crust is present. Petechiae or hemorrhage due to hemosiderin is often seen. When ulcers develop they most commonly occur overlying the medial aspect of the shin and medial malleolus. The ulcers start as small, millimeter-sized defects, frequently secondary to trauma, but can grow to several centimeters in size. Signs of venous insufficiency are present around the ulcer such as edema, fibrosis, and varicose veins. The differential for stasis dermatitis includes other dermatoses such as contact dermatitis and cellulitis. The differential diagnosis also includes other forms of ulcer such as diabetic ulcer, arterial ulcer, pyoderma gangrenosum, infectious ulcer, neoplastic ulcer, and vasculitic ulcer. Arterial ulcers are very painful, sharply demarcated, and most prominent over the lateral malleolus. Signs of arterial insufficiency are also present such as pallor, poor pulses, loss of hair, and atrophic skin. Other types of ulcers were discussed previously in the section on arterial ulcers.

Table 6.9 Treatment of pretibial myxedema

Treatment	Precautions
Universal	
Treat thyroid disease	
Compression stockings for edema	
Mild disease	
If asymptomatic no treatment necessary since may improve or resolve over time	
Mid or high potency steroid such as clobetasol (0.05% cream bid)	Monitor for steroid atrophy
Severe disease	
Steroid under occlusion	Monitor for steroid atrophy
Intralesional steroid injection	Atrophy
Excision if small lesion	

Treatment (Table 6.10)

A variety of treatments exist. Circulation can be improved with use of pressure stockings and leg elevation. Low-dose aspirin or dipyridamole has been effective in some patients. Use of occlusive dressings can also speed up the healing process. In large refractory ulcers, skin grafts may be helpful.

Table 6.10 Treatment of stasis dermatitis and ulcer

Treatment	Precautions
Universal	
Leg elevation	
Compression stockings	
Avoid topical allergens	Patients with stasis dermatis are at higher risk of developing overlying contact dermatitis
Debride any ulcer	
Mild disease	
Topical corticosteroid bid	Monitor for skin atrophy and telangiectasias
Severe disease	
Pneumatic compression	
Physical therapy with whirlpool	
Unna boot (a gauze impregnated with zinc oxide and calamine and works as a compression dressing)	
Dressings overlying ulcers	
Consider low dose aspirin or dipyridamole to improve circulation	Risk of bleeding
Consider skin grafting for ulcers	

Chapter 7 Genitalia

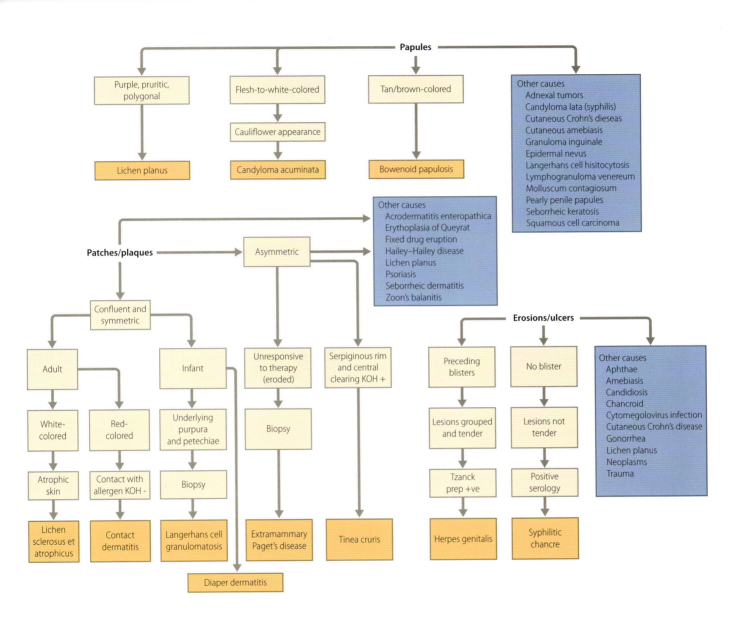

INTRODUCTION

The genital region is subject to a variety of different rashes. In adults, the genital region, not surprisingly, is the location where cutaneous manifestations of a variety of sexually transmitted diseases can be found. Other common problems found in the genital region because of its moist environment are tinea cruris and candidiasis. In babies and toddlers, the combination of diapers, wetness, friction, and incontinence of urine and stool can produce diaper dermatitis. Diaper dermatitis also needs to be distinguished from Langerhans cell granulomatosis. Although all dermatoses (e.g. seborrheic dermatitis, atopic dermatitis) can occur in the genital region, some (like lichen planus) seem to have a predilection for this site. In adults and, rarely, in children, the genital area is where the rash of lichen sclerosus et atrophicus can be most commonly found. Finally, the manifestations of extramammary Paget's disease, a malignant tumor, can mimic and be misdiagnosed as tinea cruris or dermatitis.

1. BOWENOID PAPULOSIS VERSUS CONDYLOMA ACUMINATUM

■ Features in common: warty appearing papules in genitalia

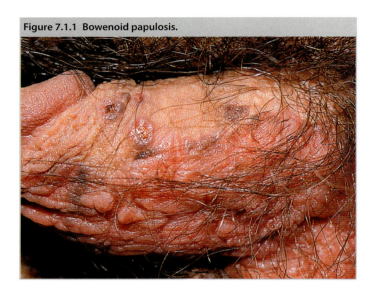

Figure 7.1.1 Bowenoid papulosis.

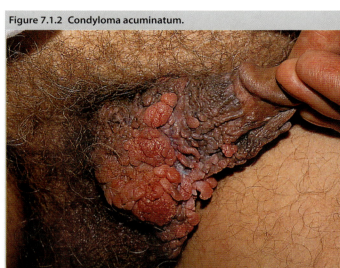

Figure 7.1.2 Condyloma acuminatum.

■ Distinguishing features

	Bowenoid papulosis	Condyloma acuminatum
Physical examination		
Morphology	Brown Papules No cauliflower-like appearance	Flesh colored Papillomatous papules and plaques Frequent cauliflower-like appearance
Distribution	Genital area	Genital area
History		
Symptoms	Asymptomatic	Asymptomatic
Exacerbating factors	None	Spread in areas of injury (Koebner's phenomenon)
Associated findings	Other sexually transmitted diseases Cervical dysplasia	Other sexually transmitted diseases Cervical dysplasia
Epidemiology	Sexually active adults	Sexually active adults
Biopsy	Yes (required for diagnosis) Epidermal acanthosis and papillomatosis; however, epidermal atypia resembling squamous cell carcinoma in situ present	No Epidermal acanthosis, papillomatosis, koilocytosis, tortuous blood vessels in dermal papilla No atypia
Laboratory	Experimental: HPV typing, HPV types 16, 18, 30, 33	Experimental: HPV typing, HPV types 6, 11, 16, 18
Outcome	Good response to therapy Duration: weeks to years Spontaneous regression may occur	Good response to therapy Duration: weeks to years Spontaneous regression may occur
HPV, human papillomavirus		

Differential diagnosis of genital papules

Common causes
- Bowenoid papulosis
- Condyloma acuminatum
- Lichen planus
- Molluscum contagiosum
- Pearly penile papules
- Seborrheic keratosis

Rarer causes
- Cutaneous amebiasis
- Cutaneous Crohn's disease
- Condyloma lata (syphilis)
- Eruptive syringoma
- Granuloma inguinale
- Langerhans cell histiocytosis
- Lymphogranuloma venereum
- Squamous cell carcinoma (giant condyloma of Buschke-Löwenstein)

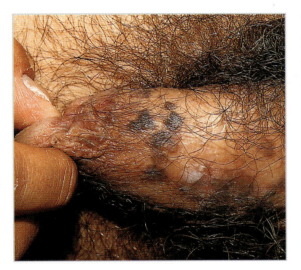

Figure 7.1.3 Bowenoid papulosis. *Clue to diagnosis:* small size of papules with brown color.

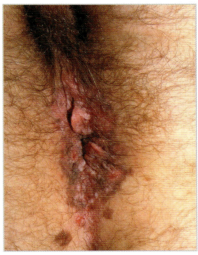

Figure 7.1.4 Bowenoid papulosis: note brown papules.

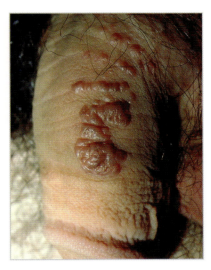

Figure 7.1.5 Bowenoid papulosis: sometimes the only way to distinguish from condyloma acuminatum is by performing a biopsy.

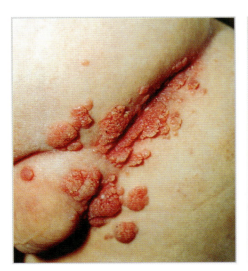

Figure 7.1.6 Condyloma acuminatum.

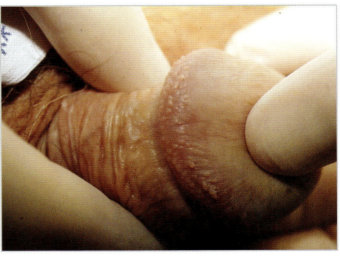

Figure 7.1.7 Pearly penile papules: normal variant seen in some men with uniform papules limited to penile corona.

2. LICHEN SCLEROSUS ET ATROPHICUS VERSUS DERMATITIS

■ **Features in common: both may present with tender white to red-coloured plaques on genitalia**

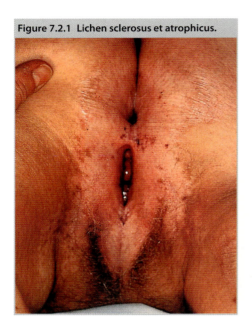
Figure 7.2.1 Lichen sclerosus et atrophicus.

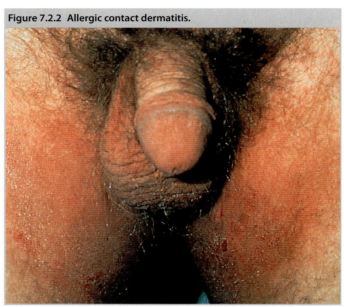
Figure 7.2.2 Allergic contact dermatitis.

■ **Distinguishing features**

	Lichen sclerosus et atrophicus	Dermatitis
Physical examination Morphology	Ivory colored Atrophy Little or no scaling Blisters rare Hemorrhage common Hourglass appearance with involvement of vulva, perineum, perianal skin	Red colored No atrophy (thickening of skin in chronic cases) Scaling prominent Blisters common Hemorrhage rare In sites of contact or irritation
Distribution	20% of time involvement elsewhere	Spares inguinal creases
History Symptoms Exacerbating factors	Soreness, dyspareunia Intercourse	Pruritus Scratching, secondary infection
Associated findings	Vitiligo, pernicious anemia, alopecia areata, systemic lupus erythematosus	None
Epidemiology	Females > males approximately 10:1 ratio; average age 45–60 years	No sex predilection, can occur at any age
Biopsy	Yes Epidermal atrophy, occasionally epidermal acanthosis, follicular plugging, homogenized collagen in upper dermis with dermal edema, bandlike lymphocytic infiltrate underneath altered collagen	No Spongiosis, parakeratosis, superficial perivascular inflammatory infiltrate
Laboratory	Usually none Experimentally: antibodies against thyroid, smooth muscle, gastric, and parietal cells	Patch testing if allergic contact dermatitis suspected
Outcome	Chronic Rarely squamous cell carcinomas develop within lesions	Good, resolves after elimination of allergens and irritants Not associated with malignancies

Differential diagnosis of genital rashes

Common causes
- Candidiasis
- Contact dermatitis
- Diaper dermatitis
- Intertrigo
- Lichen sclerosus et atrophicus
- Psoriasis
- Seborrheic dermatitis
- Tinea cruris

Rarer causes
- Acrodermatitis enteropathica
- Drug eruption or Baboon syndrome
- Granulomatous slack skin
- Intertriginous granular cell parakeratosis (probable variant of contact dermatitis)
- Hailey–Hailey disease
- Langerhans cell granulomatosis (histiocytosis-X)

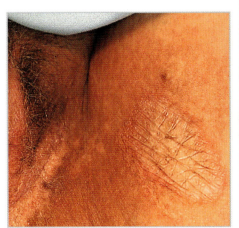

Figure 7.2.3 Lichen sclerosus et atrophicus. *Clue to diagnosis:* atrophic white patch.

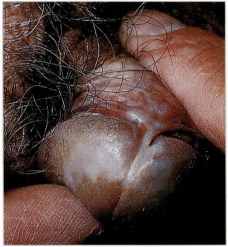

Figure 7.2.4 Balanitis xerotica obliterans (lichen sclerosus et atrophicus of the penis). *Clue to diagnosis:* porcelain white color.

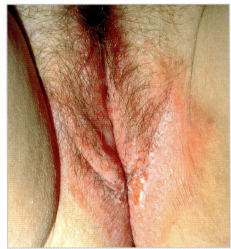

Figure 7.2.5 Lichen sclerosus et atrophicus

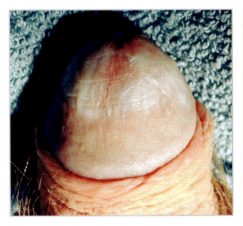

Figure 7.2.6 Balanitis xerotica obliterans

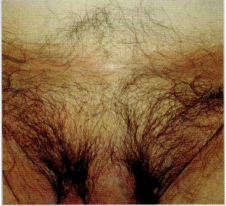

Figure 7.2.7 Chronic dermatitis (intertrigo). Brown color is due to postinflammatory pigmentary alteration.

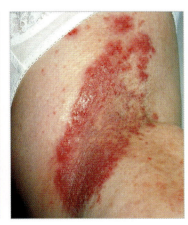

Figure 7.2.8 Hailey–Hailey (benign Familial pemphigus). *Clue to diagnosis:* family history and linear erosions.

3. HERPES GENITALIS VERSUS PRIMARY SYPHILITIC CHANCRE

Features in common: papules/erosions/ulcers in genital area

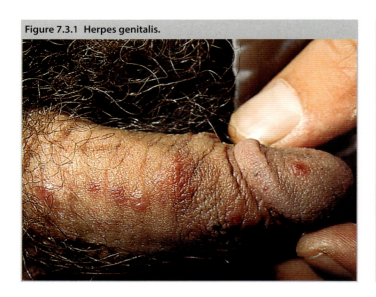

Figure 7.3.1 Herpes genitalis.

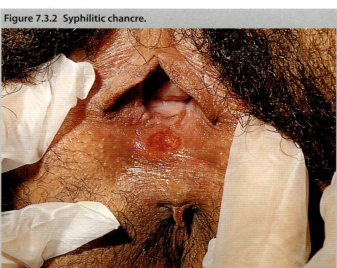

Figure 7.3.2 Syphilitic chancre.

Distinguishing features

	Herpes genitalis	Primary syphilitic chancre
Physical examination Morphology	Grouped blisters Erosions and ulcer with scalloped border Border not indurated	No grouped blisters Border smooth Border firm, indurated
Distribution	Genital area	Genital area
History Symptoms	Prodrome of burning or itching Pain	No prodrome No pain
Exacerbating factors	Immunosuppression	Immunosuppression
Associated findings	Lymphadenopathy	Lymphadenopathy Occasionally papulosquamous eruption of secondary syphilis may become evident
Epidemiology	Sexually active adults	Sexually active adults
Biopsy	No Multinucleated giant cells	No Ulcer with underlying plasma cell infiltrate, Warthin Starry stain positive for spirochetal organisms
Laboratory	Tzanck preparation positive Culture or direct immunofluorescent studies	Tzanck preparation negative Positive serology
Outcome	Chronic relapsing course	Curable with therapy; may progress to secondary or tertiary syphilis if untreated

Herpes genitalis versus primary syphilitic chancre

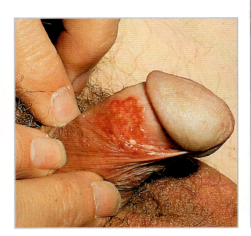
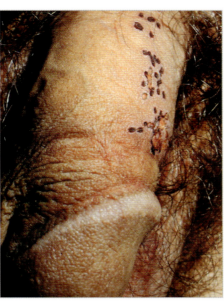
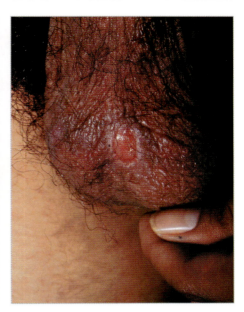

Figure 7.3.3 Herpes genitalis. *Clue to diagnosis:* erosion with scalloped borders.

Figure 7.3.4 Herpes genitalis (old lesions). *Clue to diagnosis:* grouped crusted erosions.

Figure 7.3.5 Syphilitic chancre. *Clue to diagnosis:* punched out non tender ulcer.

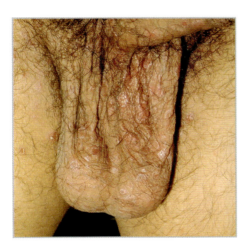
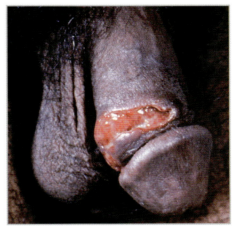

Figure 7.3.6 Secondary syphilis. *Clue to diagnosis:* pityriasiform patches in genital skin.

Figure 7.3.7 Chancroid. *Clue to diagnosis:* very tender unlike syphilitic chancre.

4. TINEA CRURIS VERSUS EXTRAMAMMARY PAGET'S DISEASE

■ Features in common: red, scaly patches/plaques in genital region

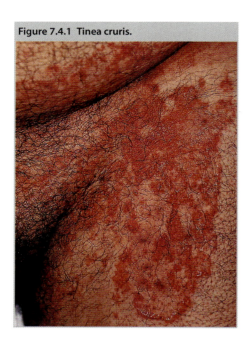

Figure 7.4.1 Tinea cruris.

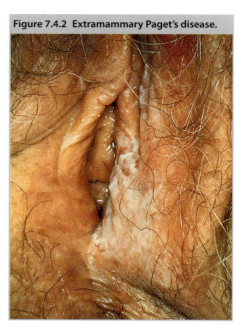

Figure 7.4.2 Extramammary Paget's disease.

■ Distinguishing features

	Tinea cruris	Extramammary paget's disease
Physical examination		
Morphology	Symmetric Serpiginous border common Central clearing Lesions flat	Asymmetric Serpiginous borders at times No central clearing Occasional elevated or nodular areas
Distribution	Genital area Spares scrotum	Genital area May involve scrotum
History		
Symptoms	Pruritus	Asymptomatic
Exacerbating factors	Topical steroid use	None
Associated findings	Tinea pedis	Internal malignancy of genitourinary or gastrointestinal tract in many cases
Epidemiology	Any age, more common in men	Elderly adults
Biopsy	No Spores and hyphae within the stratum corneum	Yes, required for diagnosis Large pale cells spreading in a pagetoid or buckshot pattern within the epidermis
Laboratory	Fungus culture KOH+	Stool guaiac, urinalysis, prostate exam for underlying malignancy Consider cystoscopy, sigmoidoscopy KOH–
Outcome	Resolves with therapy	Frequently recurs, poor prognosis if associated with internal malignancy
KOH, potassium hydroxide		

Tinea cruris versus extramammary paget's disease

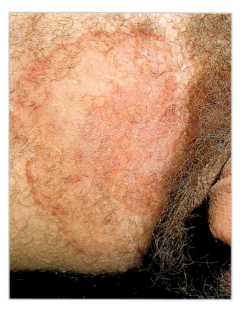

Figure 7.4.3 Tinea cruris. *Clue to diagnosis:* central clearing with peripheral scaling.

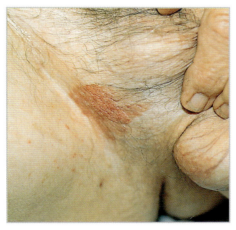

Figure 7.4.4 Extramammary Paget's disease. *Clue to diagnosis:* asymmetry and irregularly shaped borders.

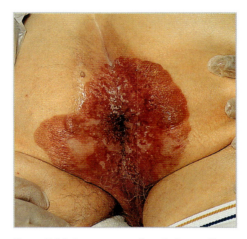

Figure 7.4.5 Extramammary Paget's disease. *Clue to diagnosis:* indurated asymmetric plaque.

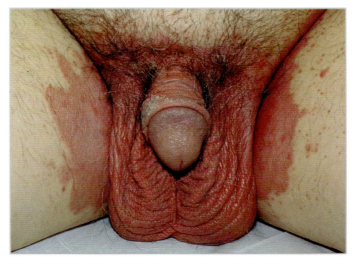

Figure 7.4.6 Candidiasis. Unlike tinea cruris, this can involve the scrotum, and is usually more bright red in color.

5. DIAPER DERMATITIS VERSUS LANGERHANS CELL GRANULOMATOSIS

■ Features in common: patches/plaques in diaper area in babies and toddlers

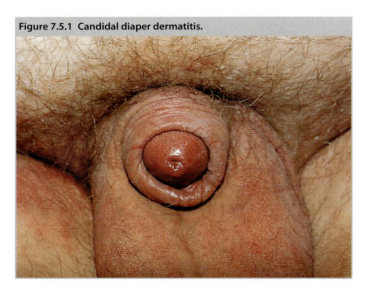

Figure 7.5.1 Candidal diaper dermatitis.

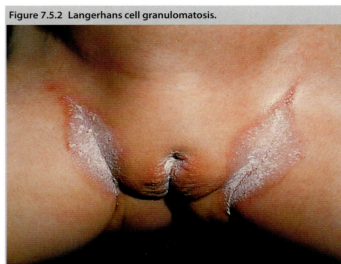

Figure 7.5.2 Langerhans cell granulomatosis.

■ Distinguishing features

	Diaper dermatitis	Langerhans cell granulomatosis
Physical examination Morphology	Erythema and scaling No papules Lichenification If Candida present: bright red erythema, satellite papules and pustules No purpura No crusts/erosions Occasional sparing of skin folds Nodules and ulcers only seen in severe cases (Jacquet's granuloma)	Erythema and scaling Brownish tan papules present No lichenification Dusky erythema No satellite papules or pustules Areas of petechiae and purpura Crusts/erosions frequently present No sparing of skin folds Occasional nodules and ulcers
Distribution	Genital area	Scalp, trunk, genital area
History Symptoms	Irritability No malaise	Irritability Generalized malaise may be present
Exacerbating factors	Infrequent diaper changes	None
Associated findings	None	Lymphadenopathy, pancytopenia, hepatosplenomegaly, pulmonary infiltrates, diabetes insipidus, exophthalmos, otitis media
Epidemiology	Infants and toddlers	Infants and toddlers, rarely adults
Biopsy	No Dermatitis with epidermal spongiosis and superficial perivascular lymphocytic infiltrate	Yes Bandlike infiltrate with 'histiocytic' appearing cells with cleaved kidney-bean shaped nucleus in dermis and extending into epidermis; foam cells, lymphocytes, and eosinophils also frequently present
Laboratory	KOH+	KOH– Complete blood count with differential, X-rays and systemic work as indicated
Outcome	Good	Variable; may resolve or occasionally may be fatal

KOH, potassium hydroxide

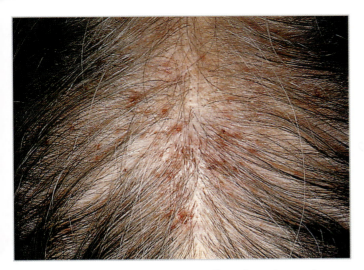

Figure 7.5.3 Langerhans cell granulomatosis. *Clue to diagnosis:* purpuric crusted papules

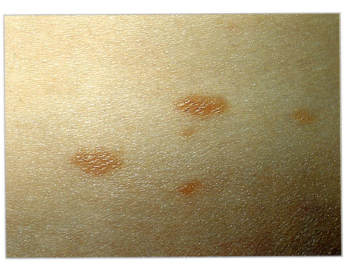

Figure 7.5.4 Langerhans cell granulomatosis. *Clue to diagnosis:* brown xanthomatous-appearing plaques.

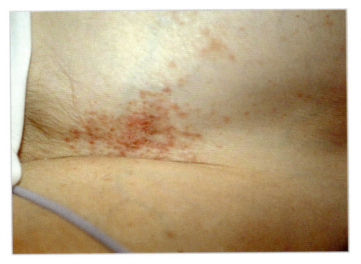

Figure 7.5.5 Langerhans cell granulomatosis. *Clue to diagnosis:* brown xanthomatous-appearing plaques.

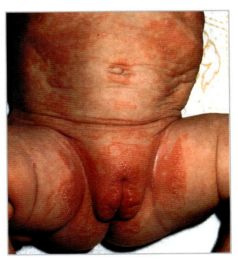

Figure 7.5.6 Diaper dermatitis: seborrheic dermatitis type. *Clue to diagnosis:* in spite of appearance rash usually asymptomatic and not bothersome to child.

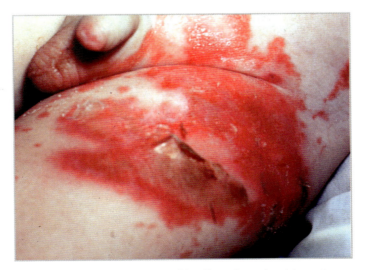

Figure 7.5.7 Acrodermatitis enteropathica. *Clue to diagnosis:* rash in newborn with low zinc levels and unresponsive to therapy.

6. LICHEN PLANUS VERSUS CONDYLOMA ACUMINATUM

■ Features in common: papules in genital area

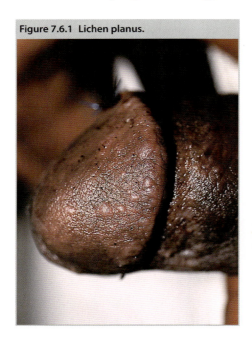

Figure 7.6.1 Lichen planus.

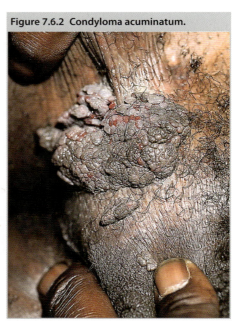

Figure 7.6.2 Condyloma acuminatum.

■ Distinguishing features

	Lichen planus	Condyloma acuminatum
Physical examination		
Morphology	Purple polygonal papules Flat topped Occasionally erosions and blisters White fine scale (Wickham's striae)	Skin-colored papules and plaques Cauliflower-like appearance No erosions or blisters No Wickham's striae
Distribution	Shaft of penis, occasionally groin flexures	Anywhere in genital area but predilection for shaft of penis and perivaginal area
History		
Symptoms	Pruritus	Asymptomatic
Exacerbating factors	Trauma, isomorphic response (e.g. Koebner's reaction: lesions develop in traumatized skin)	Trauma, isomorphic response (e.g. Koebner's reaction: lesions develop in traumatized skin)
Associated findings	Lesions on skin and in mucosa and nail dystrophy Hepatitis, rarely neoplasia Occasionally drug-induced	Other sexually transmitted diseases: syphilis, HIV infection Not drug-induced
Epidemiology	Middle-aged adults	Sexually active adults
Biopsy	Yes Bandlike (lichenoid) inflammatory infiltrate, epidermal acanthosis with sawtooth appearance, wedge-shaped hypergranulosis, colloid bodies	No Epidermal acanthosis, papillomatosis, koilocytosis, tortuous blood vessels in dermal papilla
Laboratory	Hepatitis C virus, occasionally familial	Rapid plasma reagin test HIV test, hepatitis B & C tests
Outcome	Chronic but usually self limited, variable response to therapy; isolated reports of associated squamous cell carcinoma	Curable Good response to therapy

HIV, human immunodeficiency virus

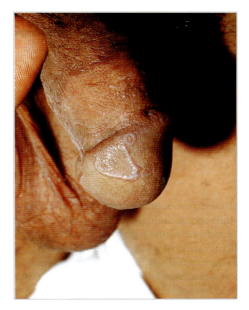 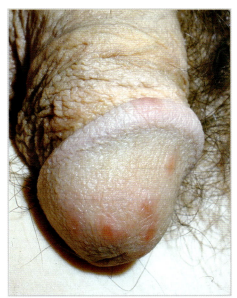

Figure 7.6.3 Lichen planus. *Clue to diagnosis:* purple color and annular configuration

Figure 7.6.4 Scabies infection. *Clue to diagnosis:* widespread itchy rash involving genital skin, and interdigital spaces.

DISEASE DISCUSSION

Bowenoid papulosis

Definition and etiology

Bowenoid papulosis is a human papillomavirus infection of the genitals in which there are warty-appearing papules that demonstrate epithelial atypia reminiscent of squamous cell carcinoma on biopsy. These lesions have also been called HSIL (high grade squamous intraepithelial lesion), but HSIL would also encompass squamous cell carcinoma in situ from which bowenoid papulosis can be clinically distinguished.

Clinical features

Multiple small (2- to 20-mm) red- to brown-colored papules and plaques that are warty, chronic, and treatment resistant are found in the genitalia most commonly in sexually active adults. Men are more frequently involved than women. Biopsy results show the changes of Bowen's disease (squamous cell carcinoma in situ). Unlike in Bowen's disease, however, the lesions of bowenoid papulosis are small and slightly brown colored, do not grow in size, and do not progress to become invasive squamous cell carcinoma. Squamous cell carcinoma is also usually a solitary lesion unlike bowenoid papulosis.

The major clinical disease in the differential diagnosis of bowenoid papulosis is condyloma acuminatum, which is caused by another human papillomavirus infection. The lesions of condyloma acuminatum are usually larger than the papules of bowenoid papulosis and are more skin-colored than the more deeply pigmented lesions of bowenoid papulosis. Atypia are also not present on biopsy of condyloma acuminatum. Lichen planus, like bowenoid papulosis, can present with colored papules in the genitalia; however, the lesions of lichen planus are very pruritic and purple colored. Lichen planus lesions are also frequently present in the oral mucosa and other skin surfaces but may occasionally be limited to genital skin. Other diseases to be considered in the differential diagnosis include psoriasis, granuloma inguinale, lymphogranuloma venereum, molluscum contagiosum, pearly penile papules (penile angiofibromas), and scabies.

Treatment (Table 7.1)

A variety of different destructive treatments can be used, such as liquid nitrogen, imiquimod, laser surgery, electrosurgical removal, excisional

Table 7.1 Treatment of Bowenoid papulosis

Treatment	Precautions
Universal	
Vaccine to prevent disease	Once disease developed vaccine not beneficial
Condoms to prevent spread	
Follow for squamous cell carcinoma development	
Mild disease	
Cryotherapy	Painful and blisters may develop
Imiquimod	May be irritating
Surgical excision	Scar, infection
Laser surgery	Pain, scarring
Electrosurgery	Scar
Severe disease	
Aminolevulinic acid photodynamic therapy	May be very painful
Intralesional interferon	May cause flu like symptoms
Topical or intralesional 5-fluorouracil	Very irritating and necrosis can develop

surgery, laser surgery, and topical 5-fluorouracil. Radical surgery is not necessary, since bowenoid papulosis biologically behaves in a benign manner.

■ Condyloma acuminatum

Definition and etiology

Condyloma acuminatum is a sexually transmitted human papillomavirus infection.

Clinical features

Sessile warty skin-colored papules and plaques in the genital area may progress to become large cauliflower-like masses. Lesions may koebnerize, or develop in sites of trauma. The major disease in the differential diagnosis is bowenoid papulosis.

Although the lesions of condyloma acuminatum are usually quite distinctive, they occasionally can be confused with skin tags, seborrheic keratoses, condyloma latum (syphilis), cutaneous Crohn's disease, cutaneous amebiasis, molluscum contagiosum, and squamous cell carcinoma. Skin tags are usually pedunculated, flesh-colored papules with a smooth surface. Seborrheic keratoses have a characteristic tan to brown color and 'stuck-on' appearance. Recent studies indicate that some clinically and histologically typical seborrheic keratoses may harbor human papilloma virus and may be 'old condylomata'. The lesions of condyloma latum (secondary syphilis) are moist, oozing, white-colored papules and always need to be considered in the differential diagnosis. In fact, since condyloma acuminatum is a sexually transmitted disease, most patients should be screened for other sexually transmitted disease such as syphilis, human immunodeficiency virus (HIV) infection, and hepatitis.

Patients with Crohn's disease may develop a combination of skin tags, fissures, fistulas, and ulcers in perianal skin. Cutaneous amebiasis occurs most frequently in patients with HIV infection and presents with perirectal ulcers, abscesses, and, occasionally, condyloma-like papules or plaques. Squamous cell carcinoma secondary to specific human papillomavirus subtypes produces large condyloma-like lesions (given the eponym *giant condyloma of Buschke–Löwenstein*). Unlike condyloma acuminatum, giant condyloma of Buschke–Löwenstein are very firm and develop fistulas and sinus tracts because of invasion into the dermis.

Treatment (Table 7.2)

A variety of destructive treatments for condyloma acuminatum exist. Liquid nitrogen is usually the first-line treatment. Other therapies include podophyllin, podophyllin toxin, imiquimod, acids, laser surgery, and intralesional or systemic interferon.

■ Contact dermatitis

Definition and etiology

Contact dermatitis is inflammation of the skin resulting from interaction between the skin and the environment. Contact dermatitis can be either an irritant type or an allergic type. Irritant contact dermatitis is a nonimmunologic reaction to a chemical that irritates the skin and causes inflammation. Conversely, allergic contact dermatitis is an individualized immunologic response to the chemical (i.e. the person who is allergic to the chemical will develop a rash when the chemical is absorbed through the skin, whereas another person who is not allergic to the chemical will not develop a rash upon contact).

Table 7.2 Treatment of condyloma acuminatum

Treatment	Precautions
Universal	
HPV vaccine to prevent disease	
Condoms to prevent transmission	
Consider checking for other venereal diseases	
Partner should be checked	High risk HPV types can produce cervical cancer in women
Mild disease	
Cryotherapy	Painful and may produce blisters
Imiquimod 5% cream 3 × a week up to 16 weeks	Irritant dermatitis very common
Podophyllin 25% solution apply q week × 4	Applied in office Irritation Rare reports of leukopenia
Podofilox 0.5% solution q12 hours × 3 days than 4 days off Repeat 1–4 weeks	Inflammation, burning, pain
Severe disease	
Intralesional or systemic interferon	Flu-like symptoms common
Aminolevulinic acid photodynamic therapy	May be painful

Irritant contact dermatitis is most frequently seen in the hands, whereas allergic contact dermatitis can occur in any part of the body in contact with the allergen.

Clinical features

In acute cases, erythema, scaling, vesicles, and swelling can be found. In patients with persistent disease, the erythema and scaling persist, but vesicles disappear and the skin becomes lichenified. It can be difficult to differentiate between irritant and allergic contact dermatitis. Since both irritant and allergic contact dermatitis can appear identical morphologically, patch testing remains the test of choice in confirming the diagnosis of allergic contact dermatitis. The differential diagnosis includes tinea cruris, diaper dermatitis, extramammary Paget's disease, Hailey–Hailey disease, and, in children, Langerhans cell granulomatosis. Tinea cruris can be excluded by a potassium hydroxide (KOH) examination of a skin scraping. The lesions of tinea cruris also have annular serpiginous borders, and some central clearing may be present. In children, allergic contact dermatitis should be considered when diaper dermatitis fails to respond to therapy. The chafing type of diaper dermatitis can be considered a type of irritant contact dermatitis. In Hailey–Hailey disease (benign familial pemphigus), the primary process is a genetically inherited blistering disease that usually presents in adolescence as maceration, erythema, and erosions in body folds. Linear erosions in a background of red patches in the axilla and groin are the characteristic findings. The rash of extramammary Paget's disease can be confused with dermatitis. The eruption is usually asymmetric, may be irregularly shaped, and may have an eroded or nodular component.

Treatment (Table 7.3)

Contact dermatitis can be cured by avoidance of the triggering allergen or irritant. Topical and oral steroids hasten the resolution of the rash.

Table 7.3 Treatment of contact dermatitis

Treatment	Precautions
Universal	
Determine and avoid allergens and/or irritants	
Mild disease	
Topical steroid such as hydrocortisone 1–2% bid	Watch for steroid atrophy
Severe disease	
Systemic steroids for 2–3 weeks Start at 40–60 mg prednisone a day for a few days	Steroid side effects: hyperglycemia, insomnia, hypertension, fluid retention. Dermatitis may flare or recur if tapered too rapidly

Table 7.4 Treatment of diaper dermatitis

Treatment	Precautions
Universal	
Frequent diaper changes	
Avoid irritants	Besides urine and feces, soap is the most common skin irritant
Barrier cream such as zinc oxide or Desitin ointment after diaper changes	
Mild disease	
Hydrocortisone 1% bid	Rare allergy
Topical antifungal cream if yeast present	Mild irritation
Severe disease	
Triamcinolone 0.1% cream or ointment bid	Follow for skin atrophy
Oral antibiotics if secondary infected as confirmed with culture	Diarrhea due to antibiotics may worsen disease

Diaper dermatitis

Definition and etiology

Diaper dermatitis is an eczematous eruption in the diaper area caused by a combination of factors, including occlusion, prolonged contact with urine and stool, bacteria, and *Candida*.

Clinical features

The clinical appearance depends on which etiologic factor is most prominent. In the irritant type of 'chafing diaper dermatitis', examination reveals erythematous lichenified plaques and patches in area of friction such as the buttocks, genitalia, and lower abdomen. The inguinal creases are commonly spared. Candidal diaper dermatitis presents with bright red plaques with overlying white scaling and satellite papules and pustules. Unlike in the chafing type of diaper dermatitis, inguinal folds are involved in candidiasis.

The differential diagnosis of diaper dermatitis includes seborrheic dermatitis, psoriasis, atopic dermatitis, tinea cruris, bullous impetigo, chronic bullous disease of childhood, acrodermatitis enteropathica, and Langerhans cell granulomatosis. In infantile and, rarely, adult seborrheic dermatitis, the diaper area develops dusky erythematous scaly plaques. Unlike the irritant or candidal type of diaper dermatitis, infants do not appear to be symptomatic. Associated findings include cradle cap and involvement of the armpits. In atopic dermatitis, the diaper area is usually spared because of the moisture produced by the occlusive diaper. Infants usually have a rash elsewhere, such as the cheeks, and they are often irritable. A family history of atopy can be elicited. Psoriasis usually spares the flexural areas and has a characteristic silver-white-colored scale. Tinea cruris primarily occurs in adults with tinea pedis. The rash is serpiginous with central clearing. KOH test results are positive for fungal elements. Acrodermatitis enteropathica may be acquired or may be inherited as an autosomal recessive disease. A sharply demarcated rash is present around the mouth, in the diaper area, and also on the distal extremities. In Langerhans cell granulomatosis, purpuric foci along with brown-colored papules may be present. A biopsy will reveal proliferation of Langerhans cells rather than the characteristic spongiosis of diaper dermatitis.

Treatment (Table 7.4)

Infants with diaper dermatitis should have their diapers changed frequently to minimize prolonged contact with urine and feces. After a diaper change, a barrier ointment should be applied. If severe inflammation is present, topical cortisone preparations are necessary. If candidiasis is present, a topical antifungal cream is also needed.

Extramammary Paget's disease

Definition and etiology

Extramammary Paget's disease (EMPD) is a rare cutaneous adenocarcinoma. The adenocarcinoma is localized to the skin in approximately one-third of cases and is secondary to an underlying adnexal adenocarcinoma in one-third of cases. It can also be secondary to an underlying internal malignancy, typically of genitourinary or gastrointestinal tract origin.

Clinical features

Physical examination reveals a sharply demarcated erythematous scaly plaque. The border may be slightly elevated, and the surface may be covered with a slight crust. EMPD frequently can be mistaken for dermatitis, tinea infection, or Bowen's disease. Dermatitis usually is symmetric, and, unless excoriated, blood or crust should not be present. Patients with tinea cruris usually also have tinea pedis. The rash is symmetric with central clearing, and the KOH test result is positive. Bowen's disease usually occurs in sun-exposed sites and does not have a raised border. When extramammary Paget's disease is suspected, a biopsy should be performed. Biopsy results reveal large clear cells scattered in a buckshot fashion throughout the epidermis.

Treatment (Table 7.5)

Small localized lesions can be treated with surgical excision. For larger lesions, treatment with CO_2 lasers has been successful. For surgically unresectable tumors or tumors with underlying adenocarcinoma, a variety of different modalities have been used such as chemotherapy, radiation therapy, and surgical approaches.

Herpes genitalis

Definition and etiology

Herpes genitalis is a sexually transmitted herpes simplex virus type II or, rarely, type I infection of the genitalia.

Clinical features

The eruption starts 2 to 10 days after exposure to herpes simplex virus. Usually, patients develop prodromal symptoms of burning, discomfort, or itching at the site of the impending eruption. In a primary episode, patients develop fever and malaise.

Table 7.5 Treatment of extramammary Paget's disease

Treatment	Precautions
Universal	
Exclude an underlying cancer of the genitourinary or gastrointestinal track	Up to one-third of patients have underlying cancer
Mild disease	
Moh's surgery or surgery	If Mohs surgery not available scouting biopsies may be helpful to evaluate extent of disease
Topical imiquimod cream reported successful	May require months of therapy. Long-term efficacy not established
Severe disease	
Chemotherapy	Numerous
Radiation therapy	Radiation dermatitis, atrophy, cancer
Laser surgery	

Table 7.6 Treatment of herpes genitalis

Treatment	Precautions
Prevention: condoms may help prevent spread	
Antivirals	
Acyclovir (200, 400, 800 mg pills) 400 mg tid for 5–10 days	Headache, nausea, diarrhea, vomiting Rare: psychosis, seizures, leukopenia, thrombocytopenia, Stevens–Johnson, TEN, etc.
Valacyclovir (500, 1000 mg pills) 2000 mg q12 × 1 day	
Famciclovir (125, 250, 500 mg) 500 mg bid × 5 to 10 days or 1500 mg × 1	

Table 7.7 Treatment of Langerhans cell histiocytosis

Treatment	Precautions
Confirm diagnosis with biopsy	Exclude mimics such as insect bite or scabies and congenital self-healing histiocytosis
Topical corticosteroids bid	Watch for steroid induced atrophy
Chemotherapy if necessary as per oncology	Numerous side effects

The lesions start out as red macules that rapidly become vesiculated and develop into widespread erosions. On closer inspection, the erosions are grouped and have scalloped borders characteristic of a herpesvirus infection. The lesions heal spontaneously in a few weeks.

The major diseases in the differential diagnosis are other sexually transmitted diseases such as syphilitic chancre, chancroid, lymphogranuloma venereum, and granuloma inguinale. Prodromal symptoms and grouped blisters do not occur in these other entities, and herpes lesions can be recurrent in some patients. Syphilitic chancres characteristically are painless ulcers with firm non-scalloped borders.

Chancroid presents with exquisitely tender ulcers with undermined borders. In granuloma inguinale, red friable papules that ulcerate are seen. In questionable cases, the diagnosis of herpes genitalis can be confirmed by finding multinucleated giant cells in a Tzanck preparation, preparing a culture, or obtaining positive results of direct immunofluorescence in a skin swab specimen.

Treatment (Table 7.6)
Oral acyclovir, valacyclovir, or famciclovir, if started during the first two days of the infection, can limit the severity and duration of disease.

Langerhans cell histiocytosis

Definition and etiology
Langerhans cell histiocytosis (histiocytosis X) is an idiopathic group of diseases caused by proliferation of Langerhans cells. Recent studies have demonstrated a mutation in BRAF V600E and MAP2K1 in about 75% of patients. Because of morphologic similarity between proliferating Langerhans cells and histiocytes, Langerhans cell granulomatosis was previously called histiocytosis X. Langerhans cell histiocytosis can present as a localized, multifocal, or generalized process. The localized form of Langerhans cell histiocytosis has been called eosinophilic granuloma. Multifocal disease with bone lesions, exophthalmos, and diabetes insipidus has been called *Hand-Schüller-Christian* disease, and the generalized form with hepatosplenomegaly, lymphadenopathy, and generalized purpura has been called *Letterer-Siwe disease*.

Clinical features
Langerhans cell histiocytosis is primarily a disease of young children but may present in adults in rare cases. Three forms are widely recognized: eosinophilic granuloma, Hand-Schüller-Christian disease, and Letterer-Siwe disease. Skin findings are most commonly seen in the Hand-Schüller-Christian and Letterer-Siwe variants and consist of small red-brown slightly scaly papules several millimeters in size. Purpura and, occasionally, larger ulcerative nodules and plaques can be present. The scalp and diaper area are most commonly involved. However, in severe cases, lesions can be found over the entire tegmentum. The cutaneous lesions of Langerhans cell granulomatosis are frequently misdiagnosed as seborrheic dermatitis or diaper dermatitis in children. Purpura should not be found in either seborrheic dermatitis or diaper dermatitis. In adults, because of their predilection for the groin and the presence of ulcers, the lesions may also be confused with hidradenitis suppurativa. The red-brown-colored papules can be confused with Darier's disease. Ultimately, a biopsy is necessary for definitive diagnosis and will reveal proliferation of Langerhans cells in the dermis. The cells have kidney-bean-shaped nuclei, stain with antibody against CD1A.

Treatment (Table 7.7)
Usually patients are treated by pediatric oncology. Recently success with B-raf inhibitor has been reported. Chemotherapeutic agents are also frequently used.

Lichen planus

Definition and etiology
Lichen planus is an idiopathic inflammatory dermatitis that can involve both glabrous and mucosal skin. The cause of lichen planus is not known. Certain drugs, such as methyldopa, ß-blockers, thiazide diuretics, gold, penicillamine, and nonsteroidal anti-inflammatory agents, can occasionally cause lichen planus.

Clinical features

Lichen planus most commonly occurs between the ages of 30 and 60 years and affects both sexes equally. Lichen planus predominantly affects the flexural surfaces of the arms and the extensor surfaces of the legs. The characteristic lesions are purple colored, flat-topped polygonal papules and are very pruritic. Wickham's striae are delicate networks of fine white-colored scales that can be seen overlying lesions.

The lesions resolve with postinflammatory hyperpigmentation. A variety of morphologic variants can be seen, such as bullous, atrophic, hypertrophic, erosive, ulcerative, erythematous, exfoliative, and follicular lichen planus. The lesions may also have annular or linear arrangements. The Koebner's phenomenon is seen, which consists of lesions occurring at sites of injury. Mucous membranes are affected in approximately half of patients with skin lesions. Thickened dystrophic nails may also be found (see Chapter 5). Patients may rarely present with scarring alopecia as the primary sign of lichen planus (see Chapter 1).

Treatment (Table 7.8)

Treatment of lichen planus is usually difficult. Any suspected causative drug should be eliminated. Drug-induced lichen planus may take a few months to subside after discontinuation of the offending drug. The most common treatment is topical steroids. Other therapies include topical or systemic retinoids.

■ Lichen sclerosus et atrophicus

Definition and etiology

Lichen sclerosus et atrophicus is an idiopathic disease in which white atrophic patches of skin develop.

Clinical features

Lichen sclerosus et atrophicus occurs most commonly in the genital skin of postmenopausal women. However, lichen sclerosus et atrophicus can also develop in children at times and in skin outside the genital area. Extragenital involvement is somewhat more common in children. In men, lichen sclerosus develops most commonly on the penis in uncircumcised individuals; genital involvement in men is called *balanitis xerotica obliterans*. Patients complain of pruritus, soreness, discomfort, oozing, and pain with intercourse. Examination reveals porcelain-white skin that is atrophic. Follicular plugging may be present. In women, the perivaginal and perirectal distribution of the patches imparts an hourglass appearance. The atrophic skin frequently becomes irritated and red, and vesicles and hemorrhage can result from trauma.

The major diseases in the differential diagnosis are contact dermatitis and vitiligo. The lesions of contact dermatitis are red, pruritic rather than painful, not atrophic, and scaly in appearance. Vitiligo is asymptomatic, and atrophy is also not present. Small, residual, pigmented macules may be seen around hair follicles in patches of vitiligo. In newly developing lesions of lichen sclerosus, a biopsy may be necessary to confirm the diagnosis, since there is less atrophy and more erythema.

Biopsy results show edema and sclerosis of the collagen bundles in the upper dermis, follicular plugging, and a bandlike lymphocytic infiltrate.

Treatment (Table 7.9)

The treatment of choice for lichen sclerosus et atrophicus is high-potency topical corticosteroids. Topical treatment with retinoids and testosterone preparations can also be effective.

■ Syphilis

Definition and etiology

Syphilis (except congenital syphilis) is a sexually transmitted disease caused by the spirochete *Treponema pallidum*. Syphilis is one of the great mimickers and can present with a variety of cutaneous and systemic manifestations.

Clinical features

The clinical features of syphilis can be subdivided into four different stages: primary, secondary, latent, and tertiary. The primary stage occurs 9–90 days after inoculation, when a painless, firm ulcer (the

Table 7.8 Treatment of lichen planus

Treatment	Precautions
Universal	
Look for underlying cause	
Mild disease	
Topical corticosteroid such as triamcinolone cream or ointment 0.1% bid or clobetasol 0.05% cream bid	Watch for steroid-induced atrophy, and steroid induced acne on face
Severe disease	
Oral prednisone	Steroid side effects: hyperglycemia, insomnia, hypertension, fluid retention
PUVA (psoralin plus ultraviolet A light)	Risk of burning and skin cancer
Acitretin 10 mg to 75 mg PO q day	Non FDA approved indication Teratogen, hypertriglyceridemia commonly seen Hair loss also relatively common

Table 7.9 Treatment of lichen sclerosus

Treatment	Precautions
Universal	
Good skin care, mild soaps	
Look for secondary yeast infection	
Periodic examination for development of squamous cell carcinoma	
Mild disease	
Class 1 topical steroid: clobetasol 0.05% bid	Although the skin may already be atrophic strong topical steroids do not worsen the problem Topical steroids may predispose to secondary fungal or yeast infection
Tacrolimus ointment 0.03% or 0.1% bid	May cause irritation
Severe disease	
Photodynamic therapy	May produce sunburn Painful
Systemic retinoids	Retinoid toxicity with dryness, increased blood lipids, liver damage, and hair loss

Table 7.10 Treatment of primary syphilis in immunocompetent host

Treatment	Precautions
Contact Department of Health as per state regulations	
Consider screening for concurrent other sexually transmitted diseases such as HIV	
Follow RPR or VDRL titers after treatment to make certain they decrease	False positive results can occur with pregnancy, autoimmune diseases, and other infections
Penicillin G 2.4 million units IM	Allergic reaction, anaphylaxis

Table 7.11 Treatment of tinea cruris

Treatment	Precautions
Universal	
Confirm diagnosis with KOH Look for and treat tinea pedis	Most patients with tinea cruris have underlying tinea pedis
Put socks on before underwear when getting dressed	
Mild/moderate disease	
Topical antifungal such as Lotrimin, econazole, terbinafine, ketoconazole	None
Severe disease	
Itraconazole 100 mg to 200 mg po q day × 2 to 4 weeks	Liver function tests at baseline Rare hepatotoxicity, watch for drug interactions
Terbinafine 250 mg po q day × 2 weeks	CBC and liver function tests at baseline Rare hepatic toxicity

chancre) usually develops in the genital region. The chancre has an indurated, round border with a fine erythematous rim.

Secondary syphilis, which occurs 8 weeks to approximately 2 years after inoculation, has protean manifestations including a truncal papular rash, moth-eaten alopecia (see Chapter 1), and white wart-like lesions in the genitalia, condyloma latum. Without treatment, the lesions of secondary syphilis resolve, and the disease evolves into a latent stage, only to erupt many years later in some patients as tertiary syphilis. The cutaneous manifestations of tertiary syphilis include nodular, psoriasiform, serpiginous plaques and gummas, which are painless, necrotic, ulcerating nodules.

The differential diagnosis of syphilitic chancre includes other sexually transmitted diseases such as herpes genitalis, chancroid, and lymphogranuloma venereum. The lesions of herpes are vesicular, scalloped, and usually multiple, in contrast to the typical syphilis chancres, which are usually single. The lesions of chancroid are very tender and have an undermined border. Granuloma inguinale presents with friable, vascular-appearing papules that ulcerate. The diagnosis in suspected cases should be confirmed by serology.

Treatment (Table 7.10)

In primary or secondary infections, 2.4 million units of intramuscular penicillin can be used. Oral tetracycline or erythromycin tablets are alternative therapies for penicillin-allergic patients.

Tinea cruris
Definition and etiology

Tinea cruris is a dermatophyte infection of the groin folds.

Clinical features

Patients with tinea cruris exhibit erythematous, serpiginous plaques with central clearing in the groin and extending down the thigh. Occasionally, if the fungus extends down into a hair follicle, a nodular component can be present. Extension onto the buttock area occurs frequently. In men, the penis and scrotum are usually spared. Tinea cruris is most commonly seen in men because of the higher incidence of tinea pedis in men, a high level of perspiration, and occlusion from clothing and from the scrotum. Tinea cruris is more common in warmer climates.

The differential diagnosis includes contact dermatitis, intertrigo, Langerhans cell granulomatosis, diaper dermatitis, seborrheic dermatitis, Hailey–Hailey disease, and extramammary Paget's disease. In contact dermatitis, vesicles may be present, and central clearing is absent. Intertrigo and diaper dermatitis are due to a combination of factors such as rubbing, moisture, bacteria, and yeast. The lesions are symmetric, and serpiginous borders are not present. In Langerhans cell granulomatosis, purpuric lesions are usually present, and a biopsy will confirm the diagnosis. Hailey-Hailey disease is an autosomal dominant blistering disease in which the primary lesion is an erosion. It most commonly will also affect the axillary area. Extramammary Paget's disease should be suspected if lesions are asymmetric and do not heal. A biopsy is required for accurate diagnosis.

Treatment (Table 7.11)

A variety of different topical or oral antifungal agents can be used. Commonly used treatments include imidazole or allylamine creams. Oral therapy with griseofulvin, terbinafine, fluconazole or itraconazole can be used in particularly severe or refractory cases in which the diagnosis has been firmly established.

Section 2

GENERALIZED RASHES

Chapter 8: Papulosquamous diseases

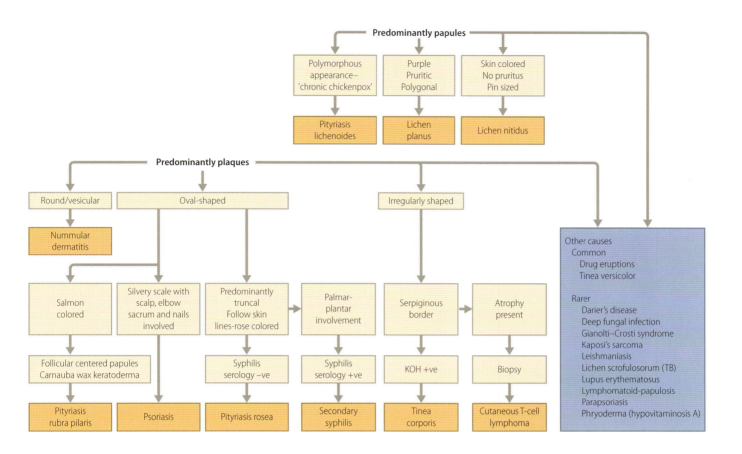

INTRODUCTION

A variety of diseases have been classified as papulosquamous disorders. These diseases have the common features of generalized scaling patches, papules, and plaques. The classic papulosquamous diseases include psoriasis, lichen planus, pityriasis rosea, pityriasis rubra pilaris, secondary syphilis, tinea corporis, and nummular dermatitis. The majority of the papulosquamous diseases can be easily diagnosed because of their morphology, distribution, and history. For example, psoriasis predominates on extensor surfaces, has a white silvery scale, and occurs symmetrically. There is often a family history of the disease. Pityriasis rosea is an acute eruption of small pink papules and plaques that follow skin lines on the trunk. The lesions of lichen planus have a purple color and a polygonal appearance and are very pruritic. Tinea corporis can be excluded if skin scrapings treated with potassium hydroxide solution are negative for hyphae. Although the rash of secondary syphilis may mimic pityriasis rosea, an accurate diagnosis can be made by the finding of palmar and plantar papules. These are not found in pityriasis rosea but are characteristic of syphilis. The sexual history, the finding of genital lesions and white mucous patches, and positive syphilis serology all help confirm the diagnosis. Nummular dermatitis usually presents in adults and is characterized by coin-sized eczematous papules and plaques. In this chapter, some uncommon papulosquamous diseases such as lichen nitidus, mycosis fungoides (cutaneous T-cell lymphoma), pityriasis rubra pilaris, and pityriasis lichenoides are also discussed and compared with the diseases they most closely mimic: lichen planus, nummular dermatitis, psoriasis, and scabies infection.

1. PSORIASIS VERSUS PITYRIASIS RUBRA PILARIS

■ Features in common: red scaly papules and plaques

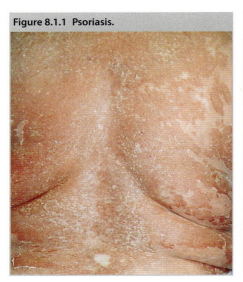

Figure 8.1.1 Psoriasis.

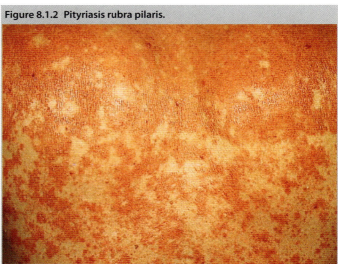

Figure 8.1.2 Pityriasis rubra pilaris.

■ Distinguishing features

	Psoriasis	Pityriasis rubra pilaris
Physical examination	Lesions red-colored	Lesions red-orange in color
	No follicular accentuation	Follicular accentuation
Morphology	When erythrodermic, no islands of normal skin are found	Islands of normal skin when erythrodermic
	Keratoderma uncommon	Keratoderma has a yellow-orange carnauba wax appearance
Distribution	Scalp and extensor surface predilection	Scalp, palmar-plantar surface, and glabrous skin; may be worse in photodistributed areas
Associated findings	Arthritis	No arthritis
	Onychodystrophy	Onychodystrophy
History	Family history in 10% to 20% of patients	Rarely autosomal dominant disorder
	Improves with sun exposure	No improvement with sun exposure
Symptoms	Asymptomatic to moderate pruritus	Asymptomatic to mild pruritus
	Arthritis in some patients	No associated arthritis
Exacerbating factors	Infections: streptococcal, HIV, and upper respiratory tract	HIV infection
	Medications: antimalarials, Angiotensin-converting enzyme inhibitors, fluoxetine, β-adrenergic blocking agents, lithium, quinidine, corticosteroid withdrawal; non- steroidal anti-inflammatory agents	
Epidemiology	Any age; no sex predilection	Any age; no sex predilection
Biopsy	Usually not necessary	Yes
	Psoriasiform epidermal hyperplasia with neutrophil microabscesses in epidermis and stratum corneum	Chronic dermatitis, parakeratotic mounds around follicular orifices, and alternating areas of parakeratosis in vertical and horizontal pattern within stratum corneum
Laboratory	None	None
Outcome	Chronic	Chronic
	Variable response to therapy	Poor response to therapy, but eventually remits
HIV, human immunodeficiency virus; PUVA, psoralen plus ultraviolet A light.		

Differential diagnosis of papulosquamous lesions

Common causes
- Drug eruption
- Lichen planus
- Nummular dermatitis
- Pityriasis rosea
- Psoriasis
- Seborrheic dermatitis
- Tinea corporis
- Tinea versicolor

Rarer causes
- Cutaneous T-cell lymphoma (mycosis fungoides)
- Darier's disease
- Deep fungal infection (coccidioidomycosis)
- Erythema annulare centrifugum
- Gianotti–Crosti syndrome
- Kaposi's sarcoma in patients with acquired immunodeficiency syndrome
- Leprosy
- Leishmaniasis
- Lichen nitidus
- Lichen spinulosus
- Lichen scrofulosorum
- Lymphomatoid papulosis
- Lupus erythematosus
- Mycosis fungoides
- Pityriasis lichenoides
- Pityriasis rubra pilaris
- Parapsoriasis
- Phrynoderma (vitamin A deficiency)
- Secondary syphilis

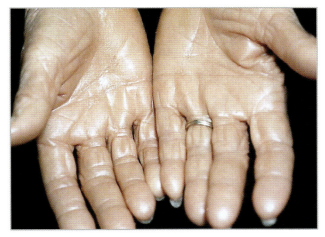

Figure 8.1.3 Pityriasis rubra pilaris. *Clue to diagnosis:* carnauba wax like keratoderma.

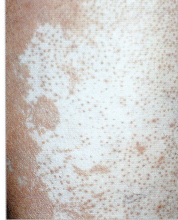

Figure 8.1.4 Pityriasis rubra pilaris. *Clue to diagnosis:* follicular based papules.

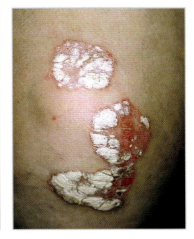

Figure 8.1.5 Psoriasis. Red plaques covered with white silvery scale.

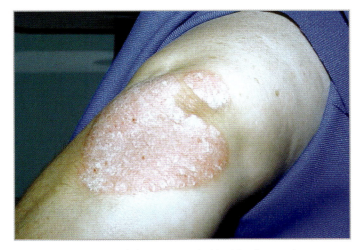

Figure 8.1.6 Psoriasis. Red plaques covered with white silvery scale.

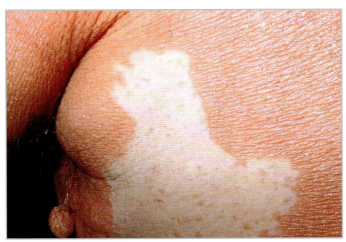

Figure 8.1.7 Pityriasis rubra pilaris. *Clue to diagnosis:* islands of normal skin in areas of erythroderma.

2. PSORIASIS VERSUS NUMMULAR DERMATITIS

■ Features in common: scaly plaques

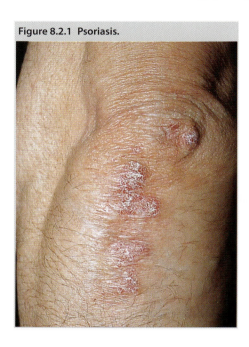

Figure 8.2.1 Psoriasis.

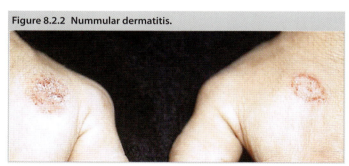

Figure 8.2.2 Nummular dermatitis.

■ Distinguishing features

Physical examination Morphology	No vesicles No crust Silvery scale Koebner's phenomenon Lesions range in size from few mm to several cm		Small vesicles and papules within plaques Crust Flesh-colored to white scale No Koebner's phenomenon Lesions the size of a quarter
Distribution	Scalp and predilection for extensor surfaces of body (elbows, knees)		Trunk and extremities
Associated findings	Arthritis Onychodystrophy (often with subungual oil spot and pits) No dry skin		No arthritis No nail dystrophy Dry skin
History Symptoms	Family history in 10–20% of patients Improves with sun exposure Asymptomatic to moderate pruritus		No family history No improvement with sun exposure More common in winter Asymptomatic to marked pruritus
Exacerbating factors	Infections: streptococcal, HIV, upper respiratory tract Medications: antimalarials, angiotensin-converting enzyme inhibitors, β-adrenergic blocking agents, lithium, quinidine, corticosteroid withdrawal, NSAIDs		Dry skin Not associated with infection No medications
Epidemiology	Any age; no sex predilection		Adult men predominate
Biopsy	Usually not necessary Epidermal hyperplasia with neutrophil micro-abscesses in epidermis and stratum corneum		No Hyperplasia of the epidermis with prominent spongiosis, scale crust, and a superficial perivascular infiltrate
Laboratory	None		None
Outcome	Chronic disease		Self-limited disease with periodic exacerbation

Drugs producing psoriasiform dermatitis or exacerbating psoriasis

- Antimalarials
- Angiotensin-converting enzyme inhibitors
- β-adrenergic receptor blocking agents
- Corticosteroid withdrawal
- Lithium
- Nonsteroidal anti-inflammatory drugs (not well established – isolated reports)
- Quinidine

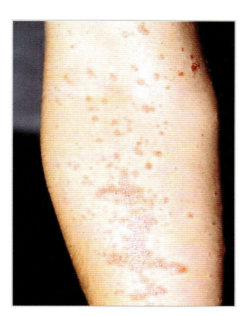

Figure 8.2.3 Psoriasis. *Clue to diagnosis:* Koebner's reaction (lesions). In this case, linear lesions developed in sites of scratching or trauma.

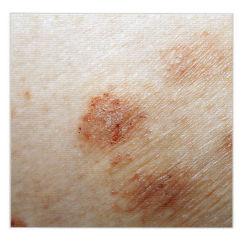

Figure 8.2.4 Nummular dermatitis. *Clue to diagnosis:* coin-sized round eczematous plaques.

3. PITYRIASIS ROSEA VERSUS SECONDARY SYPHILIS

■ Features in common: oval scaly patches and plaques on trunk

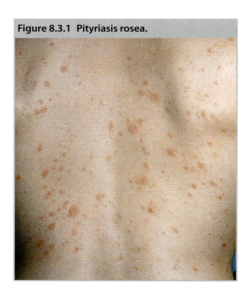

Figure 8.3.1 Pityriasis rosea.

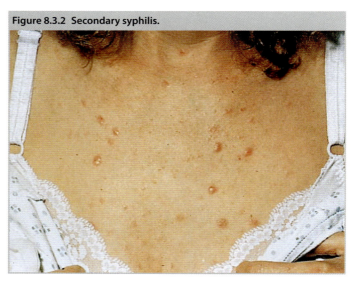

Figure 8.3.2 Secondary syphilis.

■ Distinguishing features

	Pityriasis rosea	Secondary syphilis
Physical examination	Fine white scale No palmar or plantar lesions	Minimal scale Macules and papules frequently found on palms and soles
Morphology	Disease starts as a single large patch (herald patch) No mucous patch	No herald patch White patches may be found on lips or mouth (mucous patch)
Distribution	Primarily truncal and proximal extremities	Involves entire body
History Symptoms	Not associated with sexual contact Prodrome of fever and malaise in 5% of patients	Sexual contact Generalized malaise common
Exacerbating factors	None (possibly associated with upper respiratory tract infections)	Other sexually transmitted disease Immunosuppression (human immunodeficiency virus)
Associated findings	Lymphadenopathy rare	Lymphadenopathy common Hepatitis, arthritis
Epidemiology	75% of patients between age 10 and 35; most common in fall, winter, and spring	Sexually active
Biopsy	Usually not necessary Epidermal acanthosis, spongiosis, parakeratotic mounds, and superficial perivascular lymphocytic infiltrate	Usually not done Psoriasiform hyperplasia of epidermis with superficial and deep perivascular and bandlike lymphoplasmacytic infiltrate Warthin–Starry stain positive for spirochetes in many cases
Laboratory	Syphilis serology negative	Syphilis serology positive
Outcome	Resolves spontaneously	Lesions resolve without treatment, but disease persists in a latent stage and eventually may present as tertiary syphilis

Drugs producing pityriasis-rosea-like eruption

- Barbiturates
- Captopril
- Clonidine
- Gold
- Isotretinoin
- Metronidazole
- Penicillamine

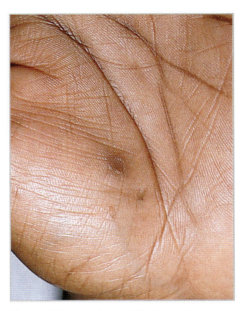

Figure 8.3.3 Secondary syphilis. *Clue to diagnosis:* palmar lesions.

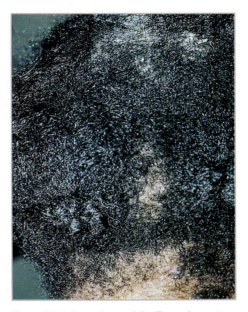

Figure 8.3.4 Secondary syphilis. *Clue to diagnosis:* moth-eaten alopecia.

4. PITYRIASIS ROSEA VERSUS GUTTATE PSORIASIS

■ Features in common: small, round, red scaly plaques and patches

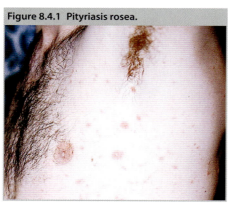

Figure 8.4.1 Pityriasis rosea.

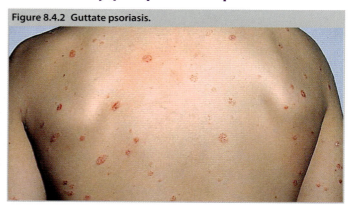

Figure 8.4.2 Guttate psoriasis.

■ Distinguishing features

	Pityriasis rosea	Guttate psoriasis
Physical examination	Pink oval plaques	Red scaly papules and plaques
	Fine white scale	Adherent silvery scale
Morphology	Disease starts as a single large patch (herald patch)	No herald patch
	Long axis of lesions follows skin lines	Lesions do not follow skin lines
	No Koebner's reaction	Koebner's reaction
Distribution	Primarily truncal and proximal extremities (elbows, knees)	Trunk and extremities favored
	Scalp and distal extremities not involved	Scalp commonly involved
History	No family history	Family history in 10–20% of patients
	Prodrome of fever and malaise in 5% of patients	Prodrome of streptococcal pharyngitis in most children
Symptoms	Asymptomatic or mild pruritus	Asymptomatic to mild pruritus
Exacerbating factors	May improve with sun exposure	Improves with sun exposure
Associated findings	No arthritis	Arthritis
	No onychodystrophy	Onychodystrophy
Epidemiology	75% of patients aged 10–35; least common in summer	Most common in children
Biopsy	Usually not necessary	Usually not necessary
	Slight epidermal acanthosis, spongiosis, parakeratotic mounds, and superficial perivascular lymphocytic infiltrate	Epidermal hyperplasia with neutrophil microabscesses in epidermis and stratum corneum
Laboratory	Syphilis serology negative	Positive anti-streptolysin-O antibody or streptozyme titer
Outcome	Resolves spontaneously	Acute or chronic disease
		In 50% of children may clear with antibiotic therapy only

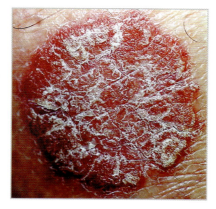

Figure 8.4.3 Psoriasis. *Clue to diagnosis:* white silvery colored scale.

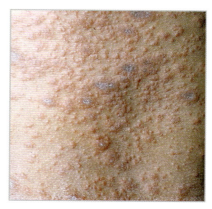

Figure 8.4.4 Pityriasis rosea. *Clue to diagnosis:* Lesions follow skin lines and have a Christmas tree-like distribution.

5. PITYRIASIS ROSEA VERSUS TINEA CORPORIS

■ Features in common: scaly papules and plaques

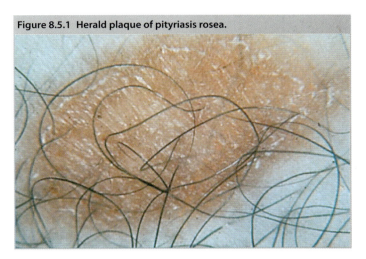

Figure 8.5.1 Herald plaque of pityriasis rosea.

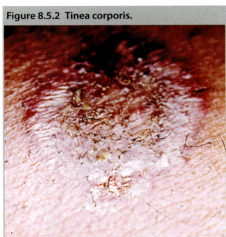

Figure 8.5.2 Tinea corporis.

■ Distinguishing features

	Pityriasis rosea	Tinea corporis
Physical examination		
Morphology	Pink oval plaques Fine white scale Disease starts as a single large patch (herald patch) Long axis of lesions follows skin lines No central clearing	Red serpiginous plaques Coarse scale No herald patch Unrelated to skin lines Central clearing
Distribution	Primarily truncal and proximal extremities	Any glabrous skin
History	Prodrome of fever and malaise in 5% of patients	No fever or malaise
Symptoms	Asymptomatic or mild pruritus	Mild to moderate pruritus
Exacerbating factors	None	Immunosuppression Corticosteroids
Associated findings	Arthritis Onychodystrophy No tinea pedis	No arthritis Onychomycosis Tinea pedis
Epidemiology	75% of patients between age 10 and 35; most common in fall, winter, and spring	Any age; more common in wrestlers, people with athlete's foot or with pets
Biopsy	No Slight epidermal acanthosis, spongiosis, parakeratotic mounds, and superficial perivascular lymphocytic infiltrate	No Neutrophilic scale crust, spongiosis, and organisms within stratum corneum
Laboratory	Rapid plasma reagin test negative	Potassium hydroxide test positive, and positive culture on DTM (dermatophyte test medium)
Outcome	Resolves spontaneously	Curable with therapy

PAPULOSQUAMOUS DISEASES

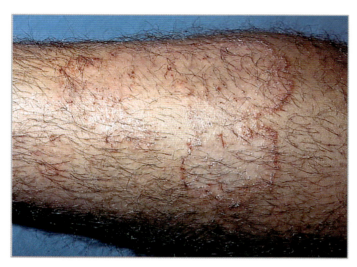

Figure 8.5.3 Tinea corporis. *Clue to diagnosis:* serpiginous borders with central clearing.

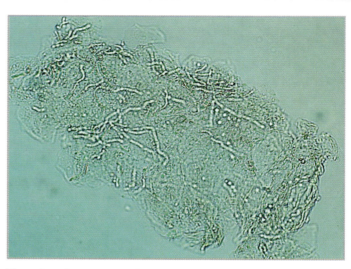

Figure 8.5.4 Tinea corporis. *Clue to diagnosis:* skin scarping treated with potassium hydroxide (KOH) solution which accentuates numerous hyphae among keratinocytes.

6. PSORIASIS VERSUS LICHEN PLANUS

Features in common: scaly papules and plaques

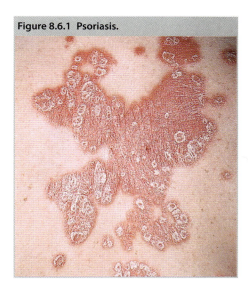

Figure 8.6.1 Psoriasis.

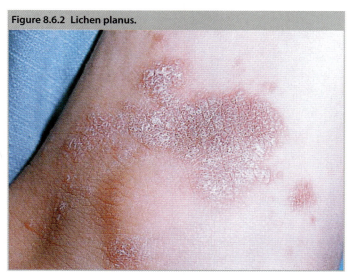

Figure 8.6.2 Lichen planus.

Distinguishing features

	Psoriasis	Lichen planus
Physical examination Morphology	Red-colored Coarse white scale	Purple color Fine white scale forming a collarette in periphery of lesions (Wickham's striae)
Distribution	Extensor surface of arms and legs (elbows, knees) Scalp involvement common	Flexural surface of forearms, extensor surface of legs Scalp involvement rare
History	Family history in 10% to 20% of patients Improves with sun exposure	No family history Gradual onset
Symptoms	Asymptomatic to moderate pruritus Arthritis in some patients	Moderate to severe pruritus No arthritis
Exacerbating factors	Infections: streptococcal, HIV and upper respiratory tract Medications: antimalarials, angiotensin-converting enzyme inhibitors, β-adrenergic blocking agents, lithium, quinidine, fluoxetine, corticosteroid withdrawal, NSAIDs	Infections: hepatitis C Medications: angiotensin-converting enzyme inhibitors, NSAIDs, sulfonylureas, gold, penicillamine, thiazides, carbamazepine, methyldopa, lithium, quinidine, quinine, β-blockers
Associated findings	Arthritis Onychodystrophy No oral lesions No associated autoimmune disease or internal malignancy	No arthritis Onychodystrophy White reticulated oral patches Rarely associated with other autoimmune diseases or malignancy
Epidemiology	Any age	Mostly middle-aged adults
Biopsy	No Psoriasiform epidermal hyperplasia with neutrophil microabscesses in epidermis and stratum corneum	Yes Irregular epidermal hyperplasia in a 'sawtoothed' pattern, colloid bodies, wedge-shaped hypergranulosis, and a dense lymphocytic infiltrate obscuring the dermal epidermal junction
Laboratory	None	None
Outcome	Chronic disease	Resolves over months to years

PAPULOSQUAMOUS DISEASES

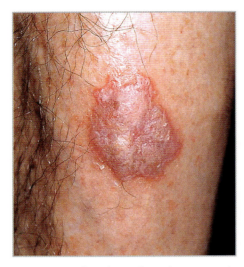

Figure 8.6.3 Lichen planus. *Clue to diagnosis:* purple color.

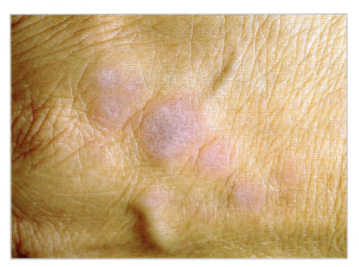

Figure 8.6.4 Lichen planus. *Clue to diagnosis:* purple pruritic polygonal papules.

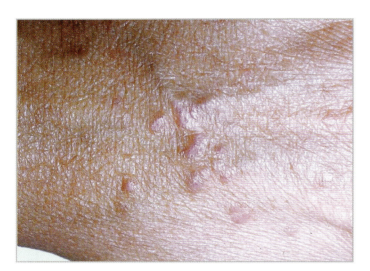

Figure 8.6.5 Lichen planus. *Clue to diagnosis:* purple pruritic polygonal papules.

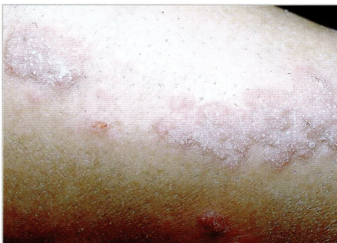

Figure 8.6.6 Lichen planus. *Clue to diagnosis:* purple pruritic polygonal papules.

7. CUTANEOUS T-CELL LYMPHOMA VERSUS DERMATITIS

Features in common: erythematous scaly plaques

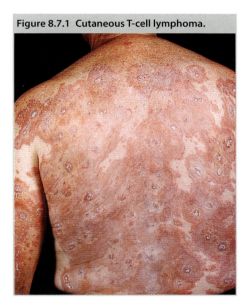

Figure 8.7.1 Cutaneous T-cell lymphoma.

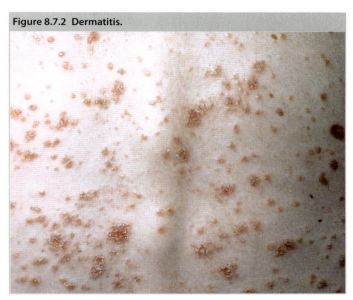

Figure 8.7.2 Dermatitis.

Distinguishing features

	Cutaneous T-cell lymphoma	Dermatitis
Physical examination	Red patches, plaques, and nodules No vesicles	Red plaques Small vesicles and papules frequently present within plaques
Morphology	No crust Scale but not prominent Lesions variable in size Lesions frequently have serpiginous borders Telangiectasias and fine wrinkling are present in patches	Crust Prominent scale Lesions the size of a quarter Lesions round No telangiectasias or wrinkling
Distribution	Trunk, extremities	Trunk, extremities
History	Chronic rash refractory to therapy	Rash worsens in winter months
Symptoms	Asymptomatic to severe pruritus	Mild to moderate pruritus
Exacerbating factors	None	Dry skin Emotional stress
Associated findings	Lymphadenopathy Hepatosplenomegaly	No lymphadenopathy No hepatosplenomegaly
Epidemiology	Adult men	Adult men
Biopsy	Yes; often nonspecific early on Bandlike infiltrate with atypical cerebriform lymphocytes extending into epidermis	No Dermatitis: psoriasiform hyperplasia of the epidermis with spongiosis, scale crust, and superficial perivascular infiltrate
Laboratory	Sézary prep for circulating atypical lymphocytes	None
Outcome	Chronic slowly progressive lymphoma; approximately 50% of patients will die of unrelated causes; occasional transformation to anaplastic lymphoma	Self-limited disease

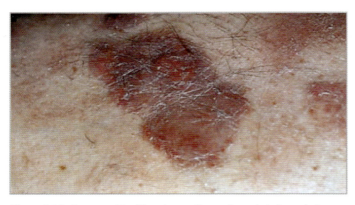

Figure 8.7.3 Cutaneous T-cell lymphoma. *Clue to diagnosis:* indurated plaques and nodules refractory to treatment.

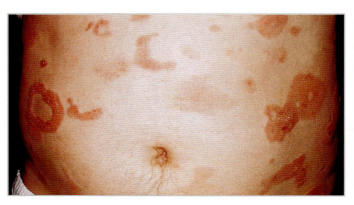

Figure 8.7.4 Cutaneous T-cell lymphoma. *Clue to diagnosis:* serpiginous annular plaques.

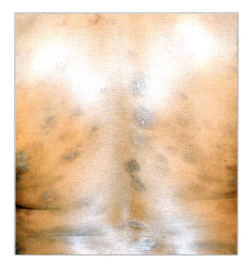

Figure 8.7.5 Cutaneous T-cell lymphoma.

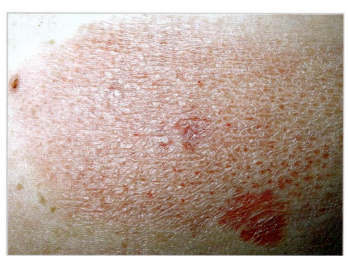

Figure 8.7.6 Cutaneous T-cell lymphoma.

8. LICHEN PLANUS VERSUS LICHEN NITIDUS

■ Features in common: small scaly papules

Figure 8.8.1 Lichen planus.

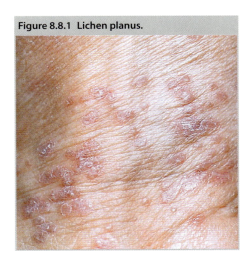

Figure 8.8.2 Lichen nitidus.

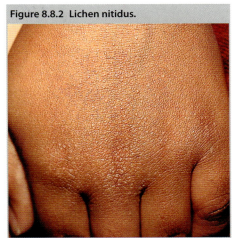

■ Distinguishing features

	Lichen nitidus	Lichen planus
Physical examination		
Morphology	Pin-sized discrete papules Skin color Minimal scale	Papules and plaques Purple color Fine white scale forming a collarette in periphery of lesions (Wickham's striae)
Distribution	Forearms, extensor surface Abdomen, chest, buttocks, and genitals commonly involved Legs less commonly involved	Forearms, flexural surface Abdomen, chest, buttocks less frequently involved Extensor surface of legs
History Symptoms Exacerbating factors	Lesions asymptomatic None	Moderate to severe pruritus Infections: hepatitis C Medications: angiotensin-converting enzyme inhibitors, nonsteroidal anti-inflammatory drugs, ß-blockers, sulfonylureas, gold, penicillamine, carbamazepine, methyldopa, lithium, quinidine, quinine
Associated findings	No onychodystrophy Mucous membrane lesions rare Occasionally associated with lichen planus Reported to be seen in Crohn's disease	Onychodystrophy White reticulated oral patches Rarely associated with other autoimmune diseases No association with Crohn's disease
Epidemiology	Children and young adults Blacks more commonly involved	Mostly middle-aged adults
Biopsy	Yes Focal lymphohistiocytic infiltrate surrounded by epidermis forming 'ball in claw' appearance	Yes Irregular epidermal hyperplasia in a 'sawtooth' pattern, colloid bodies, wedge-shaped hypergranulosis, and a dense lymphocytic infiltrate obscuring the dermal-epidermal junction
Laboratory	None	None
Outcome	May resolve within weeks or last years	Resolves over months to years

Possible etiologic factors in lichen-planus-like eruptions

- Medications
  - Angiotensin-converting enzyme inhibitors
  - Nonsteroidal anti-inflammatory drugs
  - β-Blockers
  - Sulfonylureas
  - Thiazide diuretics
  - Miscellaneous: gold, penicillamine, carbamazepine, methyldopa, lithium, quinidine, quinine
- Infections
  - Hepatitis C
- Neoplasms
- Graft vs host disease

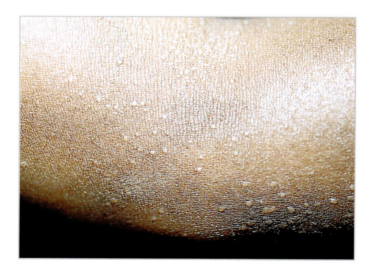

Figure 8.8.3 Lichen nitidus. *Clue to diagnosis:* small size of papules and skin colored.

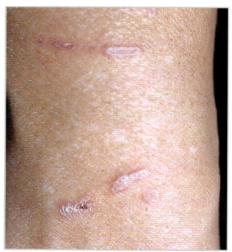

Figure 8.8.4 Lichen planus. *Clue to diagnosis:* purple color with Koebner's phenomena.

9. PSORIASIS VERSUS PITYRIASIS LICHENOIDES

Features in common: red scaly papules and plaques

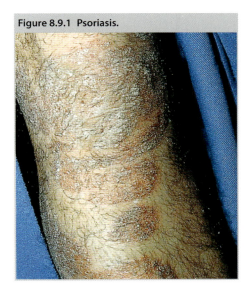

Figure 8.9.1 Psoriasis.

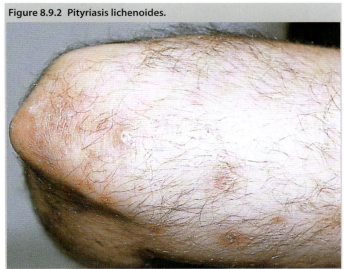

Figure 8.9.2 Pityriasis lichenoides.

Distinguishing features

		Psoriasis	Pityriasis lichenoides
Physical examination	Morphology	No vesicles Silvery scale No crust present Appearance of lesions monomorphous No scarring	Papulovesicular lesions Yellow-brown-colored micaceous-like scale Crust Appearance of lesions polymorphous Lesions heal with scar
	Distribution	Generalized: predilection for extensor surfaces of body and scalp	Generalized: trunk, thighs, upper arms; predilection for flexural surfaces
History Symptoms		Family history of psoriasis in 10–20% No fever except in pustular variants Disease usually insidious, slow onset Asymptomatic to moderate pruritus	No family history of patients may be present Occasionally fever at onset Sudden onset of lesions in crops Asymptomatic
Exacerbating factors		Infections: streptococcal, HIV, upper respiratory tract Medications: antimalarials, angiotensin-converting enzyme inhibitors, β-adrenergic blocking agents, corticosteroid withdrawal, lithium, quinidine, NSAIDs	None known
Associated findings		No associated malignancies Arthritis Onychodystrophy	Rarely associated with lymphomatoid papulosis or cutaneous T-cell lymphoma No arthritis No onychodystrophy
Epidemiology		Any age	More common in children
Biopsy		Usually not necessary Psoriasiform epidermal hyperplasia with neutrophil microabscesses in epidermis and stratum corneum	Yes Wedge-shaped lichenoid infiltrate with epidermal necrosis, scale crust, extravasated erythrocytes in epidermis and upper dermis
Laboratory		None	None
Outcome		Chronic	Acute to chronic

148 PAPULOSQUAMOUS DISEASES

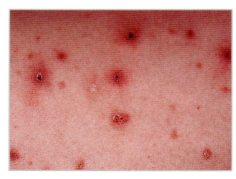

Figure 8.9.3 Pityriasis lichenoides. *Clue to diagnosis:* crusted chickenpox like papules

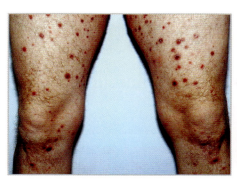

Figure 8.9.4 Pityriasis lichenoides.

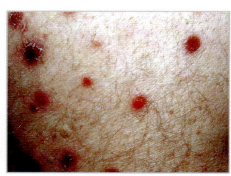

Figure 8.9.5 Pityriasis lichenoides.

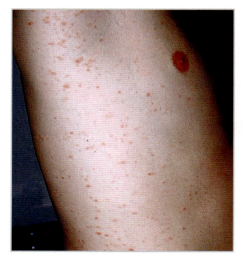

Figure 8.9.6 Pityriasis lichenoides.

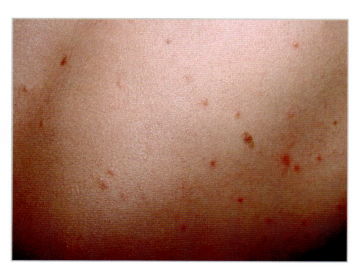

Figure 8.9.7 Pityriasis lichenoides.

10. PAPULOSQUAMOUS DISEASES: OTHER CAUSES

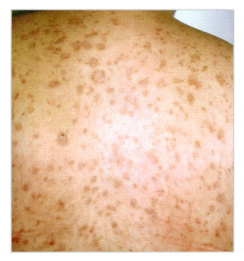

Figure 8.10.1 Lichenoid drug eruption due to gold.

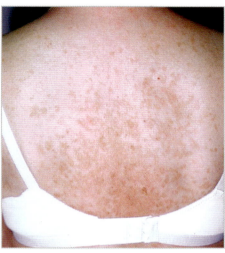

Figure 8.10.2 Tinea versicolor.

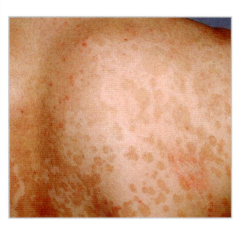

Figure 8.10.3 Tinea versicolor: note the frequent presence of hyper and hypopigmentation.

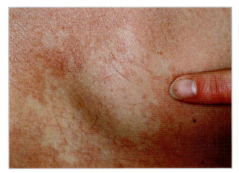

Figure 8.10.4 Tinea versicolor: note the frequent presence of hyper and hypopigmentation.

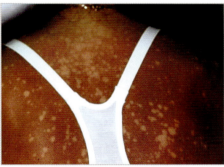

Figure 8.10.5 Tinea versicolor: note the hypopigmentation.

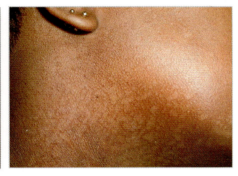

Figure 8.10.6 Cutaneous lupus erythematosus: papulosquamous lesions with scarring and on sun exposed skin.

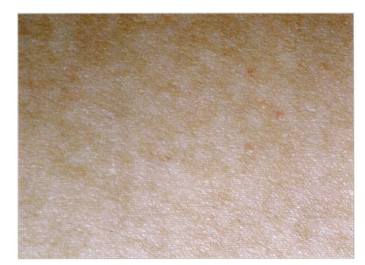

Figure 8.10.7 Cutaneous lupus erythematosus: papulosquamous lesions with scarring and on sun exposed skin.

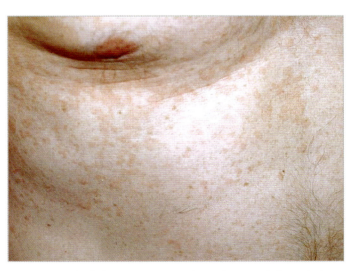

Figure 8.10.8 Small plaque parapsoriasis: digitate lesions with fine scale that fail to respond to therapy.

DISEASE DISCUSSION

Cutaneous T-cell lymphoma

Definition and etiology
Cutaneous T-cell lymphoma (mycosis fungoides) is a slowly progressive malignancy of helper T lymphocytes that have an affinity for the skin.

Clinical features
Although mycosis fungoides is not an inflammatory dermatosis, most affected individuals have scaling plaques that resemble dermatitis. The disease is often misclassified as a dermatitis for approximately 5 to 6 years before an accurate diagnosis is made. Early on, the clinical and pathologic findings are nondiagnostic. Three clinical stages of cutaneous T-cell lymphoma (mycosis fungoides) are recognized, which correspond with progressive evolution of the lymphoma: patch, plaque, and nodular stages. In the patch stage, slightly scaly, well-demarcated patches of varying sizes occur on the trunk and extremities. Lesions resemble dermatitis or psoriasis. Unlike in dermatitis or psoriasis, scaling is slight, but erythema may be prominent. There is a predilection for the chest and buttocks. Biopsy at this stage is most often nondiagnostic. On closer inspection of the skin, slight atrophy (manifested as telangiectasia and wrinkling) is present. Patches become progressively thicker, redder, and more indurated as the transition to the plaque stage occurs. Plaques frequently have a somewhat annular and serpiginous appearance. Over several years, nodules develop. Some of the nodules may ulcerate. The development of nodular lesions correlates with genetic transformation of the lymphoma to a more aggressive state.

The major diseases in the differential diagnosis include dermatitis, psoriasis, and drug eruption. Atrophy is typically a feature of at least some of the lesions of mycosis fungoides. Other lesions may be serpiginous, and scaling is on the average less than that encountered in dermatoses. When an adult has generalized dermatitis that cannot be classified as contact dermatitis, atopic dermatitis, nummular dermatitis, dermatitis medicamentosa, or seborrheic dermatitis, mycosis fungoides should be suspected. Biopsy of the lesions should be done periodically to establish a diagnosis of mycosis fungoides. Serial biopsies over time are often necessary because the histologic findings in the first few years may be nonspecific. Some pathologists have a relatively high index of suspicion for mycosis fungoides and may diagnose it with a high frequency but with false positive findings; other pathologists may diagnose mycosis fungoides with less sensitivity but with a higher rate of specificity. A biopsy diagnostic for cutaneous T-cell lymphoma will reveal a bandlike infiltrate within the dermis with extension of lymphocytes into the epidermis (epidermotropism). In psoriasis, silver-colored scaling plaques involve the scalp, elbows, and knees. Nodules do not occur. Certain drugs, especially seizure medications such as phenytoin (Dilantin), can also produce a mycosis-fungoides-like rash. Biopsy may reveal an increased number of lymphocytes trafficking in the skin, closely mimicking results seen in mycosis fungoides. A drug eruption should be suspected if the eruption starts a few weeks after a new medication is taken.

Treatment (Table 8.1)
Many different treatment options exist, but unfortunately no universally proven cure is available. For patch-stage lesions, topical treatment with nitrogen mustard (mechlorethamine) cream, ointment, or solution; psoralen plus ultraviolet A light (PUVA); or topical steroids can be used. In our experience, photochemotherapy with psoralen and ultraviolet A light is most helpful. Total-body electron-beam therapy, oral retinoids, ultraviolet B light, and combinations thereof are also effective. For advanced disease, systemic interferon therapy and conventional chemotherapy can be used. Cutaneous T-cell lymphoma is a chronic disease with a long-term survival of greater than 10 years for patients with patch- or plaque-stage disease. Approximately 50% of patients die of unrelated causes. The rest may die of sepsis or tumor burden.

Table 8.1 Treatment of cutaneous T-cell lymphoma

Treatment	Precautions
Universal	
Exclude the possibility of mycosis fungoides imitators like contact dermatitis, actinic reticuloid, and drug eruption	
Mild disease	
Topical corticosteroids bid	Atrophy with chronic application; especially intertriginous areas. Steroid acne of face. Glaucoma and cataracts if apply on eyes
Topical bexarotene 1% gel qid × 1 week then increase up to qod as tolerated	May cause irritant dermatitis, pruritus, pain, rarely leukopenia and paresthesia
Topical nitrogen mustard (mechlorethamine) 0.16% gel or compounded	May produce allergic contact dermatitis. Rare ulcerations. Not to be used under occlusive dressings
Light therapy: UVB	Burning, risk of skin cancer and photoaging
PUVA	Severe burns, increased risk of melanoma
Localized radiation therapy	Radiation dermatitis. Later long term risk of malignancies
Severe disease	
Bexarotene (systemic retinoid) 300 mg/m²	Hyperlipidemia, irritant dermatitis, nausea, xerosis, hypothyroidism
Histone deacetylase Inhibitors Romidepsin IV	Numerous adverse reactions including QR prolongation, arrhythmias, leukopenia, infections, hypotension, dermatitis
Vorinostat 400 mg PO qd	Risk of deep vein thrombosis, pulmonary embolism MI and stroke. Commonly causes fatigue, diarrhea, nausea, vomiting, and dysgeusia
Extracorporeal photopheresis	Hypotension, dizziness, light headedness and occasionally fevers
Total skin electron beam	Sun burn like reaction, long term may produce skin atrophy and loss of hairs
Methotrexate oral or IM 5 to 50 mg PO q week	Nausea, vomiting, liver cirrhosis, anemia, leukopenia, oral ulcers

# Lichen nitidus

Definition and etiology
Lichen nitidus is an uncommon, usually self-limited, inflammatory dermatosis of unknown cause characterized by flesh-colored discrete papules.

Clinical features
Pinhead-sized (1 to 2 mm) papules are seen, predominantly overlying the forearms, abdomen, chest, genitalia, and buttocks. A relationship between lichen planus and lichen nitidus has been considered, but lesions of lichen nitidus are skin colored and asymptomatic, unlike those of lichen planus. Mucosal involvement in lichen nitidus is extremely rare; when it occurs, it consists of papules and not the white reticulated patches characteristic of lichen planus. Pitting of the nails may occur but not the onychodystrophy seen in lichen planus. Occasionally, lesions of both lichen planus and lichen nitidus can be found in the same patient. The differential diagnosis includes lichen scrofulosorum, which is a now uncommon manifestation of tuberculosis infection; keratosis pilaris; phrynoderma; and lichen spinulosus. In lichen scrofulosorum, small grouped lichenoid papules develop as a hypersensitivity response to *Mycobacterium tuberculosis*. Lesions of lichen scrofulosorum are yellow to reddish-brown in color and occur predominantly on the trunk. Lesions of keratosis pilaris are follicular based and rough to palpation. Skin colored horny papules are located on the extensor surfaces of thighs and arms. Lichen spinulosus is a variant of keratosis pilaris. The horny papules in lichen spinulosus are distributed in clusters that form plaques several centimeters in diameter. Rare diseases to be considered in the differential diagnosis include phrynoderma (vitamin A deficiency), drug eruptions, lichenoid sarcoidosis, and secondary syphilis. Biopsy findings in lichen nitidus reveal focal lymphohistiocytic infiltrate in the papillary dermis surrounded by a collarette of epidermis. This configuration is often referred to as a "ball and claw" pattern.

Treatment (Table 8.2)
The natural course of lichen nitidus is variable, with disease lasting a few weeks to several years. A short course of several months is typical. Topical steroids may be of some help.

Table 8.2 Treatment of lichen nitidus

Treatment	Precautions
Universal	
Good skin care	
Mild soaps moisturizers	
Mild disease	
Topical steroid such as triamcinolone 0.1% bid	Steroid induced atrophy and acne
Topical tacrolimus (0.03% or 0.1%) bid	Occasional burning
Severe disease	
Short course oral prednisone	Hyperglycemia, hypertension, insomnia, mood change, weight gain, infection, osteoporosis
Light therapy	Sun burn, skin cancer
Acitretin 10 to 25 mg po q day	Teratogen: do not use in women of child-bearing potential. Hypertriglyceridemia and hair loss are common. Rare hepatic toxicity. Periodic lipid and liver function tests

Lichen planus

Definition and etiology
Lichen planus is an idiopathic inflammatory disease characterized by a generalized eruption of purple papules that occurs on both glabrous and mucosal skin. Certain drugs such as methyldopa, ß-blockers, thiazide diuretics, gold, penicillamine, and nonsteroidal anti-inflammatory agents can occasionally produce an eruption indistinguishable from classic idiopathic lichen planus.

Clinical features
Lesions of lichen planus most commonly occur on the flexural surface of the forearms near the wrists and on the extensor surfaces of the legs near the shin and ankle. Lichen planus can involve any glabrous skin surface. Nail and mucosal involvement is common (see Chapters 3 and 4). Diagnosis is usually possible on clinical inspection of characteristic purple polygonal papules. Lesions are most often very pruritic and covered with a fine white scale called Wickham's striae. Like psoriasis, lesions of lichen planus spread to areas of trauma (Koebner's phenomenon). Other morphologic variants of lichen planus include linear, annular, actinic, atrophic, hypertrophic, erythematous, follicular, exfoliative, and bullous types.

The major diseases in the differential diagnosis include lichen nitidus, psoriasis, lichen simplex chronicus, and lichen striatus. Lichen-planus-like lesions can be seen in patients with chronic graft-vs.-host disease and in overlap syndromes (lichen planus with lupus erythematosus, or lichen planus with bullous pemphigoid). In lichen nitidus, lesions are small pinpoint-sized papules that are skin colored and nonpruritic. The distribution of psoriasis is different than that of lichen planus, with prominent extensor surface involvement, the absence of oral lesions, and the presence of a white silvery scale. Lesions of lichen simplex chronicus are secondary to chronic rubbing. They are few and are usually located above the ankles or on the posterior neck. Examination of lichen simplex chronicus reveals thick red papules or plaques with prominent skin lines. In lichen striatus, the eruption is usually limited to a single elongated lesion composed of coalescing papules. Unlike in lichen planus, the papules and plaques are pinker than violaceous, and Wickham's striae are not present. Biopsy of lichen planus reveals irregular epidermal acanthosis with elongated and jagged rete ridges that resemble the teeth of a saw. Wedge-shaped hypergranulosis, compact orthokeratosis, colloid bodies, and a lymphocytic infiltrate that obscures the dermal-epidermal junction are all characteristic findings on biopsy of typical lesions.

Treatment (Table 8.3)
Lichen planus is difficult to treat. The use of topical corticosteroids leads to some improvement. In patients with extensive disease, a short course of oral prednisone or intramuscular corticosteroids is beneficial. Psoralen plus ultraviolet A light (PUVA) and retinoids are helpful. Griseofulvin, other oral antifungal agents, and antibiotics have been reported to be helpful, but these findings have not been confirmed by results of larger trials.

Nummular dermatitis

Definition and etiology
Nummular dermatitis is characterized by coin-shaped eczematous plaques. Precipitating factors include dry skin, irritation due to topical

Table 8.3 Treatment of lichen planus

Treatment	Precautions
Universal: remove possible cause (drug)	
Mild disease	
Hydrocortisone cream/ointment 1% bid	Rarely causes allergic contact dermatitis
Pimecrolimus cream 1% bid	Burning sensation
Moderate disease	
Triamcinolone cream/ointment 0.1% bid	Atrophy with chronic application; especially intertriginous areas Steroid acne of face Glaucoma and cataracts if apply on eyelids
Tacrolimus ointment 0.1% bid	Burning sensation
Cetirizine 10 mg bid, diphenhydramine 25–50 mg qid	Sedation
Gabapentin 100–300 mg qid	
Severe disease	
Clobetasol cream/ointment 0.5% bid	Atrophy with chronic application; especially intertriginous areas Steroid acne of face Glaucoma and cataracts if apply on eyelids
Prednisone 40–60 mg daily tapered over 2–3 weeks	Hyperglycemia, hypertension, insomnia, mood change, weight gain, infection, osteoporosis
Mycophenolate mofetil 1000–1500 mg bid	Nausea, diarrhea, bone marrow suppression, infection, birth defects
Ultraviolet light: nUVB	Burn, skin cancer
Antipruritics and baths as for moderate	
Acitretin 10 mg to 50 mg daily	Teratogen: do not use in women of child-bearing potential Hypertriglyceridemia and hair loss are common Rare hepatic toxicity

Table 8.4 Treatment of nummular dermatitis

Treatment	Precautions
Universal	
Avoid irritants Moisturizers Mild cleansing agents like Dove or Aveeno	None
Mild disease	
Hydrocortisone cream/ointment 1% bid	Rarely causes allergic contact dermatitis
Pimecrolimus cream 1% bid	Burning sensation
Moderate disease	
Triamcinolone cream/ointment 0.1% bid	Atrophy with chronic application; especially intertriginous areas Steroid acne of face Glaucoma and cataracts if apply on eyelids
Tacrolimus ointment 0.1% bid	Burning sensation
Cetirizine 10 mg bid, Diphenhydramine 25–50 mg qid Gabapentin 100–300 mg qid	Sedation
Oatmeal or tar baths Bleach bathes for skin infections: 1/4 cup in half full bathtub	None
Severe disease	
Clobetasol cream/ointment 0.05% bid	Atrophy with chronic application; especially intertriginous areas Steroid acne of face Glaucoma and cataracts if apply on eyelids
Prednisone 40–60 mg daily tapered over 2–3 weeks	Hyperglycemia, hypertension, insomnia, mood change, weight gain, infection, osteoporosis
Mycophenolate mofetil 1000–1500 mg bid	Nausea, diarrhea, bone marrow suppression, infection Birth defects
Ultraviolet light: nUVB	Burn, skin cancer
Antipruritics and baths as for moderate	

agents such as soaps, diuretics, forced air heating and secondary bacterial colonization.

Clinical features

Nummular dermatitis occurs most commonly in adult men but can also occur in children and women. The sites of predilection include the trunk, hands, forearms, and areas with the least number of sebaceous glands. The hallmark of nummular dermatitis is oval pruritic plaques. Individual plaques are discrete and well marginated. They are erythematous, scaling, and edematous; may weep serous fluid; and have overlying crust. Vesicles may be present on the surface of the plaques along with areas of oozing and crust.

The differential diagnosis includes psoriasis, pityriasis lichenoides, discoid lupus erythematosus, and other papulosquamous diseases. Isolated lesions can be confused with basal cell carcinoma or squamous cell carcinoma (see Ch. 13). Lesions of psoriasis are bright red and not dusky red in color. They are covered with silvery scale. Scalp and nail involvement does not occur in nummular dermatitis. Pityriasis lichenoides affects children most commonly and also young adults. Lesions develop in sudden crops, and papules predominate rather than plaques. The lesions have central necrosis with scale crust formation and may scar. Although lesions of discoid lupus erythematosus may also be coin shaped, lesions of cutaneous lupus have foci of atrophy, follicular plugging, hyper- and hypopigmentation, and telangiectasias. In addition, when scales are gently lifted from the skin, they have the appearance of carpet tacks.

Treatment (Table 8.4)

The mainstay of therapy for nummular dermatitis is topical steroids and emollients. In impetiginized lesions, antibiotics may also be helpful.

Pityriasis lichenoides

Definition and etiology

Pityriasis lichenoides (guttate parapsoriasis) is an idiopathic papulosquamous disease with both an acute and a chronic form. The acute variant, pityriasis lichenoides et varioliformis acuta, has also been called Mucha-Habermann disease, while pityriasis lichenoides chronica has been called guttate parapsoriasis.

Clinical features

Pityriasis lichenoides occurs mainly in adolescents and young adults. A slight male predominance has been reported. Pityriasis lichenoides acuta is characterized by the sudden onset of papules on the trunk, thigh, and upper arms. Some individuals have primarily truncal lesions, others have acral lesions, and some have a combination of both. Papules frequently have small central vesicles. With time, central necrosis and crust develop. Lesions may be purpuric. Crops of lesions develop, as in varicella.

Papules in different stages of evolution are characteristic. The polymorphous appearance and persistence of the eruption are clues to diagnosis. Scarring may occur. Patients with pityriasis lichenoides may closely resemble individuals with varicella (chickenpox). Pityriasis lichenoides chronica may develop from the acute form or de novo. Papulosquamous lesions predominate instead of vesicles or necrotic lesions. Unlike in the acute form, vesicular necrotic papules are not present. The papules and plaques are covered with a micaceous (thin-layered) platelike scale.

The differential diagnosis of pityriasis lichenoides acuta includes varicella (chickenpox), insect bites, and scabies infection. The eruption of varicella is self-limited and vesicular, and fever is present. The lesions in scabies are concentrated on the hands, axilla, umbilicus, and genitalia, and burrows are present. Insect bites predominate in exposed skin sites and may be asymmetric. Pityriasis lichenoides chronica is most commonly confused with pityriasis rosea or guttate psoriasis. No Herald patch is present in pityriasis lichenoides chronica. Scale is thicker, and the disease is chronic rather than self limiting. Pityriasis rosea does not last longer than 20 weeks. If a case of pityriasis rosea lasts longer than 20 weeks, a biopsy should be performed, which will usually show the changes of pityriasis lichenoides chronica.

Histologic changes in pityriasis lichenoides include dyskeratotic keratinocytes, bandlike lymphocytic infiltrate, scale crust, and extravasated erythrocytes.

Treatment (Table 8.5)

Pityriasis lichenoides acuta and chronica can last months to years. The acute form frequently heals after treatment with oral erythromycin or tetracycline. Ultraviolet light is helpful in severe cases.

Pityriasis rosea

Definition and etiology

Pityriasis rosea is an acute self-limiting dermatosis characterized by papulosquamous lesions on the trunk and proximal extremities. The cause is still unknown, although a virus is suspected.

Clinical features

Papules rapidly enlarge into a scaly plaque that is often several centimeters in diameter. Because this patch marks the onset of disease, it is called a herald patch. The herald patch is often misdiagnosed as tinea corporis. One to two weeks after the onset of the herald patch, additional patches and plaques develop on the trunk and proximal extremities. Plaques are oval, have a pink color, and are covered with a fine scale. An erythematous rim is present in many cases, and a brown discoloration may be seen in the center. The long axis of lesions follows skin lines. When truncal lesions are examined from a distance, one can imagine the silhouette of a Christmas tree. Pityriasis rosea resolves over a period of 6–10 weeks but may last as long as 20 weeks. Recurrences rarely occur.

The differential diagnosis includes other papulosquamous diseases such as psoriasis, nummular dermatitis, tinea versicolor, tinea corporis, secondary syphilis, and pityriasis lichenoides. Psoriasis can be diagnosed when its characteristic lesions occur on extensor surfaces and the scalp. Nail involvement with oil spots, pits, and onycholysis is a feature of psoriasis, not of pityriasis rosea. The chronic nature of psoriasis and the characteristic white-silvery scale also aid in diagnosis. Nummular dermatitis primarily affects elderly men with dry skin in the wintertime. Lesions are coin-shaped rather than oval. Vesicles may be present in nummular dermatitis but not in psoriasis. Potassium hydroxide test results will be positive in tinea versicolor and tinea corporis. The lesions of tinea versicolor usually are poorly demarcated and slightly scaly, as opposed to the well-demarcated lesions of pityriasis rosea.

Hypopigmentation and hyperpigmentation occur in tinea versicolor on the upper back and chest. Plaques of tinea corporis are serpiginous and exhibit central clearing and peripheral scaling. Secondary syphilis may be morphologically identical to pityriasis rosea. A rapid plasma reagin or other serologic test should be performed to exclude a diagnosis of syphilis. Individuals with secondary syphilis usually have palmar and plantar involvement, generalized malaise, and lymphadenopathy, features not seen in pityriasis rosea. Presence of a primary genital chancre or condyloma latum establishes a diagnosis of syphilis. Pityriasis lichenoides (guttate parapsoriasis) is chronic, unlike pityriasis rosea, which is self limited. Polymorphous papules, pityriasis rubra pilaris can also be confused with lichen spinulosus and keratosis pilaris. In these diseases, psoriasiform plaques and keratoderma do not occur.

Treatment (Table 8.6)

Pityriasis rosea is self-limited so no treatment is necessary. If the patient is complaining of pruritus a topical steroid or oral antihistamine may be helpful. There are reports of ultraviolet light phototherapy and oral erythromycin shortening the course of the disease.

Table 8.5 Treatment of pityriasis lichenoides

Treatment	Precautions
Universal	
If patient in good health and lesions not bothersome treatment may not be necessary	PLEVA type is frequently self limiting
Mild disease	
Topical corticosteroids such as triamcinolone 0.1% cream bid	Atrophy with chronic application; especially intertriginous areas. Steroid acne of face. Glaucoma and cataracts if apply on eyelids
Topical tacrolimus (0.03% or 0.1%) bid	Occasional burning
Moderate-to-severe disease	
Erythromycin 200 mg 3 to 4 × a day	Gastrointestinal upset, nausea, vomiting and diarrhea
Tetracycline 2 g daily for 2–4 weeks (minocycline and doxycycline alternatives)	Not to be used in children due to tooth discoloration. Gastrointestinal upset, nausea, vomiting and diarrhea. Causes photosensitivity. Predisposes to yeast infections
Prednisone 0.5 mg/kg/day	Hyperglycemia, hypertension, insomnia, mood change, weight gain, infection, osteoporosis
Methotrexate 7.5 mg to 20 mg q week.	Nausea, vomiting, liver cirrhosis, anemia, leukopenia, oral ulcers
Ultraviolet light: nUVB	Burn, skin cancer

Table 8.6 Treatment of pityriasis rosea

Treatment	Precautions
Universal	
No treatment necessary since self limiting	Exclude syphilis if any atypical features
Mild disease	
Topical corticosteroids such as triamcinolone 0.1% cream bid	Atrophy with chronic application; especially intertriginous areas Steroid acne of face Glaucoma and cataracts if apply on eyelids
Oral antihistamines if lesions itchy	Older antihistamines may cause drowsiness
Moderate-to-severe disease	
Erythromycin oral 500 mg po bid	Efficacy controversial and varies in different studies Gastrointestinal upset, nausea, vomiting and diarrhea
Acyclovir 400 mg tid	May only help symptoms along with erythema and scale but not speed of resolution
Ultraviolet light: nUVB	Burn, skin cancer

Psoriasis

Definition and etiology

Psoriasis is an inflammatory disease characterized by increased epidermal proliferation. The cause of psoriasis is unknown, but abnormal epidermal kinetics as well as the activation of the immune system within the skin by triggers, along with genetic factors must be taken into account.

Clinical features

Approximately one-third of patients have a family history positive for psoriasis. Psoriasis is relatively common and affects about 2% of the population of the United States. The most common age of onset is the third decade of life, but psoriasis can present at any time. Major precipitating factors include infections such as streptococcal pharyngitis or human immunodeficiency virus infection. Trauma to the skin, emotional stress, and use of drugs such as ß-blocking agents, angiotensin converting enzyme inhibitors, fluoxetine, and lithium may aggravate psoriasis.

Examination reveals bright red erythematous plaques covered with white-silvery scales. Areas of predilection include the elbows, knees, scalp, and sacrum. Pitting of the nails, oil spots, and onychodystrophy are frequently seen. Although the majority of patients with psoriasis have only a few lesions, generalized disease and even erythroderma can occur. Clinical variants of psoriasis include generalized pustular psoriasis of Von Zumbusch (see Chapter 11), palmar plantar psoriasis (see Chapter 4), guttate psoriasis, and inverse psoriasis. In guttate psoriasis, the lesions are small tear drop sized) and are commonly related to streptococcal infections. In inverse psoriasis, lesions are localized to the flexural areas of the axilla and groin instead of the extensor surfaces.

The differential diagnosis includes other papulosquamous eruptions such as nummular dermatitis, pityriasis rosea, lichen planus, pityriasis rubra pilaris, and secondary syphilis. Psoriasis is easily diagnosed if the classic symmetric distribution of red plaques with silvery-white-colored scales is present. In pityriasis rubra pilaris, follicular-based papules are present, and islands of normal skin are noted within large plaques. Plaques are salmon-orange, and palmar-plantar hyperkeratosis is more marked. Patients with secondary syphilis have lymphadenopathy, may have residual primary lesions, complain of malaise, and may have moth-eaten alopecia. Lesions are predominantly truncal and pityriasis-rosea-like. In pityriasis rosea, the presence of a herald patch, the truncal and proximal extremity disease distribution, the fine rose color, the fine peripheral scale, and the distribution of lesions along skin lines allow for a correct diagnosis. Lesions of lichen planus are distributed on flexural surfaces and have a purple color. Papules predominate and are very pruritic. Mucosal lesions may be present. Skin biopsy helps clarify the diagnosis if clinical findings are equivocal. In psoriasis, there is regular epidermal acanthosis, loss of the granular cell layer, subcorneal and intraepidermal micro pustules, and tortuous blood vessels in the dermal papillae.

Treatment (Table 8.7)

The treatment of psoriasis depends on the severity of disease. For limited involvement, topical tar preparations, calcipotriene (vitamin D3), anthralin, and topical corticosteroids may be used. For more generalized disease, ultraviolet B light or PUVA therapy is highly effective. Oral retinoids, methotrexate, and cyclosporine are helpful in refractory disease. Systemic corticosteroids should generally be avoided because they may lead to a pustular flare-up or destabilization of psoriasis upon withdrawal.

Secondary syphilis

Diagnosis and etiology

Syphilis (except for congenital syphilis) is a sexually transmitted disease caused by the spirochete *Treponema pallidum*. Syphilis is one of the great imitators and can present with a wide variety of cutaneous and systemic manifestations.

Clinical features

The clinical features of syphilis can be subdivided into four different stages: primary, secondary, latent, and tertiary syphilis. The primary stage occurs 9–90 days after inoculation, when a painless firm ulcer, the 'syphilitic chancre', develops in the genital region. Secondary syphilis occurs 8 weeks to approximately 2 years after inoculation and has protean manifestations, such as a truncal papular rash, moth-eaten alopecia (see Ch. 1), and white wartlike lesions in the genitalia known as condylomata lata. Without treatment, the lesions of secondary syphilis resolve, and the disease evolves into a latent stage, only to erupt many years later in some patients as tertiary syphilis. The cutaneous manifestations of tertiary syphilis include nodular and psoriasiform serpiginous plaques and gummas. Gummas are painless necrotic ulcerating nodules.

The scaling patches and plaques of secondary syphilis can be confused with those of any other papulosquamous disease. Like pityriasis rosea, the rash is symmetric and occurs on the trunk, and lesions follow skin lines. The rash starts out as asymptomatic non scaly red macules and develops into slightly scaly papules and patches. Older lesions have an annular appearance that mimics tinea or granuloma annulare. Clues to the diagnosis of secondary syphilis include the presence of malaise, generalized nontender lymphadenopathy, patchy moth-eaten alopecia, and condyloma latum, and involvement of the palmar-plantar surfaces with copper or ham-covered macules. The diagnosis should be confirmed with serologic testing or biopsy. Biopsy tissue may be stained with Warthin–Starry, Steiner, or Dieterle's stains to highlight spirochetes.

Treatment (Table 8.8)

Intramuscular penicillin (2.4 million units) weekly for 2 weeks cures primary or secondary syphilis. Oral tetracycline or erythromycin

Table 8.7 Treatment of psoriasis

Treatment	Precautions
Universal	
Look and eliminate trigger factors such as streptoccocal infections and medications	
Mild-to-moderate disease	
Topical steroids bid	Atrophy, steroid induced acne
Topical calcipotriene bid	Slight irritation Overuse could cause hypercalcemia
Topical tar preparations such as liquor carbonis detergens 5% bid	Irritation
Topical tazarotene 0.05%, 0.1% cream or gel	Pregnancy category X Frequently irritating
Anthralin	Stains clothing, skin and irritation
Severe disease	
TNF inhibitors Etanercept: start 50 mg SC 2 × week × 3 months than 50 mg sc q week Adalimumab Start 80 mg SC on day one then 40mg sq day eight followed by 40 mg SC q 2 weeks Infliximab 5 mg/kg IV week 0, 2 and 6 then q 8 weeks	Risk of severe infection and increased risk of malignancies especially lymphoma
IL-12, 23 blocker Ustekinumab (weight dependent dosage) for less than 100 kg: 45 mg SC ×1 on week 0 and week 4 then q 12 weeks	No black box warning, but still risk of severe infections and possibly malignancy
IL-17 blocker Secukinumab: start 300 mg SC q week × 5 than 300 mg SC q4 weeks Ixekizumab: start 160 mg SC × 1 then 80 mg SC q 2 weeks × 12 weeks. Then once a month Brodalumab: Start 210 mg SC at Weeks 0, 1 and 2, then 210 mg SC q 2 weeks	Risk of severe infection especially candidal Risk of colitis Black box warning only for brodalumab for suicidal ideation and risk
Ultraviolet light- narrow band UvB	Risk of burning and skin cancer
PUVA (psoralen plus UVA light)	Risk of burning and increased risk of skin cancer
Apremilast 30 mg PO bid	Risk of depression, diarrhea, nausea, head ache, weight loss
Methotrexate 10–25 mg q week	Risk of liver toxicity, anemia, nausea, vomiting
Acitretin 25 mg daily	Dry skin, hair loss, elevated serum lipids, birth defects Periodic liver function tests, and lipid profile Birth defects

Table 8.8 Treatment of syphilis in immunocompetent patients

Treatment	Precautions
Universal	
Contact Department of Health as per state regulations	
Consider screening for concurrent other sexually transmitted diseases such as HIV	
Follow RPR or VDRL titers after treatment to make certain they decrease	False positive results can occur with pregnancy, autoimmune diseases, and other infections
Penicillin G 2.4 milliion units IM	Allergic reaction, anaphylaxis

Table 8.9 Treatment of tinea corporis

Treatment	Precautions
Universal	
Confirm diagnosis with KOH Look for and treat tinea pedis	Most patients with tinea cruris have underlying tinea pedis
Put socks on before underwear when getting dressed	
Mild disease	
Topical antifungal such as clotrimazole (Lotrimin), econazole, terbinafine, ketoconazole	None
Severe disease	
Itraconazole 100 mg to 200 mg po q day × 2 to 4 weeks	Liver function tests at baseline Rare hepatotoxicity: watch for drug interactions
Terbinafine 250 mg PO q day × 2 weeks	CBC and liver function tests at baseline Rare hepatic toxicity

Clinical features

Patients present with irregularly shaped scaly patches and plaques. A characteristic finding is the presence of central clearing and a peripheral rim of scaling. Although tinea corporis is known as ringworm, frequently misdiagnosis can be avoided by realizing that lesions start as round symmetric papules and plaques and may over a period of weeks exhibit an irregular serpiginous or annular appearance.

The differential diagnosis includes other dermatoses such as psoriasis, pityriasis rosea and erythema annulare centrifugum. If the old dictum, "If a lesion is scaly, a KOH should be performed" is followed, an incorrect diagnosis of tinea will not be made. Erythema annulare centrifugum, is an annular idiopathic eruption that has an inner rim of trailing scale. Psoriatic and dermatitic lesions are not serpiginous and do not usually exhibit central clearing. The herald patch of pityriasis rosea is frequently misdiagnosed as tinea. This mistake would not occur if a KOH test were performed. A diagnosis of tinea corporis should not be made without identifying a possible source of disease, such as contact with another person with a dermatophyte infection (children playing with each other, wrestlers) or with a pet. Tinea corporis is more likely in an individual with onychomycosis or tinea pedis.

Treatment (Table 8.9)

For localized disease, topical therapy is usually effective in clearing the eruption.

The most effective agent currently available is terbinafine, because it has fungistatic and fungicidal activity. Also effective are numerous imidazole agents. Oral griseofulvin, itraconazole, or terbinafine can be used in cases of generalized or refractory disease.

tablets are effective in patients allergic to penicillin. Occasionally, patients with human immunodeficiency virus infection may not respond to the usual therapeutic regimens, and their serologic studies may have false-positive or false-negative results.

Tinea corporis

Definition and etiology

Tinea corporis is an infection of the skin caused by a dermatophyte.

Chapter 9 Excoriations

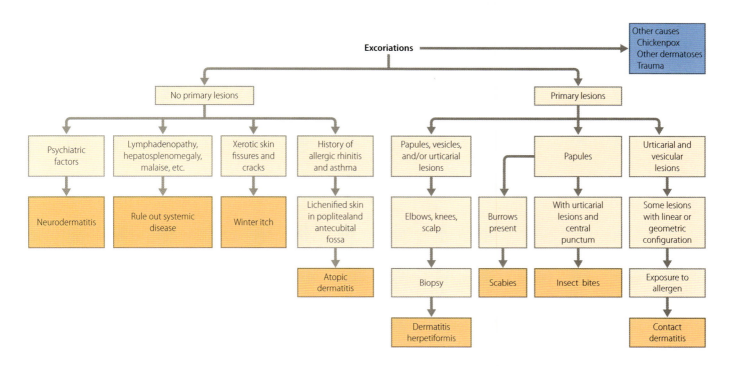

INTRODUCTION

An excoriation is an area of scratched skin. A variety of different triggers may lead to excoriations. In many cases, affected individuals already know the precipitating cause because the excoriations were due to an external factor such as contact with a pet, another person, an insect, or a prickly plant. Individuals presenting to the office for help with excoriated skin have been scratching because of severe pruritus. In some patients, the cause of the pruritus may be obvious (e.g. acute allergic contact dermatitis). Other patients who have 'sensitive skin' or atopic dermatitis are in search of relief, not a diagnosis. For patients in whom the diagnosis is not obvious, a more careful examination is necessary to rule out a systemic disease or to find the characteristic burrow and mite of scabies. Finally, excoriations may be a manifestation of a psychiatric problem or unresolved emotional conflicts or may be a response to stress.

1. SCABIES VERSUS NEURODERMATITIS

Features in common: excoriations

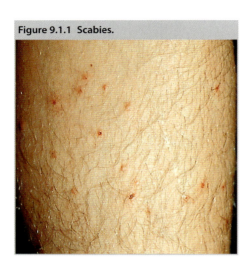

Figure 9.1.1 Scabies.

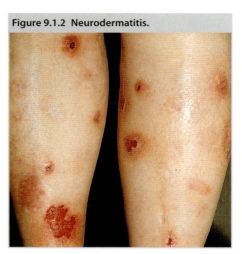

Figure 9.1.2 Neurodermatitis.

Distinguishing features

	Scabies	Neurodermatitis
Physical examination Morphology	Papules Burrows	No papules No burrows
Distribution	Generalized: lesions most prominent in finger webs, skin creases in palm and wrist, axilla, umbilicus, genitalia	Most prominent on upper extremities and upper back
History Symptoms	Severe pruritus Family members or friends may be itching too No psychiatric factors or stresses	Severe pruritus Other family members uninvolved Psychiatric factors and/or stresses present
Exacerbating factors	Immunosuppression	Stress Delusions of parasitosis
Associated findings	None	Nail biting occasionally Nails buffed owing to chronic scratching
Epidemiology	Any age; may be sexually transmitted in adults, usually transmitted through close intimate contact	Usually adults; female predominance
Biopsy	No Insect bite reaction: epidermal spongiosis eosinophils; only rarely are mites, feces, or eggs seen in the stratum corneum	No Compact stratum corneum and focal and superficial epidermal necrosis, minimal dermal inflammation
Laboratory	Scabies scraping positive for mites, eggs, or feces	Scabies preparation negative
Outcome	Curable with treatment; post-scabietic	Variable; usually chronic dermatitis may be present 1–2 weeks

Differential diagnosis of excoriations

- Atopic dermatitis
- Dermatitis herpetiformis
- Insect bites
- Scabies
- Neurodermatitis
- Pruritus of systemic disease
- Trauma
- Winter itch/eczema craquelé

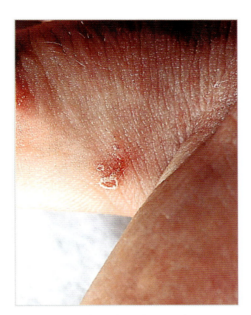

Figure 9.1.3 Scabies. *Clue to diagnosis:* burrow on finger (scabies mites measure less than 0.3 mm).

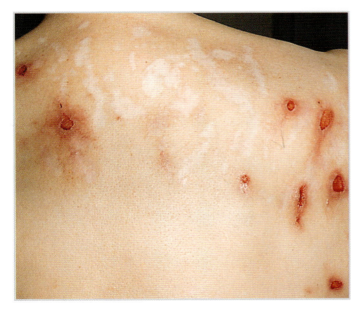

Figure 9.1.4 Neurodermatitis. *Clue to diagnosis:* excoriations only in easily accessible areas.

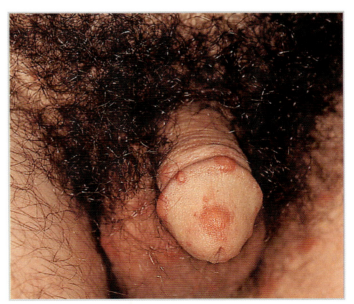

Figure 9.1.5 Scabies. *Clue to diagnosis:* papules in genital area.

2. DERMATITIS HERPETIFORMIS VERSUS ATOPIC DERMATITIS

■ Features in common: eczematous itchy rash and excoriations

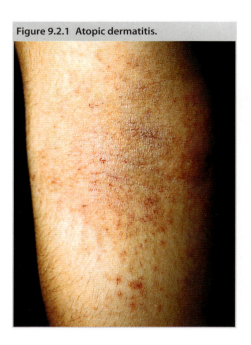

Figure 9.2.1 Atopic dermatitis.

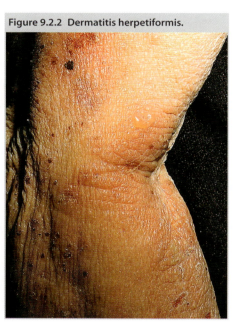

Figure 9.2.2 Dermatitis herpetiformis.

■ Distinguishing features

	Dermatitis herpetiformis	Atopic dermatitis
Physical examination	Primary lesion: papules, vesicles, or urticarial macules	No primary lesions - only manifestations of chronic rubbing or scratching
Morphology	Grouped vesicles occasionally No lichenified skin	No vesicles Lichenified skin
Distribution	Predilection for extensor surfaces: elbows, knees, buttocks, scalp	Predilection for flexural surfaces: antecubital and popliteal fossae
History Symptoms Exacerbating factors	'Burning' more than itching in some cases Gluten-rich diet Iodine in diet	Severe itching Stress, secondary infections
Associated findings	Gluten-sensitive enteropathy No family history Associated with gastrointestinal lymphoma	Asthma and allergies Dry skin, Dennie-Morgan folds, white dermatographism Family history of atopic dermatitis, asthma, or allergies frequently encountered No associated lymphoma
Epidemiology	Most common in young adults	Most common in children
Biopsy	Yes Subepidermal blister with stuffing of the dermal papillae with neutrophils	No Epidermal acanthosis, slight spongiosis, compact stratum corneum, and superficial perivascular lymphocytic infiltrate
Laboratory	Circulating antiendomysial antibodies in 80% to 100% of patients Direct immunofluorescence: granular deposition of IgA along the dermal–epidermal junction	Increased IgE levels in approximately 80% of patients Skin culture frequently positive for *Staphylococcus aureus*
Outcome	Chronic disease	Chronic disease in adults; children may outgrow

Dermatitis herpetiformis versus atopic dermatitis

Differential diagnosis of eczematous rashes

- Asteatotic dermatitis
- Atopic dermatitis
- Contact dermatitis
- Cutaneous T-cell lymphoma
- Dermatophytid
- Dyshidrotic dermatitis
- Lichen simplex chronicus
- Neurodermatitis
- Nummular dermatitis
- Psoriasis
- Scabies
- Seborrheic dermatitis

In children:
- Acrodermatitis enteropathica
- Genodermatosis
  - Ichthyosis
  - Hartnup disease
  - Phenylketonuria
  - Ectodermal dysplasia
- Immunodeficiency disease
  - Severe combined immunodeficiency
  - Omenn's syndrome
  - Job (hyper-IgE) syndrome
  - X-linked agammaglobulinemia
  - Wiskott–Aldrich syndrome
  - Langerhans cell granulomatosis

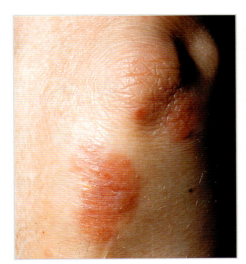

Figure 9.2.3 Dermatitis herpetiformis. *Clue to diagnosis:* lesions over elbows, knees and buttocks.

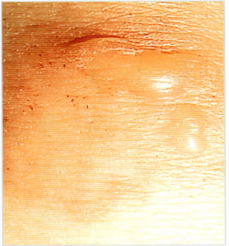

Figure 9.2.4 Dermatitis herpetiformis. *Clue to diagnosis:* grouped blisters.

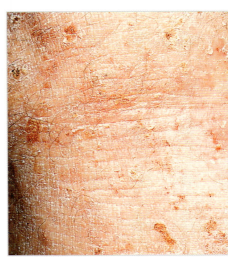

Figure 9.2.5 Atopic dermatitis. *Clue to diagnosis:* lichenified skin.

3. ATOPIC DERMATITIS VERSUS CONTACT DERMATITIS

■ Features in common: red, scaly, itchy skin

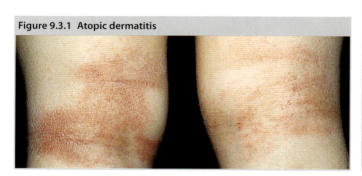

Figure 9.3.1 Atopic dermatitis

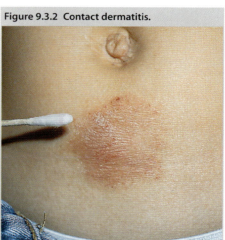

Figure 9.3.2 Contact dermatitis.

■ Distinguishing features

	Atopic dermatitis	Contact dermatitis
Physical examination	No primary lesion - rash entirely manifestation	Primary lesion vesicle or urticarial plaque of chronic rubbing or scratching
Morphology	No linear vesicles/plaques Excoriations common Lichenified skin common	Linear and geometric-shaped plaques/vesicles Few excoriations but not prominent feature No lichenified skin unless chronic and undiagnosed
Distribution	Predilection for flexural surfaces: antecubital and popliteal fossae	Areas of contact
History Symptoms Exacerbating factors	Severe itching Stress, secondary infections, dry skin	Severe itching Reexposure to allergen or exposure to additional allergens
Associated findings	Asthma and allergies Dry skin, Dennie–Morgan folds, white dermatographism	None
Epidemiology	Most common in children	Can occur at any age
Biopsy	No Nonspecific dermatitis	No Spongiotic dermatitis with eosinophils
Laboratory	Increased IgE levels in approximately 80% of patients Skin culture frequently positive for Staphylococcus aureus	Positive patch test
Outcome	Chronic disease in adults; children	Excellent

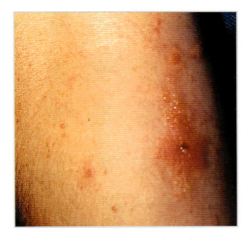

Figure 9.3.3 Contact dermatitis. *Clue to diagnosis:* linear vesicles

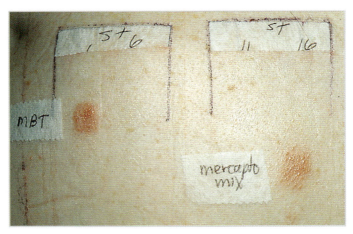

Figure 9.3.4 Contact dermatitis. *Clue to diagnosis:* positive patch tests.

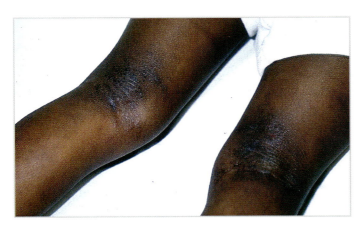

Figure 9.3.5 Atopic dermatitis. *Clue to diagnosis:* lichenified antecubital fossa.

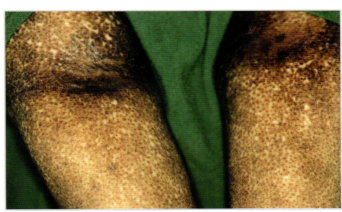

Figure 9.3.6 Atopic dermatitis. *Clue to diagnosis:* lichenified antecubital fossa.

4. PRURITUS OF SYSTEMIC DISEASE VERSUS WINTER ITCH (DRY SKIN)

■ Features in common: itchy excoriated skin with minimal rash, usually in older adults

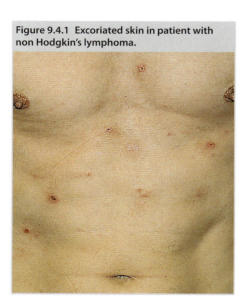

Figure 9.4.1 Excoriated skin in patient with non Hodgkin's lymphoma.

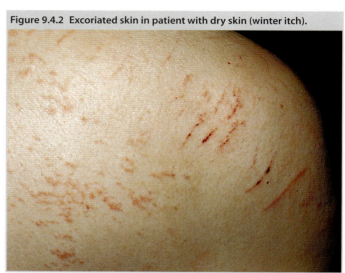

Figure 9.4.2 Excoriated skin in patient with dry skin (winter itch).

■ Distinguishing features

	Winter itch	Pruritus of systemic disease
Physical examination Morphology	Skin dry and flaky Skin in dry areas cracked and fissured with 'dried riverbed' appearance	No dry skin No fissures or cracks unless patient also has acquired ichthyosis secondary to systemic disease
Distribution	Most prominent on lower extremities and exposed surfaces	Generalized
History Symptoms	Pruritus relieved by scratching	Pruritus unrelieved by scratching Patients may feel that the itching is coming from below the skin
Exacerbating factors	Atopic dermatitis Frequent bathing Harsh soaps	Not applicable
Associated findings	Lichenified skin secondary to chronic rubbing, changes	Dependent on systemic disease Lymphoma: fever, night sweats, weight loss, lymphadenopathy Metabolic: hair loss in thyroid disease Liver: jaundice
Epidemiology	Any age, but more prevalent in elderly	Increases with age
Biopsy	No Normal skin; epidermal necrosis due to scratching	No Normal skin; epidermal necrosis due to scratching
Laboratory	Normal	Chest X-ray, liver function tests, complete blood count with differential, renal and thyroid function tests Other tests as per clinical suspicion
Outcome	Resolves with therapy	Variable; depends on underlying disease

Systemic causes of pruritus

- Iatrogenic: drug allergy, opiates
- Renal disease
- Hepatic disease
- Hematologic: anemia, polycythemia vera, paraproteinemia
- Malignancies: most commonly lymphoma
- Infections: parasites
- Metabolic: diabetes, thyroid disease, carcinoid
- Miscellaneous: pregnancy
- Psychiatric: stress, delusions of parasitosis

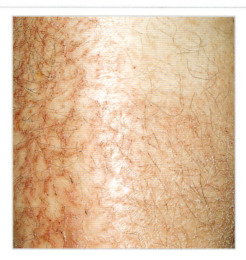

Figure 9.4.3 Winter itch. *Clue to diagnosis:* cracked fissured skin with a 'dried riverbed'-like appearance.

5. OTHER EXAMPLES

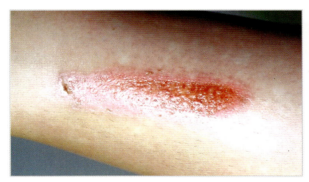

Figure 9.5.1 Scratch.

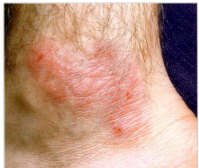

Figure 9.5.2 Lichen simplex chronicus: lichenified skin usually localized over ankle or neck from chronic rubbing (localized neurodermatitis).

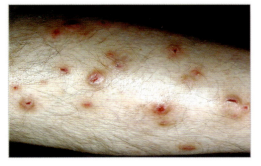

Figure 9.5.3 Prurigo nodularis: variant of neurodermatitis where nodules develop.

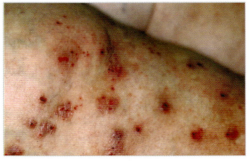

Figure 9.5.4 Prurigo nodularis: variant of neurodermatitis where nodules develop.

DISEASE DISCUSSION

Atopic dermatitis

Definition and etiology

Atopic dermatitis is a form of chronic dermatitis (usually starting in childhood) in patients with a familial predisposition for dermatitis, hay fever, and asthma. Patients with atopic dermatitis are born with 'sensitive skin'.

Clinical features

Early on, a slight amount of macular erythema may be present, but the primary skin manifestations are the result of chronic rubbing and excoriation of skin. Examination reveals lichenified erythematous scaly patches and plaques, with the rash most prominent in the antecubital area and popliteal fossa. In adults, the primary manifestation of atopic dermatitis may be hand dermatitis. Because of the morphologic similarity between atopic dermatitis and other dermatoses, guidelines for diagnosis have been established. Three of the major features and three or more minor features must be present for the diagnosis to be made.

Major features
- Pruritus
- Eczematous rash
- Chronic rash
- Flexural distribution in adults, facial and extensor involvement in infants
- Personal or family history of atopy (dermatitis, asthma, allergic rhinitis)

Minor features
- Xerosis
- Ichthyosis
- Keratosis pilaris
- Childhood onset
- Intolerance of wool cloths
- Dennie–Morgan infraorbital fold
- Food intolerance
- White dermatographism
- Susceptibility to cutaneous infections
- Elevated serum IgE level
- Early-onset cataracts
- Itch aggravated by sweating
- Pityriasis alba

Using these criteria, it is usually possible to make an accurate diagnosis of atopic dermatitis. The major differential diagnostic considerations would be other dermatoses, such as scabies, and neurodermatitis. In acute contact dermatitis, vesicles are present. In chronic contact dermatitis, the distribution, history, and results of patch testing will lead to an accurate diagnosis. In scabies, papules and burrows are present, and the rash has a predilection for the finger webs, wrists, axillae, umbilicus, and genitalia. Other family members or friends may also be itching. Neurodermatitis primarily affects adults, and excoriations and scarring occur predominantly on the arms and upper back, areas easily accessible to scratching. Psychologic stresses are also usually readily apparent. In babies and infants, atopic-like dermatoses can also be associated with a variety of immunodeficiency states. The signs of immunodeficiency are usually readily apparent (e.g. frequent infections, failure to thrive, and diarrhea). A skin biopsy is not necessary to make the diagnosis of atopic dermatitis.

Biopsy results would be identical to those in any other chronic dermatosis, revealing epidermal acanthosis, slight spongiosis, parakeratosis, and a superficial perivascular lymphocytic infiltrate.

Treatment (Table 9.1)

The mainstay of treatment of atopic dermatitis includes avoidance of irritants, moisturization of the skin, and judicious use of topical steroids as well as antihistamines. Steroid free alternatives include crisaborole ointment (a phospodiesterase type 4 inhibitor) or tacrolimus and pimecroliums ointment/creams (calcineurin inhibitors) applied twice a day. Oral antibiotics effective against *Staphylococcus aureus* are helpful when evidence of secondary infection is present, such as pustules, fissures, and yellow crusting. In exceptional cases, ultraviolet phototherapy, systemic steroids, and immunomodulators may be necessary. Recently weekly subcutaneous injections with an Il-4 and Il-13 inhibitor have been approved for patients with severe atopic dermatitis.

Contact dermatitis

Definition and etiology

Contact dermatitis is inflammation of the skin resulting from the interaction between the skin and chemicals. Contact dermatitis can

Table 9.1 Treatment of atopic dermatitis

Treatment	Precautions
Universal	
Avoid irritants Moisturizers Mild cleansing agents like Dove or Aveeno	None
Mild disease	
Hydrocortisone cream/ointment 1% bid	Rarely causes allergic contact dermatitis
Pimecrolimus cream 1% bid	Burning sensation
Moderate disease	
Triamcinolone cream/ointment 0.1% bid	Atrophy with chronic application; especially intertriginous areas Steroid acne of face Glaucoma and cataracts if apply on eyelids
Tacrolimus ointment 0.1% bid	Burning sensation
Crisaborole 2% ointment bid	Occasional burning stinging upon application
Cetirizine 10 mg bid Diphenhydramine 25–50 mg qid Gabapentin 100–300 mg qid	Sedation
Oatmeal or tar baths Bleach bathes for skin infections: 1/4 cup in half full bathtub	None
Severe disease	
Dupilumab 600 mg SC x 1 then 300 mg SC q week (precautions: injection site reaction, cold sores, conjunctivitis and keratitis)	
Clobetasol cream/ointment 0.5% bid	
Prednisone 40–60 mg daily tapered over 2–3 weeks	
Mycophenolate mofetil 1000–1500 mg bid	

be either an irritant type or an allergic type. Irritant contact dermatitis is a nonimmunologic reaction to a chemical that irritates the skin and causes inflammation. Conversely, allergic contact dermatitis is an individualized immunologic response to the chemical (i.e. the person who is allergic to the chemical will develop a rash when the chemical is absorbed through the skin, whereas another person who is not allergic to the chemical will not develop a rash upon contact). Irritant contact dermatitis is most frequently seen on the hands, whereas allergic contact dermatitis can occur in any part of the body in contact with the allergen.

Clinical features

In acute cases, erythema, scaling, vesicles, and swelling can be found. In patients with persistent disease, the erythema and scaling persist but vesicles can no longer be found and the skin becomes lichenified. The rash is severely pruritic, and patients may present with numerous excoriations. The most common cause of acute allergic contact dermatitis is contact with poison ivy, poison oak, or poison sumac. The first exposure to the allergen requires sensitization by the immune system, and the eruption does not appear until 7 to 10 days later. Upon subsequent exposures, however, the rash will develop within 12–72 hours. The area of greatest contact with the offending allergen will develop vesicular and urticarial lesions first, with other lesions developing within the next week. A characteristic finding in allergic contact dermatitis secondary to exposure to plants is linear vesicles in spots where the skin brushed against the plant. Common allergens other than plants include nickel, rubber components, chromates, fragrances, and preservatives (e.g. ethylenediamine, formaldehyde, quaternium 15, and bronopol).

The differential diagnosis of contact dermatitis depends on the location of the rash (see Chapters 2 and 4). In cases of generalized eruption with prominent excoriations, the differential diagnosis could include neurodermatitis, scabies, pruritus of systemic disease, atopic dermatitis, and winter itch. To make the correct diagnosis, a high index of suspicion is required. Individuals must be asked about possible antigen exposure and patch testing performed. In none of these other diseases are vesicles routinely found (see discussion on atopic dermatitis). The diagnosis of contact dermatitis can be made clinically or by patch testing. A biopsy, usually not necessary, would show only epidermal spongiosis, and a superficial perivascular infiltrate as in other dermatoses.

Treatment (Table 9.2)

Re-exposure to the allergen or irritant should be avoided. In severe cases, 2 weeks of systemic steroids may be helpful. Shorter courses of steroids should generally be avoided, since patients may suffer from a rebound rash if the steroid is tapered too quickly. In milder cases, strong topical steroids can be used. Oral antihistamines are helpful for itching. Topical antihistamines should be avoided, since they occasionally can also produce an allergic contact type of dermatitis. Topical doxepin cream has found to be a frequent sensitizer.

Dermatitis herpetiformis

Definition and etiology

Dermatitis herpetiformis is a chronic, intensely pruritic autoimmune blistering disease. The pathogenesis of dermatitis herpetiformis involves deposition of IgA immune complexes in dermal papillae. The IgA deposition may be triggered by gluten, since approximately three-fourths of patients with dermatitis herpetiformis have asymptomatic gluten-sensitive enteropathy. If patients with dermatitis herpetiformis avoid all gluten, a ubiquitous protein found in wheat products, IgA complexes eventually will no longer be detected in the skin, and the disease will remit.

Clinical features

An intensely pruritic burning sensation is the hallmark of dermatitis herpetiformis. The gluten-sensitive enteropathy is usually asymptomatic. The disease most often begins in adulthood and may be misdiagnosed for years as a form of dermatitis. Sometimes patients will note a flare-up of disease activity after eating foods containing a high amount of gluten.

Symmetrically distributed grouped vesicles typically occur on the elbows, knees, buttocks, low back, and shoulders and are typical of dermatitis herpetiformis. Because of intense itching, however, crusts and excoriations may be the only signs of previous blisters. In most patients, the vesicles are hard to detect. Dermatitis-like changes or excoriations may be the predominant feature. In such patients, dermatitis herpetiformis can be confused with scabies, neurodermatitis, or pruritus of systemic disease. In scabies, burrows are seen, and other family members often are also infested. Neurodermatitis primarily involves the extremities and upper back. In pruritus of systemic disease, no primary lesions or blisters are seen. In suspected cases of dermatitis herpetiformis, the diagnosis should always be confirmed or excluded based on skin biopsy of lesions. Biopsy results reveal subepidermal blistering with neutrophilic infiltrates, and immunofluorescence reveals granular deposition of IgA along the basement membrane in perilesional normal skin. Indirect immunofluorescence reveals circulating antibodies to endomysium in a sizable proportion of cases.

Treatment (Table 9.3)

The skin lesions of dermatitis herpetiformis clear and patients characteristically become asymptomatic quite rapidly after the institution of oral dapsone therapy. Although difficult to maintain, a gluten-free diet should be followed if possible. The beneficial effects of a gluten-free diet are unfortunately not seen for months after institution of the diet; however, the diet is helpful in bringing dermatitis herpetiformis under long-term control.

Neurodermatitis

Definition and etiology

Neurodermatitis is a term used to describe dermatitis in individuals who present with pruritic excoriated skin but in whom no underlying cause (except for psychologic factors and stress) can be found.

Table 9.2 Treatment of allergic contact dermatitis

Treatment	Precautions
Universal	
Determine and avoid allergen	
Mild disease	
Topical steroid such as clobetasol 0.05% cream bid	Avoid in intertriginous areas because of risk of atrophy Avoid on face since can produce steroid acne
Severe disease	
Systemic steroids for 2 weeks. Start at 40–60 mg prednisone a day for few days	Steroid side effects: hyperglycemia, insomnia, hypertension, fluid retention, etc. Dermatitis may flare or recur if tapered too rapidly

Table 9.3 Treatment of dermatitis herpetiformis

Treatment	Precautions
Universal	
Gluten-free diet	Gluten is found in numerous foods containing wheat, barley and rye Diet may take a few weeks to be effective and is difficult to follow
Mild disease	
Topical corticosteroids bid may help	Avoid in intertriginous areas because of risk of atrophy Avoid on face since can produce steroid acne
Severe disease	
Dapsone 25 mg to 100 q day	Patients will see improvement within a few days Monitor for anemia and methemoglobinemia

Table 9.4 Treatment of neurodermatitis

Treatment	Precautions
Universal	
Avoid irritants, such as harsh soaps Moisturize skin Keep fingernails cut short	
Mild disease	
Topical corticosteroids bid	Avoid in intertriginous areas because of risk of atrophy Avoid on face since can produce steroid acne
Anti-itch creams Sarna, oatmeal, pramoxine	
Oatmeal baths	
Severe disease	
Short course of systemic corticosteroids	
Gabapentin 300–1200 mg tid	May cause drowsiness, dizziness, ataxia, fatigue and depression
Behavioral modification	
Phototherapy	

Clinical features

The predominant features are numerous excoriations and scars in areas easily accessible to scratching. Primary lesions are not found. Owing to chronic rubbing, the skin may become thickened (lichenified) with prominent skin markings. Patients may have other associated habits such as nail biting or trichotillomania (pulling out of hairs). The differential diagnosis includes other dermatoses such as atopic dermatitis, scabies infection, winter itch, and pruritus of systemic disease. Usually, patients with neurodermatitis will readily admit to scratching their skin and to underlying psychologic stresses. In scabies, burrows and papules should be found. Primary lesions are also not seen in pruritus of systemic disease, atopic dermatitis, and winter itch. In winter itch, patients have very dry skin, and the rash is usually worse in the lower extremity. Atopic dermatitis usually starts in childhood. Patients have a history of atopy, and the lesions are more prominent in the flexural and popliteal fossae. The pruritus of systemic disease is a generalized unrelenting process.

Treatment (Table 9.4)

Treatment is difficult. Counseling or psychiatric help to relieve underlying stress may be helpful. Patients should be instructed to cut their nails short to minimize possible damage to the skin due to scratching. If the lesions have become impetiginized, a short course of oral antibiotics may be helpful. Other helpful therapies include topical steroids, neuroleptics, antipruritic medications, and covering of lesions with occlusive bandages or dressings that expedite the natural healing process and protect affected areas from manipulation.

Pruritus of systemic disease

Definition and etiology

A variety of systemic diseases can produce pruritus by a wide range of mechanisms.

Clinical features

Occasionally, patients present with a chief complaint of pruritic skin. Sometimes no clinical lesions can be seen. Other patients have pruritus with generalized excoriations. If no apparent dermatologic disease is causing the pruritus, a variety of systemic diseases should be excluded. Patients with liver disease, renal disease, blood diseases, internal malignancies, endocrine diseases, allergies, or parasitic infections all may suffer from pruritus. In our experience, patients with pruritus secondary to an underlying lymphoma may state that the pruritus seems to be coming from underneath the skin and, unlike in other causes of pruritus, is not relieved by scratching. Our routine work-up includes a complete blood count with differential to exclude iron deficiency anemia, polycythemia, and leukemia. Liver and renal function tests are done to exclude liver and renal disease. Thyroid function is tested to exclude hyper- or hypothyroidism. Fasting blood glucose testing is ordered to exclude diabetes. Stool is checked for ova and parasites. In elderly patients, an erythrocyte sedimentation rate, chest x-ray, mammogram, and stool guaiac test should be obtained to help exclude malignancies. A thorough drug and allergy history should be undertaken.

Table 9.5 Treatment of pruritus

Treatment	Precautions
Universal	
Avoid irritants; use mild soap, moisturizers	
Treat systemic disease	
Mild disease	
Topical triamcinolone 0.1% bid	May cause atrophy, steroid induced acne Avoid in intertriginous areas, and around eye and face
Antihistamines Hydroxyzine 10 mg to 25 mg PO qid Cetirizine 10 mg q day	May cause drowsiness
Severe disease	
Gabapentin 300–1200 mg tid	May cause drowsiness, dizziness, ataxia, fatigue and depression
Ultraviolet light	Sun burn, and increased risk of skin cancer

Treatment (Table 9.5)

The underlying disease should be treated. If this is not possible, symptomatic treatments include antihistamines, topical or oral doxepin, topical steroids, psoralen plus ultraviolet A light (PUVA) and activated charcoal.

Human scabies infection

Definition and etiology
Scabies is a mite infestation affecting mammals. Human scabies is caused by *Sarcoptes scabiei var. hominis*. The mite lives, reproduces, and feeds in the stratum corneum layer of human skin, thereby producing an extremely pruritic rash.

Clinical features
Patients with scabies complain of a very itchy rash that frequently is worse at night, preventing sleep. The infection is contagious through direct contact, and other family members, close friends, roommates, and playmates may also complain of an itchy rash. The characteristic lesion of scabies is the burrow, a linear papule with a small black punctum at one end where the mite is located. Burrows can be found in the finger webs, the skin creases of the wrists, the axillae, the periumbilical areas, the genitalia, and the feet. Burrows can be overshadowed by generalized excoriations, urticarial papules, and eczematous plaques. The latter two lesions result from a generalized hypersensitivity response to the mite.

Whenever scabies infection is suspected, the burrows and papules should be scraped, and the scrapings should be examined under the microscope for mite parts or scybala (feces and eggs). Burrows and mites can also be detected by dermoscopy. Burrows are not seen in any other disease. Although animal mites can infest humans, they do not produce burrows. In children, scabies infection can be mistaken for atopic dermatitis, but the latter is a chronic disease characterized by lichenified plaques with prominent involvement of the flexural surfaces. Unlike atopic dermatitis, scabies infection does not involve the face and scalp. In adults, the differential diagnosis also includes winter itch and pruritus of systemic disease. If a patient has a 'scabies-like' rash that persists a number of weeks, and no one else who has been in close contact is itching, a systemic disease, not scabies, should be suspected, since scabies infection is contagious.

Treatment (Table 9.6)
The patient and any close contacts are treated with oral ivermectin or topical permethrin cream or lindane lotion from the neck downward. The entire body, especially under the fingernails, is treated. Most patients should be retreated in 2 weeks to ensure that any mites that may have hatched from eggs are killed. Lindane is second line therapy since potential neurotoxin and is less effective as an ovicidal agent than permethrin. All recently used clothing and linen should be washed to kill any mites that have fallen off the skin.

Winter itch

Definition and etiology
Winter itch (asteatotic dermatitis) is a pruritic eruption most commonly seen in the elderly. It is caused by dryness of the skin.

Clinical features
With age, the skin becomes thinner, contains less collagen and less ground substance, and functions as a less effective barrier. It also becomes dryer. These factors make the skin more susceptible to environmental insults. In the winter, the dry skin can be very pruritic and inflamed. Patients complain most frequently of itchy skin rather than skin changes. If the skin is very dry, it can be fissured and cracked and can develop some eczematous changes. These findings are termed 'eczema craquelé'. Usually, the dryness is most accentuated in the lower legs. Exacerbating factors include dry weather, harsh soaps, and forced air heating. The diagnosis can be readily made by palpating the patient's skin and noting its dry, rough feel. Unlike in pruritus of systemic disease, the patient's symptoms are relatively mild and respond well to simple therapy.

Treatment (Figure 9.7)
Patients should avoid harsh soaps. The length of baths or showers should be less than 15 minutes, and a moisturizer should be applied immediately after the skin has been patted dry. Creams are generally more effective than lotions. Some of the newer moisturizers containing lactic acid or glycolic acids not only may prevent evaporation of water from the skin but also can draw water into the skin from the blood. A short course of antihistamines may also help with the itching.

Table 9.6 Treatment of scabies

Treatment	Precautions
Universal	
Confirm the diagnosis with scabies prep or via dermoscopy of burrow Treat everyone in close contact Wash or isolate clothing for 3 days	
Treatment options	
Ivermectin 0.2 mg/kg ×1 repeat in 2 weeks	Rare reports of hypotension, tachycardia, and seizures
Permethrin 5% cream ×1 repeat in 2 weeks	Apply to entire body from neck down May cause burning, pruritus, erythema, and numbness
Lindane 1% lotion	Apply to entire body from neck down Rare reports of seizures, death and neurotoxicity Caution in infants and children

Table 9.7 Treatment of winter itch

Treatment	Precautions
Universal	
Avoid irritants, mild soap, moisturizers	
Mild disease	
Topical triamcinolone 0.1% bid	May cause atrophy, steroid induced acne Avoid in intertriginous areas, and around eyes and face
Antihistamines Hydroxyzine 10–25 mg PO qid Cetirizine 10 mg q day	May cause drowsiness
Gabapentin 300–1200 mg tid	May cause drowsiness, dizziness, ataxia, fatigue and depression
Severe disease	
Ultraviolet light	Risk of burning and skin cancer

Chapter 10: Vesicular and bullous diseases

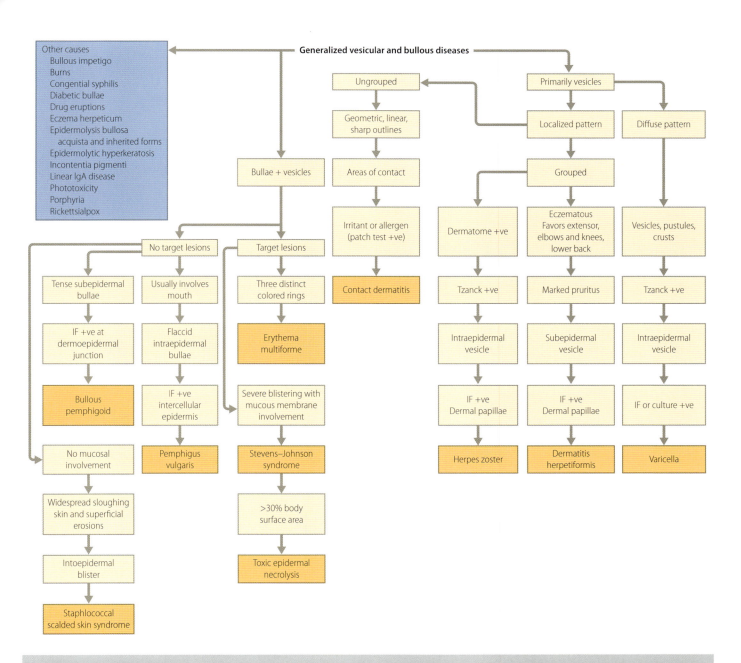

INTRODUCTION

Vesicles and bullae are easily recognized primary lesions that when ruptured produce erosions, crusting, and weeping. A number of diseases are characterized by the presence of blisters. The clinician should rule out common diseases such as contact dermatitis or varicella before considering rare diseases such as bullous pemphigoid or pemphigus vulgaris. If the physical examination is not distinctive (e.g. target lesions diagnostic of erythema multiforme), then laboratory tests such as the Tzanck smear or skin biopsy are quite helpful in differentiating these diseases. Depending on the disease, blister formation characteristically occurs within the epidermis or subepidermis. For example, herpes infections, contact dermatitis, and pemphigus vulgaris occur intraepidermally. Bullous pemphigoid, dermatitis herpetiformis, and erythema multiforme occur beneath the epidermis. The autoimmune diseases have characteristic immunofluorescence findings that are distinctive and important in making the diagnosis. Thus, the clinical features plus the pathologic findings allow the clinician to formulate a definite diagnosis and appropriate therapy.

1. CONTACT DERMATITIS VERSUS BULLOUS PEMPHIGOID

■ Features in common: scattered vesicles and bullae

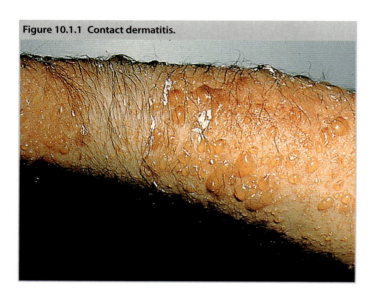

Figure 10.1.1 Contact dermatitis.

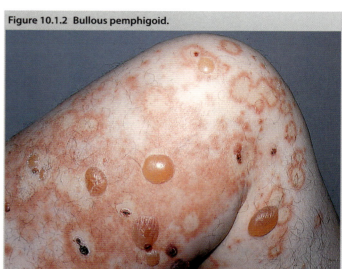

Figure 10.1.2 Bullous pemphigoid.

■ Distinguishing features

	Contact dermatitis	Bullous pemphigoid
Physical examination		
Morphology	Vesicles predominate, bullae occasionally Lichenified plaques Asymmetric	Tense bullae No lichenified plaques Symmetric
Distribution	Areas of contact – geometric, linear configuration	Groin, axillae, flexor extremities
History		
Symptoms	Pruritus	Pruritus
Exacerbating factors	Exposure to allergen or irritant	No exposure to allergen or irritant Medications: furosemide
Associated findings	No oral involvement	Oral involvement in 1/3
Epidemiology	Common All ages	Rare Elderly
Biopsy	Intraepidermal blister Spongiosis	Subepidermal blister with eosinophils
Laboratory	Immunofluorescence negative Patch test positive	Direct and indirect immunofluorescence positive Patch test negative
Outcome	Curable; remove contactant	Chronic; low mortality

Differential diagnosis of scattered vesicles and bullae

- Dermatitis herpetiformis
- Erythema multiforme
- Disseminated herpes simplex and herpes zoster
- Impetigo
- Varicella
- Linear IgA disease
- Epidermolysis bullosa
- Drug eruption
- Bullous insect bite eruption
- Burn
- Contact dermatitis
- Bullous pemphigoid

Common allergens

- Plants
  - Poison ivy and oak
  - Primrose
- Metals
  - Nickel
  - Chromate
- Cosmetics
  - Fragrances
  - Preservatives
  - Paraphenylenediamine
  - Lanolin
- Gloves/shoes
  - Rubber chemicals
- Medicaments
  - Benzocaine
  - Neomycin
  - Bacitracin
- Resins
  - Epoxy
  - Colophony

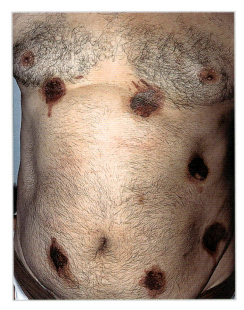

Figure 10.1.3 Contact dermatitis. *Clue to diagnosis:* geometric outlines where there is contact.

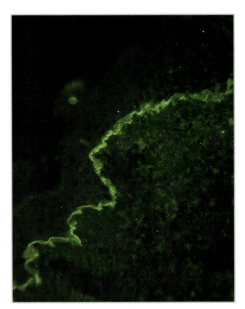

Figure 10.1.4 Bullous pemphigoid. *Clue to diagnosis:* positive immunofluorescent staining shows linear deposit at dermal-epidermal junction.

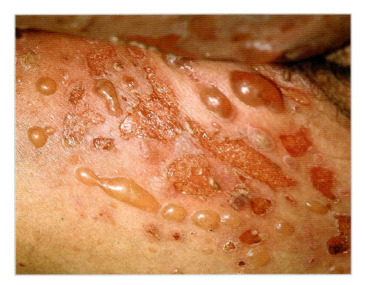
Figure 10.1.5 Bullous pemphigoid.

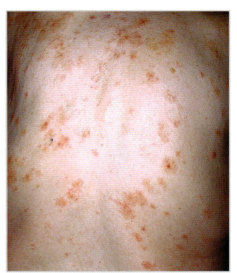
Figure 10.1.6 Bullous pemphigoid.

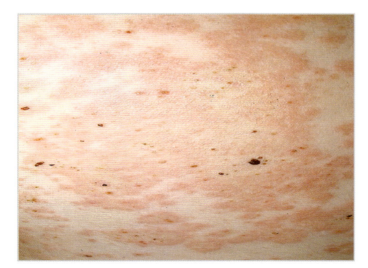
Figure 10.1.7 Bullous pemphigoid.

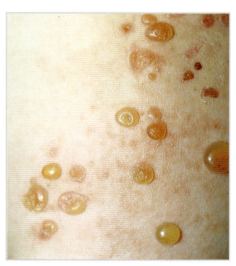
Figure 10.1.8 Bullous pemphigoid.

2. BULLOUS PEMPHIGOID VERSUS PEMPHIGUS VULGARIS

Features in common: generalized bullae

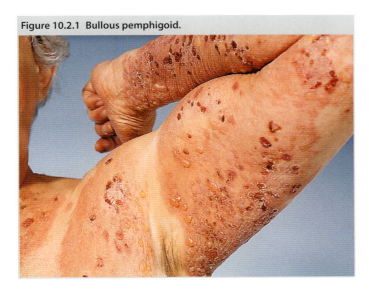

Figure 10.2.1 Bullous pemphigoid.

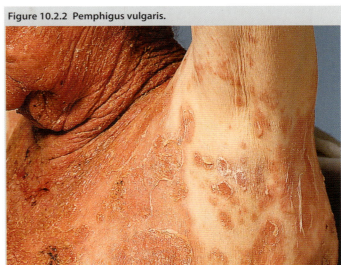

Figure 10.2.2 Pemphigus vulgaris.

Distinguishing features

	Bullous pemphigoid	Pemphigus vulgaris
Physical examination		
Morphology	Tense bullae Harder to rupture Smaller erosions	Flaccid bullae Easily ruptured Large erosions
Distribution	Nikolsky's sign negative Generalized, flexural areas	Nikolsky's sign positive Generalized, no flexural accentuation
History Symptoms Exacerbating factors	Pruritus Medications: furosemide	Pain Medications: penicillamine, captopril
Associated findings	Oral involvement in 33%	Oral involvement in 95%
Epidemiology	Rare Elderly	Rare Middle-aged
Biopsy	Subepidermal blister No acantholysis	Intraepidermal blister Acantholysis
Laboratory	Immunofluorescence: linear stain at dermal-epidermal junction	Immunofluorescence: intercellular staining of epidermis
Outcome	Chronic; low mortality	Chronic; high mortality if untreated

Differential diagnosis of generalized bullae

- Contact dermatitis
- Dermatitis herpetiformis
- Erythema multiforme
- Impetigo
- Varicella
- Disseminated zoster
- Kaposi's varioliform eruption
- Rickettsialpox
- Staphylococcal scalded skin syndrome
- Pemphigoid
- Pemphigus
- Epidermolysis bullosa acquisita

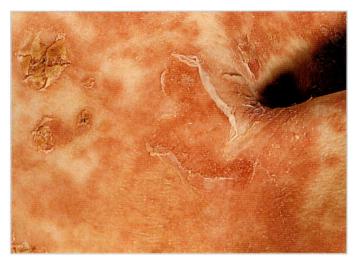

Figure 10.2.3 Pemphigus vulgaris. *Clue to diagnosis:* Nikolsky's sign.

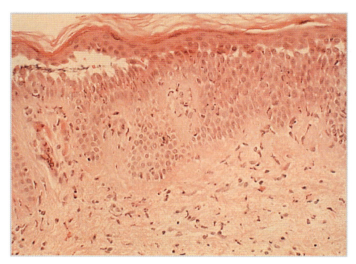

Figure 10.2.4 Pemphigus vulgaris. *Clue to diagnosis:* biopsy reveals intraepidermal blister with acantholysis.

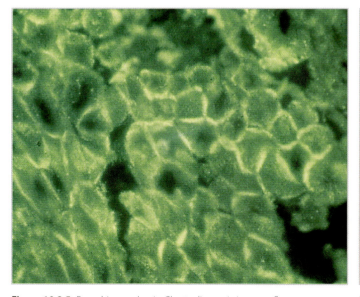

Figure 10.2.5 Pemphigus vulgaris. *Clue to diagnosis:* immunofluorescence shows intercellular staining in the epidermis.

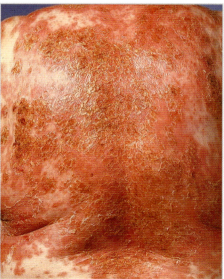

Figure 10.2.6 Pemphigus vulgaris.

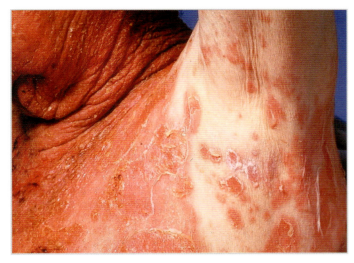
Figure 10.2.7 Pemphigus vulgaris.

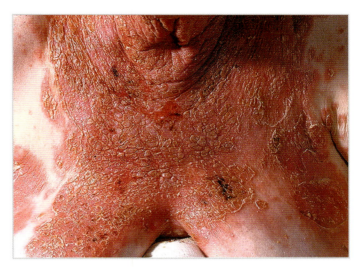
Figure 10.2.8 Pemphigus vulgaris.

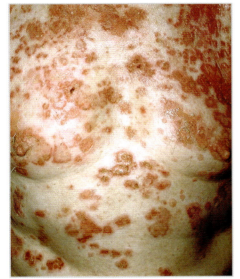
Figure 10.2.9 Pemphigus vulgaris.

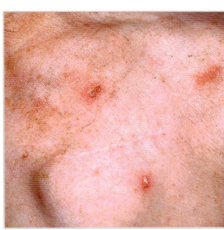
Figure 10.2.10 Pemphigus vulgaris.

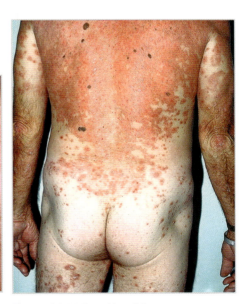
Figure 10.2.11 Pemphigus foliaceus.

3. ERYTHEMA MULTIFORME VERSUS BULLOUS PEMPHIGOID

Features in common: Generalized bullae with vesicles

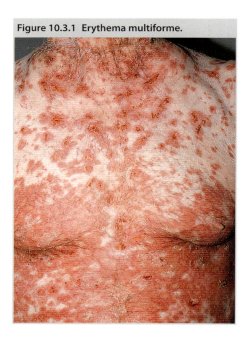

Figure 10.3.1 Erythema multiforme.

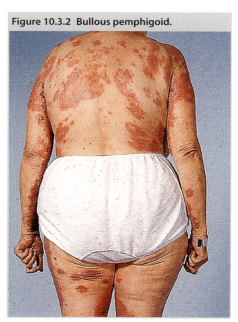

Figure 10.3.2 Bullous pemphigoid.

Distinguishing features

	Erythema multiforme	Bullous pemphigoid
Physical examination		
Morphology	Target lesions Tense bullae Urticarial papules and plaques	No target lesions Tense bullae Few urticarial papules and plaques
Distribution	Symmetric, favors extremities	Groin, axillae, flexor extremities
History		
Symptoms	Systemically ill Little pruritus	Not systemically ill Pruritus
Exacerbating factors	Infections: viral, bacterial, fungal. Less commonly, drugs: antibiotics, anticonvulsants, non-steroidal anti-inflammatory drugs	Drugs: furosemide No infection
Associated findings	Mucous membranes of mouth, eyes, nose, genitalia involved	Oral involvement in 33%
Epidemiology	Uncommon All ages	Rare Elderly
Biopsy	Epidermal necrosis Subepidermal blister with lymphocytes	No necrosis Subepidermal blister with eosinophils
Laboratory	Immunofluorescence negative	Direct and indirect immunofluorescence positive
Outcome	Acute Minor: spontaneously resolves in a couple weeks Major: Stevens–Johnson syndrome-like oral mucosal involvement	Chronic; low mortality

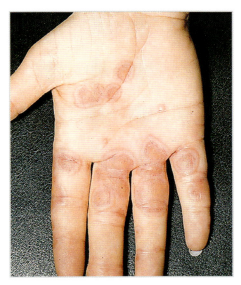

Figure 10.3.3 Erythema multiforme. *Clue to diagnosis:* target lesion with three distinct zones of color.

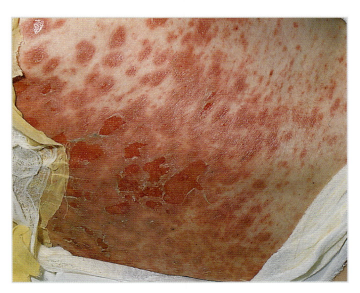

Figure 10.3.4 Erythema multiforme major.

4. TOXIC EPIDERMAL NECROLYSIS VERSUS STAPHYLOCOCCAL SCALDED SKIN SYNDROME

■ Features in common: generalized bullae

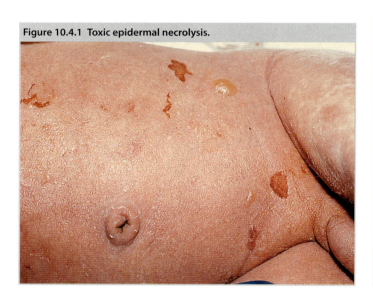

Figure 10.4.1 Toxic epidermal necrolysis.

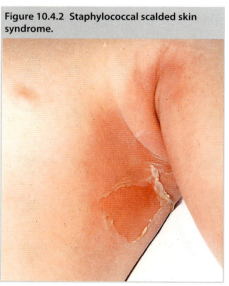

Figure 10.4.2 Staphylococcal scalded skin syndrome.

■ Distinguishing features

	Toxic epidermal necrolysis	Staphylococcal scalded skin syndrome
Physical examination		
Morphology	Tense bullae Deeper erosions	Flaccid bullae Superficial erosions
Distribution	Generalized	Face, neck, groin, axillae
History		
Symptoms	Extremely ill	Mildly ill
Exacerbating factors	Drugs No *Staphylococcus aureus* infection	No drugs *Staphylococcus aureus* infection
Associated findings	Mucous membranes affected	Mucous membranes not affected
Epidemiology	Rare; adults or children	Rare; children, adults with renal failure
Biopsy	Subepidermal blister Necrotic epidermis	Subcorneal blister No necrosis
Laboratory	Culture negative	Culture positive for *Staphylococcus aureus*
Outcome	Frequently fatal (20–50%)	Not fatal

Drugs causing toxic epidermal necrolysis

- Sulfonamides
- Anticonvulsants
- Nonsteroidal anti-inflammatory drugs
- Allopurinol

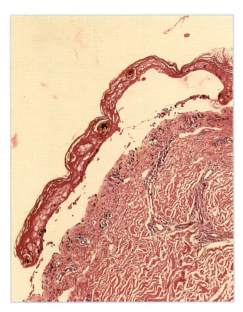

Figure 10.4.3 Toxic epidermal necrolysis. *Clue to diagnosis:* subepidermal blister and necrotic epidermis.

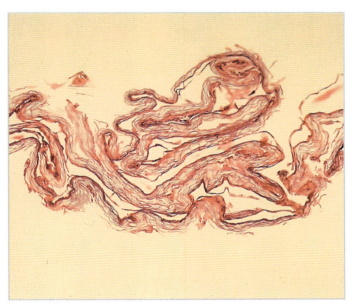

Figure 10.4.4 Staphylococcal scalded skin syndrome. *Clue to diagnosis:* intraepidermal blister.

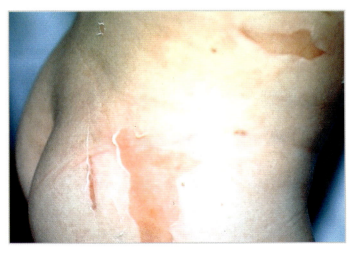

Figure 10.4.5 Staphylococcal scalded skin syndrome.

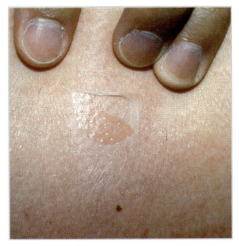

Figure 10.4.6 Staphylococcal scalded skin syndrome: positive Nikolsky's sign.

5. DERMATITIS HERPETIFORMIS VERSUS VARICELLA

Features in common: generalized vesicles

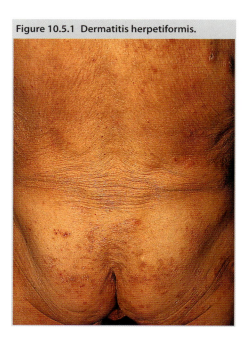

Figure 10.5.1 Dermatitis herpetiformis.

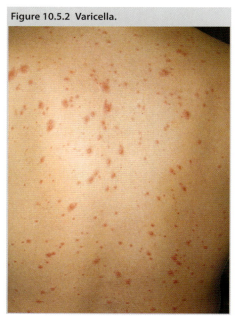

Figure 10.5.2 Varicella.

Distinguishing features

	Dermatitis herpetiformis	Varicella
Physical examination		
Morphology	Vesicles rare, secondary to excoriations Grouped vesicles or erosions Eczematous plaques	Vesicles common Individual vesicles Lesions in different stages: vesicles, papules, pustules, crusts No eczematous lesions
Distribution	Localized: elbows, knees, buttocks, low back, shoulders	Generalized
History		
Symptoms	No fever No systemic symptoms	Fever Systemic symptoms
Exacerbating factors	Gluten Iodine	Adulthood, pregnancy, immunosuppression
Associated findings	Gluten-sensitive enteropathy	No enteropathy
	No pneumonia, hepatitis, encephalitis	Pneumonia, hepatitis, encephalitis occasionally
Epidemiology	Rare Young adults, male predominance 2:1	Common Children
Biopsy	Subepidermal blister with neutrophils	Intraepidermal blister, ballooning degeneration Multinucleated giant cells
	Tzanck negative	Tzanck positive
Laboratory	Culture negative	Culture often negative
	Immunofluorescence: granular IgA in dermal papillae Circulating antiendomysial antibody	Immunofluorescence: herpes, varicella-zoster
Outcome	Chronic	Acute

Dermatitis herpetiformis versus varicella

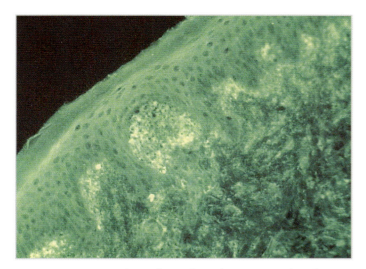

Figure 10.5.3 Dermatitis herpetiformis. *Clue to diagnosis:* IgA in dermal papillae on immunofluorescence.

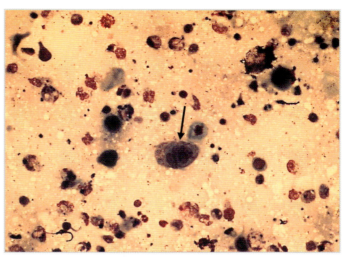

Figure 10.5.4 Varicella. *Clue to diagnosis:* positive Tzanck test results showing multinucleated giant cells (arrow).

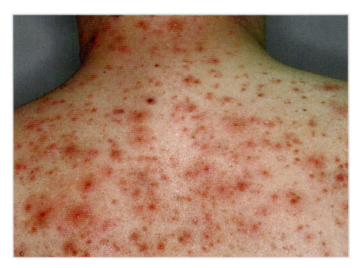

Figure 10.5.5 Varicella.

6. VARICELLA VERSUS DISSEMINATED HERPES ZOSTER

Features in common: generalized vesicles

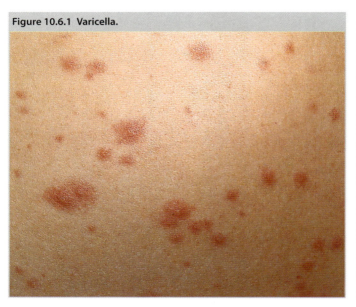

Figure 10.6.1 Varicella.

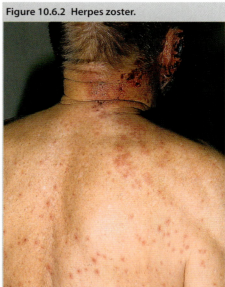

Figure 10.6.2 Herpes zoster.

Distinguishing features

	Varicella	Herpes zoster disseminated
Physical examination		
Morphology	Lesions not grouped Lesions in different stages: vesicles, papules, pustules, crusts	Lesions grouped Lesions in different stages: vesicles, papules pustules, crusts
Distribution	Not dermatomal Generalized	Dermatomal initially Generalized
History		
Symptoms	No pain Marked pruritus Fever Systemic symptoms	Pain Little pruritus Little fever Few systemic symptoms
Exacerbating factors	Adulthood Immunosuppression, pregnancy	Immunosuppression, pregnancy
Associated findings	Pneumonia, hepatitis, encephalitis occasionally No cancer, AIDS	Pneumonia, hepatitis, encephalitis occasionally Cancer, AIDS
Epidemiology	Common Children	Common Adults
Biopsy	Intraepidermal blister Ballooning degeneration Multinucleated giant cells Tzanck results positive	Intraepidermal blister Ballooning degeneration Multinucleated giant cells Tzanck results positive
Laboratory	Culture often negative Immunofluorescence: herpes, varicella-zoster	Culture often negative Immunofluorescence: herpes, varicella-zoster
Outcome	Acute Rarely fatal No residual pain	Acute Rarely fatal Postherpetic neuralgia
AIDS, acquired immunodeficiency syndrome		

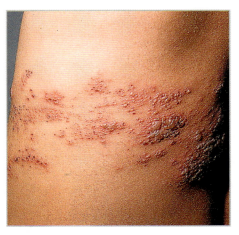

Figure 10.6.3 Herpes zoster. *Clue to diagnosis:* initial dermatomal involvement.

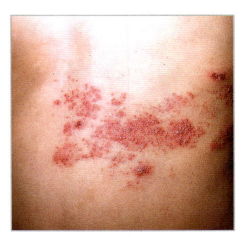

Figure 10.6.4 Herpes zoster.

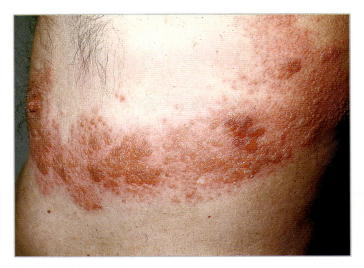

Figure 10.6.5 Herpes zoster.

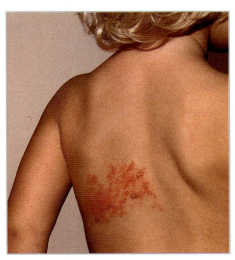

Figure 10.6.6 Herpes zoster.

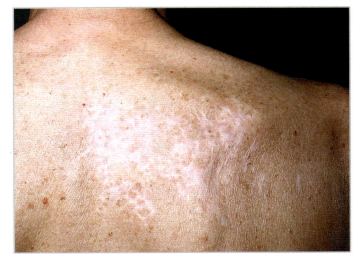

Figure 10.6.7 Herpes zoster (post-herpetic scarring).

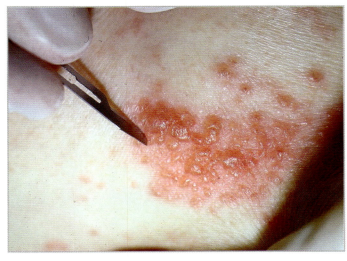

Figure 10.6.8 Herpes zoster (Tzanck preparation).

7. OTHER CAUSES

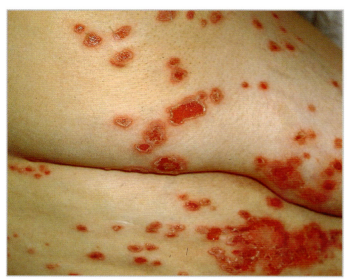

Figure 10.7.1 Linear IgA disease.

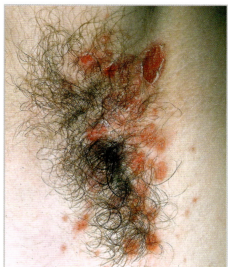

Figure 10.7.2 Bullous impetigo.

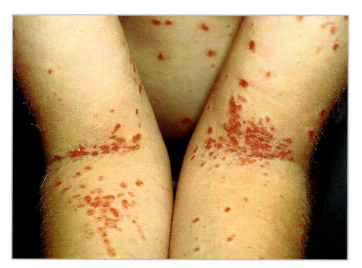

Figure 10.7.3 Bullous impetigo.

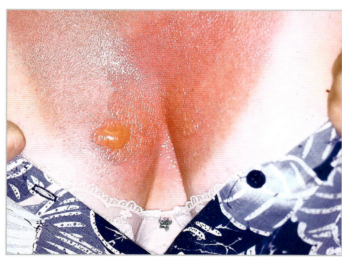

Figure 10.7.4 Sunburn.

8. OTHER EXAMPLES

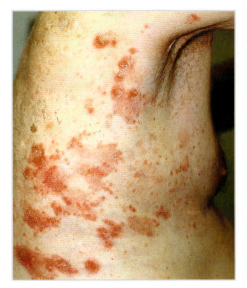

Figure 10.8.1 Sneddon-Wilkinson disease.

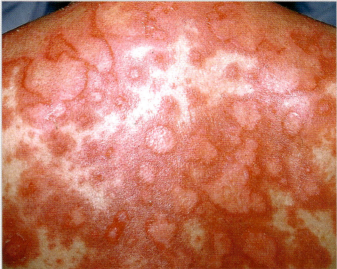

Figure 10.8.2 Bullous acute cutaneous lupus erythematosus.

DISEASE DISCUSSION

■ Bullous pemphigoid

Definition and etiology
Bullous pemphigoid is an autoimmune disease characterized by tense subepidermal bullae.

Clinical features
Bullous pemphigoid occurs predominantly in the elderly. Pruritus is a significant symptom, as is the discomfort caused by oozing and weeping blisters. Sometimes an urticarial eruption with or without blisters may predominate. Immunoglobulin G autoantibodies directed against the bullous pemphigoid antigen found in the basement membrane zone cause the blistering process. These antibodies can be detected along with C3 antigen in direct and indirect immunofluorescence studies.

The large tense blisters of bullous pemphigoid occur on normal or erythematous appearing skin. They can occur anywhere on the head, trunk, and extremities but have a preferred distribution in the groin, axilla, and antecubital and popliteal fossae. The blisters of bullous pemphigoid are usually not fragile and heal without scarring. About one-third of patients have oral mucous membrane involvement.

The differential diagnosis of bullous pemphigoid includes any of the chronic blistering diseases, particularly pemphigus vulgaris, dermatitis herpetiformis, erythema multiforme, and contact dermatitis. Before immunofluorescence studies, pemphigus and bullous pemphigoid were considered to be the same disease; therefore, differentiation based on morphology alone can be very difficult. In contact dermatitis, possible exposure to allergens should be present, and the lesions have symmetric, linear, and geometric patterns. In erythema multiforme, blisters are less prominent, and target lesions are present.

Treatment (Table 10.1)
Because the blistering skin of bullous pemphigoid has a tendency to heal, the prognosis is excellent with a low mortality rate. Bullous pemphigoid, however, may last months or years, and the morbidity caused by widespread blistering usually requires treatment with immunosuppressive agents such as systemic steroids, azathioprine, methotrexate, mycophenolate mofetil, and/or rituximab. In some cases, doxycycline has been effective.

■ Contact dermatitis

Definition and etiology
Contact dermatitis is an inflammatory reaction to an exogenous chemical, irritant, or allergen that comes in contact with the skin. Irritant contact dermatitis is precipitated by a substance that has direct toxic properties, whereas allergic contact dermatitis is triggered by a delayed-type hypersensitivity reaction. Irritating chemicals include acids, alkalies, solvents, and detergents. There are numerous allergens, including plants (poison ivy and oak), metals (nickel), rubber chemicals, cosmetic ingredients (fragrances and preservatives), and topical medicines (neomycin and bacitracin).

Clinical features
Contact dermatitis varies from acute to chronic, which results in varying appearances. Acute contact dermatitis has marked epidermal edema, or spongiosis.

This causes vesicles and bullae to rupture, resulting in oozing and crusting. The hallmark of chronic contact dermatitis is lichenification or thickening of the epidermis associated with scaling and

VESICULAR AND BULLOUS DISEASES

Table 10.1 Treatment of bullous pemphigoid

Treatment	Precautions
Universal	
Good wound care: wash daily and cover with a non-adherent dressing	
Mild/moderate disease	
Clobetasol cream/ointment 0.5% bid	Atrophy with chronic application; especially intertriginous areas Steroid acne of face Glaucoma and cataracts if apply on eyelids
Severe disease	
Prednisone 40–60 mg daily tapered as warranted by clinical response	Hyperglycemia, hypertension, insomnia, mood change, weight gain, infection, osteoporosis
Immunosuppressants: azathioprine, mycophenolate mofetil, methotrexate	Numerous
Rituximab 1000 mg infusion × 2 separated by 2 weeks	Severe infusion and mucocutaneous reactions, reactivation of hepatis B virus, progressive multifocal leukoencephalopathy
Doxycycline 100 mg bid or Tetracycline 500 mg bid (some physicians add nicotinamide)	Photosensitivity, gastrointestinal upset

Table 10.2 Treatment of irritant and allergic contact dermatitidis

Treatment	Precautions
Universal	
Avoid irritant or allergen	None
Mild disease: irritant	For allergic, stronger topical steroids necessary
Hydrocortisone cream/ointment 1% bid	Rarely causes allergic contact dermatitis
Pimecrolimus cream 1% bid	Burning sensation
Moderate disease	
Triamcinolone cream/ointment 0.1% bid	Atrophy with chronic application; especially intertriginous areas Steroid acne of face Glaucoma and cataracts if applied on eyelids chronically
Tacrolimus ointment 0.1% bid	Burning sensation
Cetirizine 10 mg bid, Diphenhydramine 25–50 mg qid Gabapentin 100–300 mg qid	Sedation
Oatmeal or tar baths	None
Severe disease	
Clobetasol cream/ointment 0.5% bid	Atrophy with chronic application; especially intertriginous areas Steroid acne of face Glaucoma and cataracts if apply on eyelids
Prednisone 40–60 mg daily tapered over 2–3 weeks	Hyperglycemia, hypertension, insomnia, mood change, weight gain, infection, osteoporosis
Mycophenolate mofetil 1000–1500 mg bid	Nausea, diarrhea, bone marrow suppression, infection Birth defects
Ultraviolet light: nUVB	Burn, skin cancer
Antipruritics as for moderate	

fissuring. The distribution of contact dermatitis corresponds with the area of contact. Streaks, geometric outlines, and sharp margins typically occur where there has been application of the contactant or brushing by the leaf or stem of poison ivy or oak. The diagnosis of acute contact dermatitis is usually straightforward. In the case of an irritant, patients develop symptoms quite quickly and know they have come in contact with a caustic material. For an allergen, this may not be so obvious, since it takes one or two days after exposure for the blistering to develop. A history of outdoor activity, however, and finding of a typical configuration make the diagnosis of allergic contact dermatitis to poison ivy or oak easy to establish. For other allergens, patch testing is often required to identify the cause. Results of a skin biopsy, if needed, reveal an intraepidermal spongiotic blister. It is important to remember, that the biopsy cannot distinguish between allergic and irritant contact dermatitis as well as other dermatitis such as atopic.

Treatment (Table 10.2)

The management of contact dermatitis should emphasize prevention and complete avoidance of the offending irritants or allergens. This may require a change in occupation or lifestyle. The principal treatment is topical steroids; for those individuals with severe or widespread contact dermatitis, a short course of systemic steroids is indicated. Ultraviolet light and /or mycophenolate mofetil can reduce the need for systemic steroids. Colloidal oatmeal or tar baths reduce inflammation and itching. Antihistamines or gabapentin are also used to reduce itching.

Dermatitis herpetiformis

Definition and etiology

Dermatitis herpetiformis is a chronic, intensely pruritic autoimmune vesicular disease. The pathogenesis of dermatitis herpetiformis is related to IgA immune complex deposition in the dermal papillae. The IgA deposition may be related to gluten, since approximately three-fourths of patients with dermatitis herpetiformis have asymptomatic gluten-sensitive enteropathy. When patients with dermatitis herpetiformis avoid gluten, IgA complexes are not detected in the skin, and the blistering remits.

Clinical features

Intense pruritus and burning are the hallmarks of dermatitis herpetiformis. Although gluten-sensitive enteropathy typically occurs in these patients, it is usually asymptomatic. Disease activity usually begins in early adulthood, and often years elapse before a definitive diagnosis is made. Sometimes, patients will note a flare-up of disease activity after eating foods containing a high amount of gluten.

Symmetrically distributed grouped vesicles, typically occur on the elbows, knees, buttocks, low back, and shoulders. Because of intense itching, crusting and excoriation may be the only sign of the previous vesicle. In many patients, the vesicles are hard to detect, and, as the name implies, dermatitic changes are prominent.

The differential diagnosis of dermatitis herpetiformis initially includes a number of other blistering disorders such as varicella or dermatitis. The skin biopsy, which reveals a subepidermal blister with collections of neutrophils in the papillary dermis, along with immunofluorescence findings revealing granular IgA deposits in the dermal

Table 10.3 Treatment of dermatitis herpetiformis

Treatment	Precautions
Gluten-free diet	Difficult to follow Consider dietitian consult
Dapsone 50–300 mg daily	Hematologic: hemolysis, dyscrasias, methemoglobinemia, G6PD deficiency, rare neuropathy

papilla, confirms the diagnosis of dermatitis herpetiformis. Eighty per cent of patients also have antiendomysial antibody in their serum.

Treatment (Table 10.3)

Characteristically, dermatitis herpetiformis clears and becomes asymptomatic quite rapidly after the institution of dapsone or sulfapyridine therapy. Although difficult to maintain, a gluten-free diet should be initiated. The beneficial effects of a gluten-free diet, however, are not seen for months.

Erythema multiforme

Definition and etiology

Erythema multiforme is a characteristic inflammatory reaction in the skin secondary to a wide variety of causes. The most common are medications and infections such as herpes simplex virus or *Mycoplasma pneumoniae* infection. Other causes include neoplasms, connective tissue diseases, physical agents, foods, and topical agents.

Clinical features

Erythema multiforme ranges in severity from the self-limited minor form, which spontaneously resolves in a couple of weeks, to a severe major form, which may be fatal. Recurrent erythema multiforme minor is usually secondary to herpes labialis or herpes genitalis. Another common infectious cause is *Mycoplasma pneumoniae*.

The examination of the skin reveals a characteristically symmetric eruption that favors the extremities. The lesions, being multiform, vary from urticarial papules and plaques to large bullae. The target or iris lesion is diagnostic of erythema multiforme and has three zones of color:
- a central dark erythematous area or blister
- a surrounding pale erythematous zone
- a peripheral erythematous ring.

Widespread blistering and erosions of the skin and mucous membranes occur in erythema multiforme major, Stevens–Johnson syndrome, and toxic epidermal necrolysis. These patients are systemically ill with fever, arthralgias, and severe malaise. Death can occur owing to secondary infection or electrolyte imbalance.

The differential diagnosis of erythema multiforme is usually not difficult if characteristic target lesions are present. The acute onset usually differentiates it from other widespread blistering diseases such as bullous pemphigoid and pemphigus vulgaris. Contact dermatitis, with its asymmetric distribution and geometric and linear configuration, should be relatively easy to distinguish from erythema multiforme. If a skin biopsy is needed, findings will show the characteristic signs of necrotic keratinocytes, interface lymphocytic inflammation, and a subepidermal blister.

Treatment (Table 10.4)

Erythema multiforme usually resolves spontaneously after the precipitating factor has been eliminated. Within the first few days of disease onset, systemic steroids have been used, but their efficacy has been controversial. Prolonged steroid use is not advised because of the possibility of their masking the signs of infection.

An ophthalmologist should be consulted if there is eye involvement to prevent scarring. Topical dressings may help heal the erosions. In severe cases, the patient should be treated in a burn unit, where infection and electrolyte and fluid balance can be closely monitored.

Table 10.4 Treatment of erythema multiforme

Treatment	Precaution
Universal	
Remove/treat precipitating factor: infection, drug	
Supportive care	
Mild/moderate disease	
Clobetasol cream/ointment 0.05% bid	None if used for short course – 2 weeks
Severe disease	
Prednisone 40–60 mg daily tapered over 2–3 weeks	Hyperglycemia, hypertension, insomnia, mood change, weight gain, infection, osteoporosis
Intravenous immunoglobulin (IVIG)	Controversial, expensive, risk of an allergic reaction and rare cases of anaphylaxis in IgA deficiency

Herpes zoster

Definition and etiology

Herpes zoster is caused by the recrudescence of latent varicella-zoster virus in individuals who have had varicella. The vesicular dermatomal eruption is distinctive, and on occasion cutaneous dissemination occurs.

Clinical features

Herpes zoster occurs in both normal and immunosuppressed individuals. It may be the presenting sign of acquired immunodeficiency syndrome or lymphoma, particularly if there is dissemination. Typically, the eruption is preceded by a painful prodrome, which may be confused with a migraine, pleurisy, myocardial infarction, or appendicitis.

The examination characteristically reveals grouped vesicles on an erythematous base distributed unilaterally along a dermatome. When cutaneous dissemination occurs, individual papules, vesicles, and pustules are found widely scattered on the trunk, extremities, and head.

The dermatomal distribution of herpes zoster is diagnostic and rarely causes confusion. Varicella is not characterized by this distinctive dermatomal focus of vesicles. Herpes simplex virus infection may rarely occur in a dermatomal fashion but would be recurrent, in contrast to herpes zoster, which uncommonly recurs. Since varicella and herpes zoster are caused by the same virus, the Tzanck preparation results, immunofluorescence findings, and culture results are identical.

Treatment (Table 10.5)

Herpes zoster in the immunocompetent patient who is younger than 50 years of age need not be treated. For those older than 50 years of age, immunocompromised patients, and patients with disseminated

Table 10.5 Treatment of herpes zoster

Treatment	Precautions
Prevention	
Vaccine for adults 60-year-old or greater	Immunosuppressed
Ophthalmology consult when nasal tip is involved	Eye damage
Moderate-severe disease	
Valacyclovir 1000 mg tid for 7 days	Rarely psychosis, seizures, leukopenia, thrombocytopenia, Stevens–Johnson, toxic epidermal necrolysis
Adults 50-year-old or greater, 72 hours or less since start of rash	Headache, nausea, diarrhea, vomiting
Famciclovir 500 mg tid for 7 days	Same as for valacyclovir
Acyclovir 800 mg five time daily for 7 days	Same as for valacyclovir
Prednisone controversial to prevent post-herpetic neuralgia	

Table 10.6 Treatment of pemphigus vulgaris

Treatment	Precautions
Universal	
Good wound care: wash daily and cover with a non-adherent dressing. If widespread, consider a burn unit. Monitor fluid and electrolyte status	
Mild/moderate disease	
Clobetasol cream/ointment 0.5% bid	Atrophy with chronic application; especially intertriginous areas. Steroid acne of face. Glaucoma and cataracts if apply on eyelids
Severe	
Prednisone 40-80 mg daily tapered as warranted by clinical response. If hospitalized, IV methylprednisolone (Solu-Medrol)	Hyperglycemia, hypertension, insomnia, mood change, weight gain, infection, osteoporosis
Immunosuppressants – azathioprine, mycophenolate mofetil, methotrexate	Numerous
Rituximab 1000 mg infusion × 2 separated by 2 weeks	Severe infusion and mucocutaneous reactions, reactivation of hepatis B virus, progressive multifocal leukoencephalopathy
Dapsone 50–300 mg daily	Hematologic: hemolysis, dyscrasias, methemoglobinemia, G6PD deficiency, rare neuropathy

herpes zoster, antiviral therapy with acyclovir, valacyclovir, or famciclovir should be instituted to lessen the amount of postherpetic neuralgia and prevent further disease progression or dissemination. Prevention with the zoster vaccine is indicated in individuals older than 60 years.

Pemphigus vulgaris

Definition and etiology

Pemphigus vulgaris is an autoimmune blistering disease that affects the skin and mucous membranes. The bullae occur intraepidermally, where autoantibodies against desmoglein 3 of the keratinocyte cell junction are deposited. This results in loss of adhesion between keratinocytes with the formation of acantholysis and blisters.

Clinical features

Pemphigus vulgaris is a rare blistering disease. The oral mucosa is almost always involved and frequently is the presenting site. The examination reveals generalized blistering of the skin. The bullae are flaccid and superficial, range in size from 1 centimeter to several centimeters, and are fragile, leaving large denuded, bleeding, weeping, and crusted erosions. Extension of the bulla laterally with application of peripheral pressure is characteristic of pemphigus vulgaris; this is called *Nikolsky's sign*. Involvement of the oral cavity is frequent and may be severe with widespread erosions (see Chapter 3).

The differential diagnosis of pemphigus vulgaris mainly includes autoimmune chronic blistering diseases such as bullous pemphigoid, dermatitis herpetiformis, epidermolysis bullosa acquisita, linear IgA bullous dermatosis, paraneoplastic pemphigus and the other forms of pemphigus (vegetans, foliaceus, and erythematosus). A skin biopsy and immunofluorescence studies help separate pemphigus from the other autoimmune diseases. The blister occurs intraepidermally just above the basal layer with loss of cohesion between epidermal cells (acantholysis). Results of direct and indirect immunofluorescence studies are positive, showing deposits of immunoglobulins (usually IgG) and complement in the intracellular spaces between keratinocytes.

Treatment (Table 10.6)

The treatment of choice for pemphigus vulgaris is systemic steroids. Once blistering has subsided and disease activity has been controlled, other immunosuppressive agents such as azathioprine, mycophenolate mofetil, methotrexate, and rituximab may be added for their steroid sparing effect. Before systemic corticosteroids were available, pemphigus vulgaris had a high mortality rate because of widespread blistering with resultant fluid and electrolyte imbalance and infection.

Staphylococcal scalded skin syndrome

Definition and etiology

Staphylococcal scalded skin syndrome is a widespread superficial blistering disease caused by an exfoliative toxin produced by certain strains of *Staphylococcus aureus*, usually group II.

Clinical features

Staphylococcal scalded skin syndrome occurs predominantly in young children but may also affect immunosuppressed adults with renal failure. Although febrile and irritable, the patient is usually not very ill. Characteristically, the skin is tender and erythematous. Superficial vesicles and bullae occur on the face, neck, axilla, and groin. This leads to widespread sloughing of the skin, leaving a red, slightly weeping, moist base and a scalded appearance.

The diagnosis of staphylococcal scalded skin syndrome is usually straightforward, since it has the characteristic appearance of scalded skin. At one time, it was thought to be a form of toxic epidermal necrolysis, but the clinical features, skin biopsy results, and etiologic factors clearly separate these two entities. Although a biopsy is not usually necessary, biopsy findings reveal an intraepidermal blister just below the stratum corneum. The infection is not within the bullae, as in bullous impetigo, but is found in a distant focus such as the nasal mucosa or is localized. Culture results from the widespread blisters will be negative, since blisters are a result of the exfoliative toxin.

Table 10.7 Treatment of staphylococcal scalded skin syndrome

Treatment	Precautions
Eliminate focus of infection	
Good skin care	
Analgesics as necessary	
IV nafcillin or oxacillin if MRSA Vancomycin	Numerous

Treatment (Table 10.7)

Antistaphylococcal antibiotics that eradicate the toxin-producing organisms are commonly used but have not been shown to affect the outcome of the skin rash. Topical antibiotics and dressings can be used, as in routine wound care.

■ Toxic epidermal necrolysis

Definition and etiology

Toxic epidermal necrolysis (TEN) was formerly felt to be the most severe form of erythema multiforme. However, most agree that TEN is a distinct disease. It is usually secondary to drug use, especially anticonvulsants and antibiotics.

Clinical features

The sudden onset of widespread blistering of the skin and mucous membranes in a gravely ill patient makes this disease a dermatologic emergency. Fortunately, it is relatively rare. The examination shows widespread blistering and sloughing of the epidermis and mucous membranes of the mouth, nose, eyes, and genitalia with greater than 30% body surface area affected. Large erosions leaving raw red dermis develop in patients who are severely ill. Toxic epidermal necrolysis should be easily distinguished from staphylococcal scalded skin syndrome. Results of a skin biopsy reveal full-thickness epidermal necrosis with subepidermal blister formation.

Treatment (Table 10.8)

Discontinuation of the precipitating drug is paramount. Although controversial, systemic steroids or intravenous immunoglobulin are frequently used. Most important are supportive measures, which require specialized nursing care in a burn unit to avoid sepsis and fluid and electrolyte imbalances. Death may occur in up to 50% of patients with toxic epidermal necrolysis.

■ Varicella

Definition and etiology

Varicella, or chickenpox, is an acute highly contagious infection caused by the varicella-zoster virus.

Clinical features

Varicella is predominantly a childhood disease. A 2–3-week incubation period occurs after exposure. The first signs and symptoms of the disease are a 2–3-day prodrome of chills, fever, malaise, headache, sore throat, anorexia, and dry cough. The characteristically pruritic vesicular eruptions then occur. The patient is infectious for approximately 1 week, from a couple of days before the rash develops until all the vesicles have become crusted.

Table 10.8 Treatment of toxic epidermal necrolysis

Treatment	Precautions
Universal	
Remove offending drug	
Good wound care – wash daily and cover with a non-adherent dressing Consider a burn unit Monitor fluid and electrolyte status	
Systemic steroids, cyclosporine, and intravenous gammaglobulin (IVIG) are controversial	

Varicella is a markedly pruritic vesicular eruption affecting all regions of the body, including the mucous membranes of the mouth and the conjunctiva. Characteristically, there are crops of rapidly progressive lesions beginning with macules, which evolve into papules, vesicles, and pustules. Crusting and necrosis follow. A typical lesion has been described as a 'dew drop on a rose petal'. Typically, all these types of lesions are present at the same time.

The differential diagnosis of varicella once included smallpox before eradication of that disease. The acute onset, limited duration, and occurrence in childhood separate varicella from dermatitis herpetiformis. Disseminated herpes zoster and varicella are caused by the same virus. Disseminated herpes zoster, however, has distinctive dermatomal involvement. Other diseases that might be considered in the differential diagnosis are disseminated herpes simplex, coxsackievirus, echovirus, monkeypox, and rickettsialpox. The diagnosis of varicella is usually straightforward. A Tzanck preparation reveals multinucleated giant cells typical of a herpesvirus infection. Direct immunofluorescence is the most sensitive and specific way of confirming the diagnosis.

Treatment (Table 10.9)

Treatment of chickenpox in the normal child is largely symptomatic, with use of antihistamines and topical agents to reduce itching. In adults and immunosuppressed patients, acyclovir reduces disease length, severity, and complications such as pneumonia, encephalitis, and hepatitis. The live attenuated varicella vaccine appears to be safe and moderately effective and is recommended for those in good health who have no history of clinical varicella and who are older than 1 year of age. Immunodeficient patients who are exposed to varicella may be immunized with varicella-zoster immune globulin (VZIG) prophylactically, but not for active disease.

Table 10.9 Treatment of varicella

Treatment	Precautions
Prevention	
Varicella virus vaccine	
Varicella-zoster immune globulin	
Immunosuppressed individuals, adults, severe infection	
Acyclovir 10 mg/kg IV every 8 hours or 20 mg/kg (800 mg max) orally qid	Headache, nausea, diarrhea, vomiting Rarely psychosis, seizures, leukopenia, thrombocytopenia, Stevens–Johnson, toxic epidermal necrolysis

Chapter 11: Macular and urticarial rashes

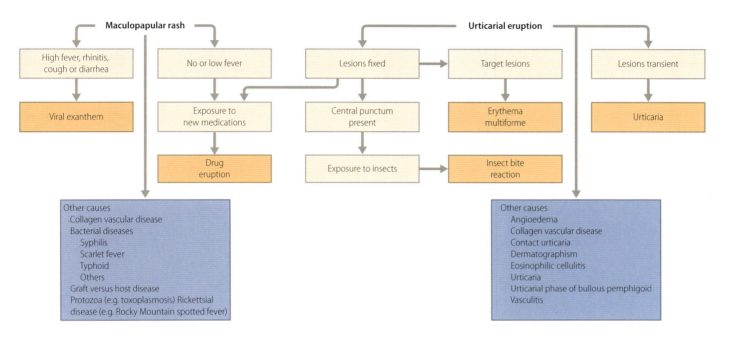

INTRODUCTION

Maculopapular and urticarial rashes are perhaps morphologically the most easily recognizable type of skin rash. Unfortunately, recognition of the eruption does not immediately unveil its cause. A maculopapular drug rash is morphologically indistinguishable from a maculopapular viral exanthem. Correct diagnosis is made possible only by taking a careful history, looking for ancillary findings, observing symptoms, and obtaining blood tests. Ultimately, the clinical course will confirm a correct diagnosis.

Urticarial eruptions can be seen in patients with urticaria or erythema multiforme and after insect bites. In these eruptions, a careful history, a skin biopsy, and careful inspection of the skin will result in the correct diagnosis.

1. MACULOPAPULAR DRUG ERUPTION VERSUS VIRAL EXANTHEM

■ Features in common: symmetric red macules and papules on the trunk and extremities

Figure 11.1.1 Drug eruption.

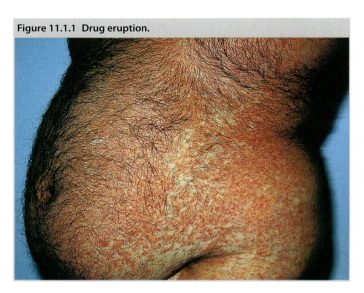

Figure 11.1.2 Viral exanthema.

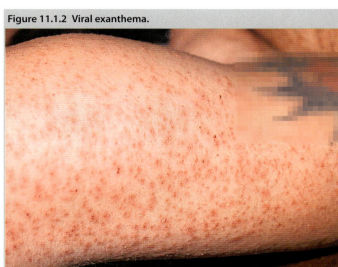

■ Distinguishing features

	Maculopapular drug eruption	Viral exanthem
Physical examination Morphology	May be identical: symmetric and confluent macules and papules on trunk No Koplik's spots or slapped-cheek appearance	May be identical: symmetric and confluent macules and papules on the trunk Koplik's spots in measles (white grainy papules on a red base, usually on buccal mucosa) Slapped-cheek appearance in erythema infectiosum
Distribution	Trunk and extremities	Trunk and extremities
History Symptoms	No or low-grade fever Starts 1–10 days after starting medication No other patients with similar complaints Pruritus	Low- to high-grade fever No new medication Other patients with similar symptoms in community Minimal or no pruritus
Exacerbating factors	None	Immunosuppression
Associated findings	No systemic symptoms	Systemic symptoms usually present (malaise, myalgia, rhinorrhea, diarrhea, risk of miscarriage in erythema infectiosum)
Epidemiology	Any age	Most common in children
Biopsy	No, nonspecific Superficial nonspecific lymphocytic infiltrate	No, nonspecific Superficial nonspecific lymphocytic infiltrate
Laboratory	Occasionally peripheral eosinophilia	Lymphocytosis or lymphopenia may be present
Outcome	Resolves	Resolves

Differential diagnosis of maculopapular eruptions

- Viral exanthem
  - Measles (rubeola) (paramyxovirus)
  - German measles (rubella)
  - Erythema infectiosum (parvovirus)
  - Roseola infantum (herpesvirus 6)
  - Infectious mononucleosis (Epstein–Barr virus)
  - Hepatitis
  - Human immunodeficiency virus (retrovirus)
  - Miscellaneous viruses: echovirus, adenovirus, dengue
- Drug eruption
- Urticaria
- Collagen vascular diseases
  - Still's disease
- Syphilis
- Toxoplasmosis
- Bacterial diseases
  - Brucellosis
  - Scarlet fever
  - Typhoid
- Rickettsial diseases
  - Rocky mountain spotted fever
  - Typhus
- Kawasaki's disease

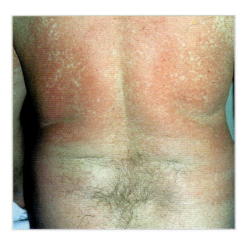

Figure 11.1.3 Drug eruption due to nafcillin.

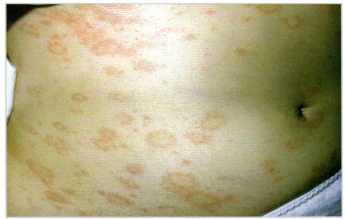

Figure 11.1.4 Drug eruption due to amoxicillin in patient with infectious mononucleosis.

2. URTICARIA VERSUS ERYTHEMA MULTIFORME

■ Features in common: urticarial plaques

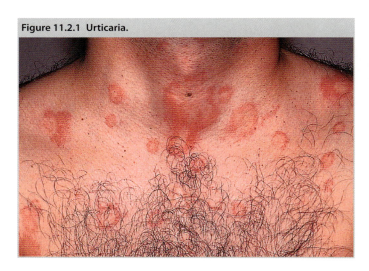

Figure 11.2.1 Urticaria.

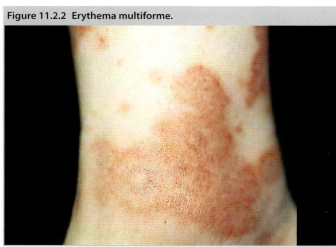

Figure 11.2.2 Erythema multiforme.

■ Distinguishing features

	Urticaria	Erythema multiforme
Physical examination Morphology	No target lesions Lesions transient and move around No mucous membrane lesions	Target lesions Lesions fixed Mucous membrane lesions
Distribution	Generalized, no acral predominance; lesions rare on hands/feet	Generalized, but acral predominance with lesions on hands and feet
History Symptoms	Occasional prodromal upper respiratory tract infection Ingestion of new medication No fevers No problem eating or drinking No pain and discomfort Severe pruritus	Occasional prodromal upper respiratory tract infection Ingestion of new medication Fever rarely presents, more common in prodrome, malaise Can't eat or drink Pain and discomfort No pruritus
Exacerbating factors	Aspirin, salicylates, NSAIDs	None
Associated findings	Occasionally angioedema Usually idiopathic Numerous associations Infections: streptococcal, sinus, urinary tract, parasitic Most medications Associated with neoplasm Tissue disease Physical factors: cold, sunlight, vibration Not associated with physical factors	No angioedema Rarely idiopathic Numerous associations Infections: *Mycoplasma pneumoniae*, viral, herpes simplex Most common medications: nonsteroidal Rarely anti-inflammatory agents, antibiotics, or connective barbiturates Rarely associated with neoplasm factors: or connective tissue disease Not associated with physical factors pressure, exercise, water
Epidemiology	Young adults	Young adults
Biopsy	No No epidermal necrosis; sparse perivascular inflammatory infiltrate composed of lymphocytes, neutrophils, and eosinophils	Yes Epidermal necrosis with underlying mixed lymphocytic infiltrate
Laboratory	Work-up usually not necessary except as directed by symptoms or if urticaria becomes chronic	Work-up usually required for underlying cause
Outcome	Good, usually resolves spontaneously by 6–8 weeks	Good; usually resolves over 4–6 weeks, rarely fatal if sepsis occurs

Differential diagnosis of urticarial lesions

- Angioedema (acquired and inherited C1 esterase inhibitor deficiency)
- Collagen vascular disease
- Contact urticaria
- Dermatographism
- Drug eruption
- Eosinophilic cellulitis
- Insect bite reaction
- Urticaria
  - Cold
  - Pressure
  - Heat
  - Cholinergic
  - Exercise
  - Aquagenic
  - Vibratory
  - Solar
  - Familial
- Urticaria multiforme
- Urticarial phase of bullous pemphigoid
- Vasculitis

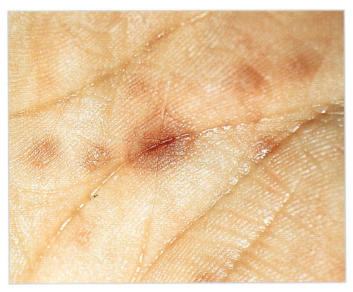

Figure 11.2.3 Erythema multiforme. *Clue to diagnosis:* target lesion.

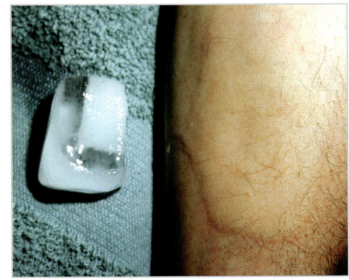

Figure 11.2.5 Cold urticaria induced by ice cube.

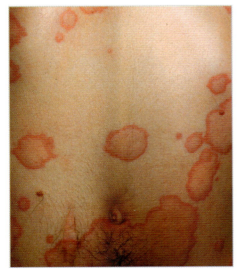

Figure 11.2.4 Urticaria.

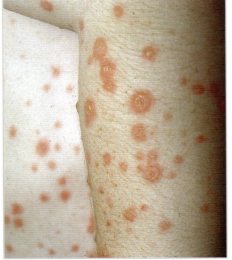

Figure 11.2.6 Erythema multiforme.

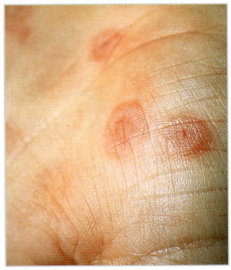

Figure 11.2.7 Erythema multiforme.

3. URTICARIA VERSUS INSECT BITE REACTION

Features in common: urticarial plaques or papules

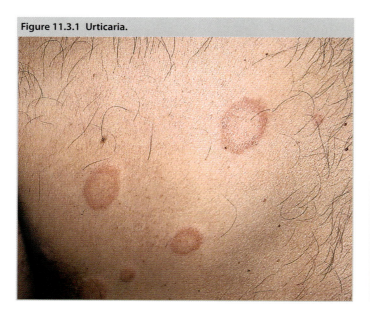

Figure 11.3.1 Urticaria.

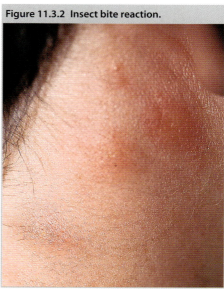

Figure 11.3.2 Insect bite reaction.

Distinguishing features

	Urticaria	Insect bite reaction
Physical examination		
Morphology	Lesion transient No vesicles No central punctum	Lesions fixed Vesicles may be present Central punctum or necrosis may be present
Distribution	Generalized Lesions not grouped	Localized, usually to exposed surfaces Lesions may be grouped (breakfast, lunch and dinner)
History		
Symptoms	Occasional prodromal upper respiratory tract infection Occasionally new medication Pruritus	No prodromal symptoms No new medication Pruritus
Exacerbating factors	Aspirin, salicylates, and nonsteroidal anti-inflammatory agents	None
Associated findings	No angioedema except in patients with acquired or inherited C1 esterase inhibitor deficiency Usually idiopathic Numerous associations Infections: streptococcal, sinus, urinary tract, viral, parasitic Medications Rarely associated with neoplasm or connective tissue disease Occasionally associated with physical factors: cold, sunlight, vibration, pressure, exercise, water	In highly allergic patients, angioedema and shock may occur Source of insects: usually outdoor exposure or pets Numerous possible insects: fleas, mites, spiders, mosquitoes No associated diseases No history of medication intake May be associated with outdoor activities
Epidemiology	Young adults	Any age
Biopsy	No Sparse perivascular mixed inflammatory infiltrate composed of lymphocytes, neutrophils, and eosinophils	Occasionally Wedge-shaped mixed inflammatory infiltrate usually composed of lymphocytes and eosinophils
Laboratory	Work-up usually not necessary except as directed by symptoms or if urticaria becomes chronic	None necessary
Outcome	Good; usually resolves spontaneously in 6–8 weeks	Good; resolves spontaneously within 1–3 weeks

Urticaria versus insect bite reaction

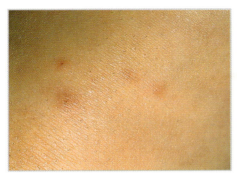

Figure 11.3.3 Insect bite reaction. *Clue to diagnosis:* central punctum.

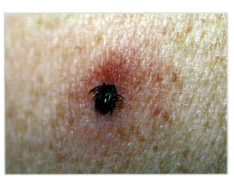

Figure 11.3.4 Tick bite.

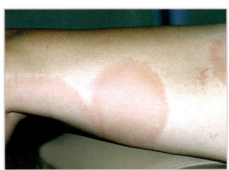

Figure 11.3.5 Erythema migrans (lyme disease). *Clue to diagnosis:* large expanding urticarial macules.

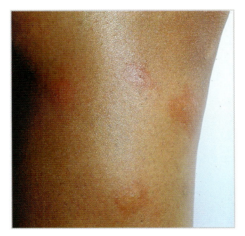

Figure 11.3.6 Urticaria.

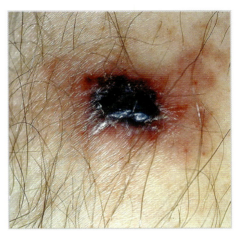

Figure 11.3.7 Brown reclose spider bite. *Clue to diagnosis:* hemorrhagic plaque

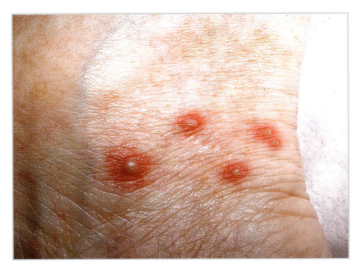

Figure 11.3.8 Insect bites.

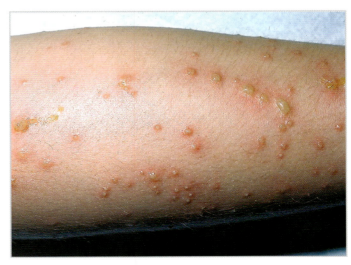

Figure 11.3.9 Insect bites.

4. OTHER CAUSES

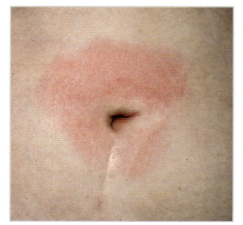

Figure 11.4.1 Cellulitis.

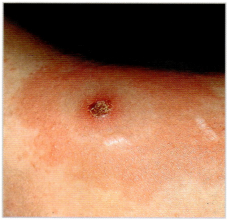

Figure 11.4.2 Cellulitis.

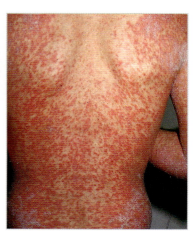

Figure 11.4.3 Graft versus host disease.

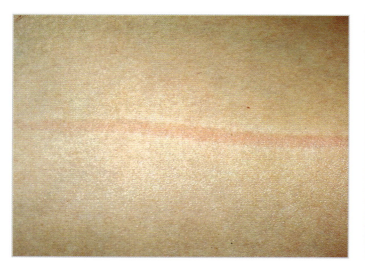

Figure 11.4.4 Dermatographism (urticarial plaque in area of rubbing).

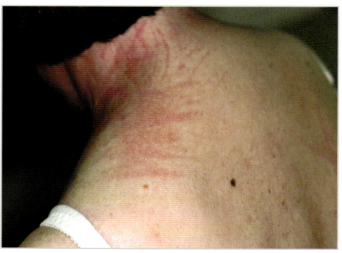

Figure 11.4.5 Dermatographism (urticarial plaque in area of rubbing).

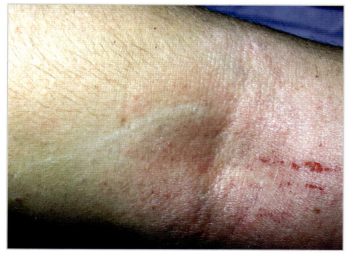

Figure 11.4.6 White dermatographism in patient with atopic dermatitis.

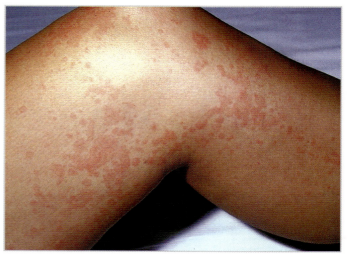

Figure 11.4.7 Still's disease.

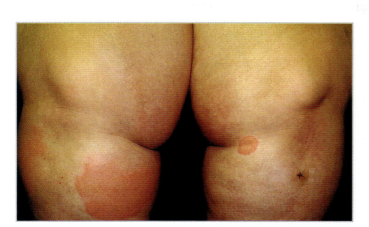

Figure 11.4.8 Eosinophilic cellulitis.

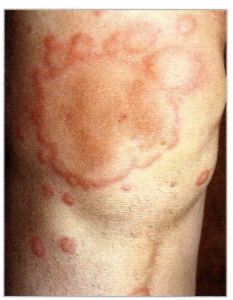

Figure 11.4.9 Urticarial vasculitis.

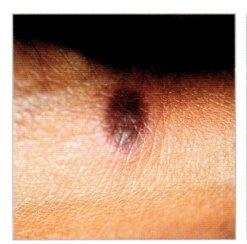

Figure 11.4.10 Fixed drug eruption.

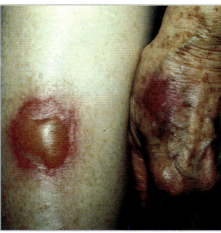

Figure 11.4.11 Fixed drug eruption.

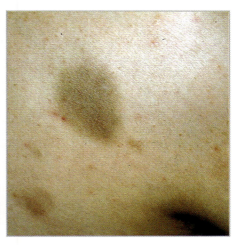

Figure 11.4.12 Fixed drug eruption.

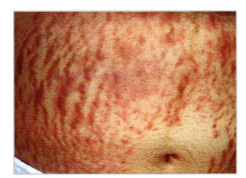

Figure 11.4.13 Pruritic urticarial papules and plaques of pregnancy (polymorphic eruption of pregnancy). *Clue to diagnosis:* predilection for stretch marks.

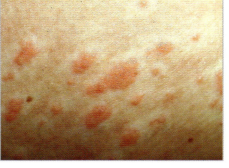

Figure 11.4.14 Pruritic urticarial papules and plaques of pregnancy (polymorphic eruption of pregnancy). *Clue to diagnosis:* predilection for stretch marks.

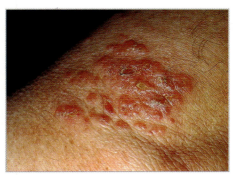

Figure 11.4.15 Hydatoid sting.

DISEASE DISCUSSION

Acute urticaria

Definition and etiology

Urticaria is commonly known as hives. Urticaria is a transient pruritic swelling of the skin due to histamine and other vasoactive substances released in the skin. Histamine release can be mediated by immunoglobulin E (IgE) or complement or effected through a direct mast-cell-releasing agent. Acute urticaria most commonly is idiopathic but can have a number of causes, including infections and medications.

Clinical features

Urticaria is easily recognized because of the characteristic transient, pink, edematous, non-scaling swelling of the skin. Lesions are not fixed; they disappear and reappear in different locations throughout the day. Urticaria can be subdivided into acute and chronic cases. Episodes lasting less than 6 weeks are considered acute. In both acute and chronic cases of urticaria, an underlying cause is found in only a minority of patients. In acute cases of urticaria, work-up is rarely indicated, and diagnosis should be based on history and symptoms. Some causes include foods, salicylates, medications (e.g. penicillin, sulfonamides, morphine, codeine), and infections such as streptococcal sore throat, viruses, sinusitis, and urinary tract infection. Patients should also be asked if the urticaria can be induced by physical factors such as exercise, sunlight, cold, heat, vibration, pressure, and water.

The differential diagnosis includes insect bites, erythema multiforme, urticarial vasculitis, and the urticarial phase of bullous pemphigoid. In these diseases, lesions are not transient. Target lesions, mucosal lesions, and lesions on the hands and feet are common in erythema multiforme. The lesions of insect bites are usually papular and asymmetric and may be vesicular or have a central punctum or necrotic area. Urticaria is predominantly a disease of young individuals, whereas bullous pemphigoid occurs in elderly adults. The lesions of bullous pemphigoid ultimately will blister and are more prominent on flexural surfaces. In urticarial vasculitis, a variant of leukocytoclastic vasculitis, the lesions stay in one area longer than 24 to 48 hours and frequently are purpuric. A biopsy will also distinguish between the two. In urticaria, a sparse mixed perivascular infiltrate is present, whereas in urticarial vasculitis, vasculitis involving postcapillary venules is present.

Treatment (Table 11.1)

Any possible underlying causes should be eliminated. Since most cases of urticaria are acute and therefore self-limited, overly aggressive therapy and workup should be minimized. The mainstay of therapy is antihistamines. Oral prednisone is occasionally necessary; however, it should be avoided if possible in cases of chronic urticaria because of its side effects.

Drug eruption

Definition and etiology

Drug eruptions are produced after parenteral or percutaneous absorption of a medication. They may be an allergic or a toxic reaction to virtually any medication.

Clinical features

Medications can produce a wide variety of cutaneous eruptions. Almost any cutaneous reaction pattern can be produced by medications. Eruptions that are exanthematous, urticarial, psoriasiform, pityriasis-rosea-like, blistering, lichenoid, vasculitic, lymphomatoid, photosensitive, or granulomatous can be produced by medications. Other possibilities include alopecia, pigmentary abnormalities, and nail dystrophy. One of the most common types of rash is the exanthematous or maculopapular eruption. This eruption may start 1 to 2 days after onset of medication administration if the patient has had prior exposure; it may begin in 7 to 10 days if the medication is taken for the first time. The most common drugs producing exanthematous eruptions are antibiotics in the penicillin, cephalosporin, and sulfonamide families. However, almost any drug can be the culprit.

The major differential diagnostic consideration is viral exanthem. Viral exanthems usually occur in children and are uncommon in adults. The timing of onset of the rash (after starting a new medication) and the lack of systemic symptoms such as myalgia, high fever, rhinorrhea, and diarrhea (which could be caused by a viral infection) help clarify the diagnosis. In some of the childhood exanthems, ancillary physical findings (such as Koplik's spots in measles or a slapped-cheek appearance in erythema infectiosum) help in establishing a precise diagnosis.

Treatment (Table 11.2)

Drug eruptions clear within a couple of days to 2 weeks after discontinuing the medication. Occasionally, the rash can resolve even if the drug is continued owing to desensitization of the immune system by continued exposure. Antihistamines and topical steroids are helpful for pruritus.

Erythema multiforme

Definition and etiology

Erythema multiforme is a reactive inflammatory skin disease secondary to a wide variety of stimuli. Common causes include medications and infections, most commonly caused by *Mycoplasma pneumoniae*

Table 11.1 Treatment of acute urticaria

Treatment	Precautions
Universal	
Avoid and eliminate any possible triggers	
Mild disease	
No treatment necessary	
Antihistamines as needed	Usually start with non-sedating antihistamines (loratadine, cetirizine, fexofenadine)
Severe disease	
Consider short course of prednisone	
Maximize antihistamine dose and combinations of first and second generation antihistamines may be used (first generation antihistamines: cyproheptadine, diphenhydramine, hydroxyzine, and doxepin)	First generation antihistamines cause drowsiness
IM epinephrine if angioedema	Tachycardia, nausea, vomiting, tremor, headaches, and rarely arrhythmias, hypertension

Table 11.2 Treatment of urticarial or maculopapular drug eruption (see also erythema multiforme/toxic epidermal necrolysis and pustular drug eruption)

Treatment	Precautions
Universal	
Stop the potential culprit	
Antihistamines as needed	
Topical corticosteroid as needed	
Moderate-to-severe reactions	
Consider prednisone 40–80 mg for 1–2 weeks	Avoid in diabetic patients Hyperglycaemia, hypertension, insomnia, mood change, weight gain, osteoporosis and risk infection
IVIG	Controversial, expensive Risk of allergic reaction Rare cases of anaphylaxis in IgA deficiency

Table 11.3 Treatment of erythema multiforme

Treatment	Precautions
Universal	
Eliminate any potential causative agents or factors: drug and infection	
Mild disease	
Topical corticosteroids bid	May produce steroid acne on face, or atrophy
Severe disease (Stevens–Johnson syndrome)	
Consider prednisone 40–80 mg for 1–2 weeks	Avoid in diabetic patients Hyperglycaemia, hypertension, insomnia, mood change, weight gain, osteoporosis and risk infection
IVIG	Controversial, expensive Risk of allergic reaction Rare cases of anaphylaxis in IgA deficiency

or herpes simplex. Other possibilities include infections (viral, bacterial, mycobacterial, fungal, protozoal), medications (sulfonamides, penicillins, nonsteroidal anti-inflammatory agents, barbiturates, phenytoin), neoplasms (especially lymphoma), connective tissue diseases, physical agents (radiation therapy), foods, topical agents, and miscellaneous causes (pregnancy, sarcoidosis, inflammatory bowel disease).

Clinical features

Erythema multiforme commonly involves both mucosal and glabrous skin. In the mucosa, generalized erosions with pseudomembrane and crust formation are seen. Sometimes mucosal involvement can precede skin findings, which include symmetric urticarial macules and papules. Rarely, mucosal involvement is the only manifestation of erythema multiforme. Within the first few days, some of the lesions develop concentric color changes owing to necrosis, producing the characteristic 'target' or 'iris' lesions. Blisters may also develop. The lesions appear first on extremities and then extend onto the trunk. Patients complain of pain due to the mucosal involvement along with mild malaise or itching. In the severe form (erythema multiforme major), fever, arthralgia, severe malaise, and even death due to secondary infection can occur. Erythema multiforme major characteristically has mucous membrane involvement (oral, nasal, ocular) as well as severe and widespread skin disease (Stevens–Johnson syndrome). The relationship between erythema multiforme and toxic epidermal necrolysis (TEN), a disease with widespread tissue desquamation, continues to be debated. In TEN, target lesions are not present. In addition to TEN, the major disease in the differential diagnosis is urticaria or urticaria multiforme in children. Unlike in urticaria, the lesions of erythema multiforme are fixed and have a tendency to involve the hands and feet. Also, oral lesions, blisters, and necrotic lesions are not seen in urticaria. Urticaria multiforme is a rare hypersensitivity reaction in children with polycyclic lesions resembling targets. Acral edema like erythema multiforme is frequently present. Like urticaria the lesions are transient, and there is a good clinical response to antihistamines. Children also usually do not appear sick. In some cases, a biopsy may be necessary to establish the diagnosis of erythema multiforme. Typical pathologic findings in erythema multiforme include scattered dyskeratotic keratinocytes, dermal edema, and an interface lymphocytic infiltrate.

Treatment (Table 11.3)

Erythema multiforme usually resolves spontaneously with supportive care if the precipitating factor has been eliminated. Some physicians advocate the use of systemic steroids in the first few days of involvement, but their efficacy has been controversial. Prolonged steroid use is not advised, since signs of underlying infection may be missed. Ophthalmologic consultation should be obtained if eye involvement is suspected to prevent synechia formation or scarring. Topical dressings may help lesions to heal. In severe cases, patients should be treated in a burn unit, and electrolyte and fluid balance should be closely monitored.

Insect bite reaction

Definition and etiology

Arthropods include both carnivorous spiders and eight-legged insects. Arthropods frequently bite humans, which produces a variety of cutaneous reactions ranging from necrotic ulcers and blisters to urticarial papules and plaques. Urticarial lesions, the most common insect bite reaction, are commonly seen after bee, black fly, and mosquito bites. Papular urticarial lesions can be produced after flea, mite, and bedbug bites.

Clinical features

Arthropod bite reactions can be very difficult to diagnose, since the insect usually goes unnoticed. A clue to the diagnosis of an insect bite is the finding of pruritic lesions distributed haphazardly on exposed sites. Often, in the center of the urticarial papules or plaques, a small punctum from the bite can be found. Unlike in idiopathic urticaria, lesions are fixed and not transitory, lasting a few weeks.

Treatment

The patient needs to avoid the source of exposure to the insect, or the area needs to be fumigated. Strong topical steroids can be used to minimize inflammation. If the patient has a severe reaction with systemic symptoms (hives, hypotension and dizziness) and there is a danger of anaphylaxis, epinephrine should be given. Epinephrine kits also exist for home use (e.g. ANA-kit, epi-pen). Oral antihistamines help alleviate the pruritus.

Table 11.5 Classical childhood exanthems (number based on order of description)

1st disease	Measles due to paramyxovirus
2nd disease	Scarlet fever (not viral due to *Streptococcus*)
3rd disease	Rubella (German measles) – RNA togavirus
4th disease	Duke's disease (Scarlet fever variant)
5th disease	Erythema infectiosum: Parvovirus B17 (also cause of some cases of papular purpuric gloves and socks syndrome)
6th disease	Roseola infantum (exanthem subitum): HHV6 or HHV-7

Table 11.6 Treatment of viral exanthems

Treatment	Precautions
Universal	
Supportive care Nonsteroidal antiinflammatory or Tylenol in children for fever	Aspirin in children can produce Reye's syndrome (swelling in liver and brain)
Determine if an antiviral agent is needed (i.e. testing for HIV, hepatitis as per clinical suspicion)	

■ Viral exanthem

Definition and etiology
A variety of viruses can produce an exanthematous maculopapular morbilliform (measles like) eruption.

Clinical features (Table 11.5)
Viral exanthems are most commonly encountered in children but can occur in adults. A viral eruption may be morphologically indistinguishable from a drug rash. Certain viral exanthems do, however, have recognizable features. Children with erythema infectiosum infection (caused by parvovirus B19) often have a 'slapped cheek' appearance because of prominent facial erythema. Patients with measles have white grainy papules on an erythematous base on the buccal mucosa, the so-called 'Koplik's spots'. Frequently, the diagnosis can be made only when other features such as cough and coryza are present (as in measles). Other common symptoms of viral infections include rhinorrhea, diarrhea, and myalgia. The fever of a viral infection is often higher than the fever encountered in drug reactions.

Treatment (Table 11.6)
Childhood viral exanthems are self-limited and do not require treatment. Some infections, such as those due to human immunodeficiency virus or hepatitis, require prolonged antiviral therapy.

Chapter 12: Generalized pustular eruptions

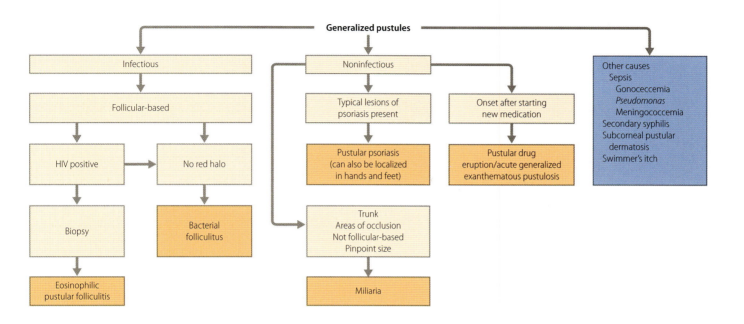

INTRODUCTION

A pustule is a circumscribed 'blister' of the skin containing pus. Microscopic evaluation reveals a focal collection of neutrophils or eosinophils. Pustular eruptions can be subdivided into either localized or generalized eruptions. Pustules can also be categorized according to cause (infectious versus noninfectious). The most common localized noninfectious form of pustular eruptions is acne, which is discussed in Chapter 2. Causes of localized infectious pustules such as impetigo and candidiasis are also discussed in Chapters 2 and 3.

Generalized non-infectious pustular eruptions include pustular psoriasis, acute generalized exanthematous pustulosis, and miliaria. The diagnosis is usually relatively straightforward, since patients with pustular psoriasis most often have classic psoriatic lesions elsewhere. Acute generalized exanthematous pustulosis start after the onset of administration of a drug, and miliaria occurs in occluded areas in patients who have been sweating. Generalized infectious pustular eruptions include eosinophilic pustular folliculitis (Ofuji's disease), which is likely due to an as-yet-unidentified organism, and bacterial folliculitis.

1. EOSINOPHILIC PUSTULAR FOLLICULITIS VERSUS BACTERIAL FOLLICULITIS

Features in common: follicular papules and pustules

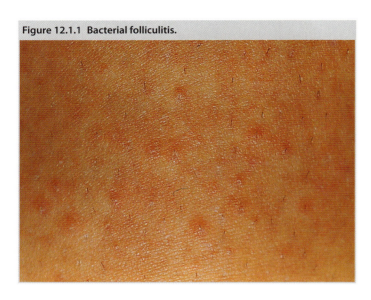

Figure 12.1.1 Bacterial folliculitis.

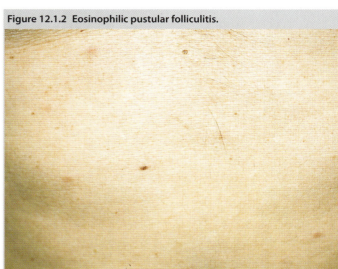

Figure 12.1.2 Eosinophilic pustular folliculitis.

Distinguishing features

	Bacterial folliculitis	Eosinophilic pustular folliculitis
Physical examination		
Morphology	No surrounding halo (except in pseudomonal folliculitis, also known as hot-tub folliculitis)	Red halo surrounding pustules
	No urticarial papules	Urticarial papules
Distribution	Trunk, buttocks, and thighs	Trunk and proximal extremities favored
	Face rarely involved	Face may be involved
History		
Symptoms	Pruritus	Pruritus
Exacerbating factors	Diabetes	None known
Associated findings	None	None
Epidemiology	No age or sex predilection	Most common in patients with acquired immunodeficiency syndrome or individuals of Japanese heritage
	Most commonly seen in normal population but can also occur in patients with human immunodeficiency virus disease	Rarely seen in normal population
Biopsy	No	Yes
	Pustule filled with neutrophils connected to hair follicle	Pustule filled with eosinophils connected to hair follicle
Laboratory	Culture positive for *Staphylococcus aureus*	Culture negative
Outcome	Good	Chronic

Differential diagnosis of follicular based papules and pustules

- Acne vulgaris
- Acneiform drug eruption
- Bacterial folliculitis (*Staphylococcus, Pseudomonas*)
- Eosinophilic pustular folliculitis
- Folliculitis decalvans
- Fox Fordyce disease
- Herpes simplex/zoster
- Hidradenitis suppurativa
- Insect bites
- Keratosis pilaris
- Lichen planus/lichen planopilaris
- Lupus miliaria disseminatum faciei
- Majocchi's granuloma
- Miliaria (should be eccrine based)
- Newborn
  - Candidiasis
  - Erythema toxicum neonatorum
  - Pustular melanosis of infancy
- Pyoderma gangrenosa
- Scurvy
- Sycosis barbae

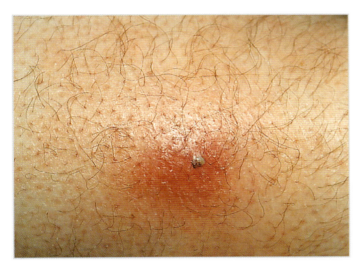

Figure 12.1.3 Bacterial folliculitis. *Clue to diagnosis:* furuncle (follicular based abscess).

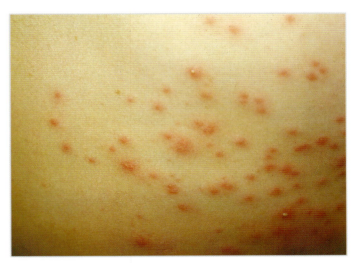

Figure 12.1.4 Bacterial/*Pseudomonas* folliculitis. *Clue to diagnosis:* hot tub use.

2. MILIARIA RUBRA VERSUS BACTERIAL FOLLICULITIS

Features in common: generalized papules and pustules

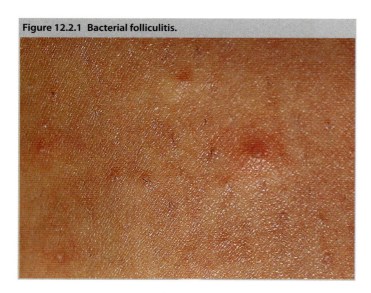

Figure 12.2.1 Bacterial folliculitis.

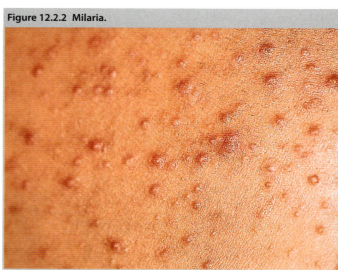

Figure 12.2.2 Milaria.

Distinguishing features

	Bacterial folliculitis	Miliaria rubra
Physical examination Morphology	Primary lesion: pustule, no vesicles Excoriations common	Primary lesion: small papules and vesicles (pustules secondary finding) Excoriations rare
Distribution	Trunk, buttocks, and thighs	Trunk or in areas of occlusion like diaper area in children
History Symptoms	Pruritus	No pruritus
Exacerbating factors	Use of hot tub in *Pseudomonas* folliculitis None	No hot tub use Occlusive clothing Hot humid climate
Associated findings	Diabetes	Fever, profuse sweating
Epidemiology	No age or sex predilection	Most common in babies and infants
Biopsy	No Pustule filled with neutrophils connected to hair follicle	No Dilated and obstructed eccrine duct
Laboratory	Culture positive for *Staphylococcus aureus*	Culture negative
Outcome	Good	Good

Differential diagnosis of generalized pustular eruptions

- Common causes
  - Folliculitis
  - Impetigo
  - Miliaria
  - Pustular drug eruption/acute generalized exanthematous pustulosis
  - Pustular psoriasis
  - Transient neonatal pustular melanosis
- Rarer causes
  - Ecthyma gangrenosum
  - Eosinophilic pustular folliculitis (Ofuji's disease)
  - Erythema toxicum neonatorum
  - Gonococcemia
  - IgA pemphigus
  - Impetigo herpetiformis
  - Pyoderma gangrenosum
  - Reiter's disease
  - Secondary syphilis
  - Subcorneal pustular dermatosis
  - Swimmer's itch

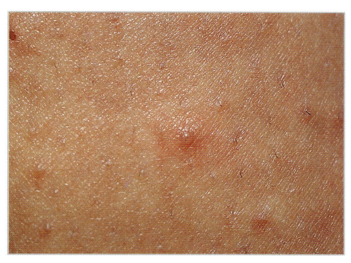

Figure 12.2.3 Bacterial folliculitis. *Clue to diagnosis:* follicular based pustule.

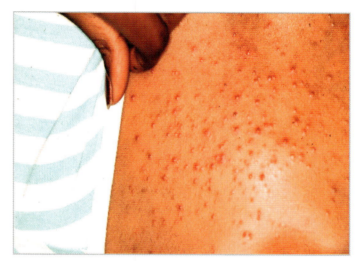

Figure 12.2.4 Miliaria rubra: red bumps localized to eccrine orifices.

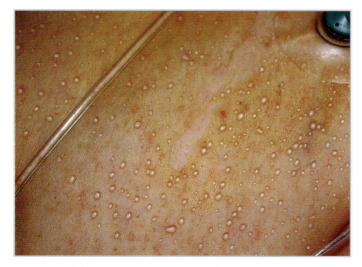

Figure 12.2.5 Miliaria pustulosa: pustules localized to eccrine orifices.

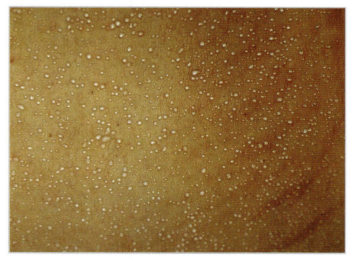

Figure 12.2.6 Miliaria crystalline: clear fluid filled papules.

3. PUSTULAR PSORIASIS VERSUS ACUTE GENERALIZED EXANTHEMATOUS PUSTULOSIS

Features in common: generalized pustules

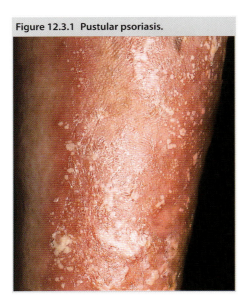

Figure 12.3.1 Pustular psoriasis.

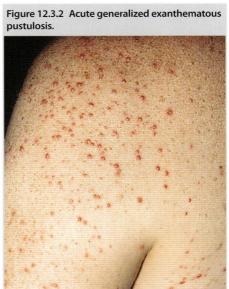

Figure 12.3.2 Acute generalized exanthematous pustulosis.

Distinguishing features

	Pustular psoriasis	Acute generalized exanthematous pustulosis
Physical examination Morphology	Red papules and plaques Silvery-colored scale Pustules not follicular based Annular plaques/patches with peripheral pustules may be present	No plaques No scale Pustules may be follicular based No annular lesions
Distribution	Scalp and predilection for extensor surfaces of body	Truncal, no predilection for extensor surfaces
History Symptoms	No new drug Fever	New drug Fever rare
Exacerbating factors	Tapering of oral steroids, infections, pregnancy, medications, irritating topical medications, sunburn	None
Associated findings	Positive family history in 10–20% of patients Improves with sun exposure Arthritis in some patients Onychodystrophy	No family history of psoriasis No relationship to sun exposure No arthritis No onychodystrophy
Epidemiology	Any age, no sex predilection	Usually adults
Biopsy	Yes Psoriasiform epidermal hyperplasia with neutrophil microabscesses in epidermis and stratum corneum	Sometimes Subcorneal pustule Occasionally vasculitis Eosinophils usually present
Laboratory	Increased erythrocyte sedimentation rate (ESR) Leukocytosis Hypocalcemia	Slight leukocytosis
Outcome	Chronic disease	Resolves after drug is discontinued

Common drugs causing acute generalized exanthematous pustulosis

- Antibiotics
- Calcium channel blockers
- Carbamazepine
- Hydroxychloroquine
- Sulphonamides
- Terbinafine

DISEASE DISCUSSION

Acneiform drug eruptions

Definition and etiology
A variety of medications can produce an acneiform eruption resembling acne (see next).

Drugs causing acneiform eruption
- Androgens
- Anti-seizure medications
- Corticosteroids
- Cyclosporine
- Epidermal growth factor inhibitors
- Isoniazid
- Lithium
- Halogens (iodide, bromide)
- Sirolimus
- Tricyclic antidepressants
- Tyrosine kinase inhibitors
- Vitamin B_{12}

Clinical features
Acneiform pustular drug eruptions resemble acne except that lesions are predominantly monomorphous pustules and comedones are rarely found. Acneiform drug eruptions are most commonly produced by androgens, oral corticosteroids, isoniazid, lithium, halogens, and epidermal growth factor inhibitors. Onset of acneiform eruption in an elderly person or acne unresponsive to therapy should raise the suspicion of possible drug being the culprit.

Treatment (Table 12.1)
Since the medications causing the acneiform rash often need to be continued, therapy is similar to treatment of acne vulgaris.

Bacterial folliculitis

Definition and etiology
Bacterial folliculitis is an infection of hair follicles, most often due to *Staphylococcus aureus* but also sometimes due to *Pseudomonas aeruginosa*. *Pseudomonas* folliculitis is most commonly seen in patients who have been using hot tubs.

Bacterial folliculitis can occur on anybody site that has hair follicles. Folliculitis decalvans and dissecting cellulitis are specific variants that occur on the scalp. Sycosis barbae is a form that occurs on the beard area. The most common sites of bacterial folliculitis are the legs, thighs, and trunk. Examination reveals follicular-based papules and pustules that often have a central hair. The lesions are highly pruritic

Table 12.1 Treatment acneiform drug eruptions

Treatment	Precautions
Universal	
Stop or change the medication if possible	No always possible in some patients if medication is medically necessary such as in EGF inhibitors for cancer treatment
Mild-to-moderate disease	Treat as regular acne
Mild disease	
Tretinoin cream (0.025, 0.05, 0.1%) Tretinoin gel (0.01, 0.025%) Adapalene cream (0.1%) Adapalene gel (0.1, 0.3%)	May be too irritating for elderly patients Apply on dry skin and small amount or may be too irritation Apply at nighttime since light may inactivate Do not pimple dab since trying to prevent new lesions
Moderate disease	
Use one of above and add benzyl peroxide and/or topical antibiotics Clindamycin Erythromycin	May be irritating Rare allergic reactions
Severe disease	
Add oral antibiotics	
Minocycline Doxycycline	Photosensitivity, Can produce blue discoloration of gums and skin Rare lupus like syndrome with fevers, malaise, rash Photosensitivity Esophagitis Vaginal yeast infections
Other considerations for women	
Oral contraception	Risk of stroke, thrombus especially in smokers and older women
Spironolactone 50–100 mg q day	Avoid pregnancy
Miscellaneous treatments	
Isotretinoin	Class X: causes birth defects Rare cases of depression and suicide Rare cases of coexistent or worsening of inflammatory bowel disease
Azelaic acid 20% cream	Only treatment that is class B and can safely be used during pregnancy
Dapsone 5% gel	Alternative topical if allergic to others

and often excoriated. Because of chronic scratching, eczematous changes may be present.

The differential diagnosis includes miliaria pustulosa, acne, dermatitis herpetiformis, *Pityrosporum* folliculitis, and Grover's disease (transient acantholytic dermatosis). Unlike in acne, comedones are not present in folliculitis, and the distribution of lesions is usually different. Miliaria pustulosa is caused by occlusion of eccrine glands. Miliaria most commonly occurs suddenly after an episode of severe sweating in sites of occlusion, such as the trunk. The lesions are usually smaller than lesions of folliculitis, and small vesicles and pustules are present. Grover's disease is a very pruritic, nondescript papular truncal eruption (pustules are usually absent) that is predominantly found in adult men. *Pityrosporum* folliculitis is morphologically identical to bacterial folliculitis but is due to *Pityrosporum orbiculare*, a commensal yeast. It occurs more commonly in immunosuppressed individuals and may uncommonly be a presenting sign of underlying disease, such as Hodgkin's disease. The diagnosis is made clinically, and positive culture results are confirmatory. In most cases of folliculitis, a biopsy is not necessary.

Treatment (Table 12.2)

Occlusive clothing should be avoided. In severe cases, oral antibiotics effective against *Staphylococcus aureus* should be used. In milder cases, topical antibiotics and antibiotic soaps are effective. In some cases, recurrence is common and the disease difficult to eradicate despite use of appropriate antibiotics and antibacterial soaps. Work-up for immune deficiency or diabetes, however, is usually still negative

Eosinophilic pustular folliculitis

Definition and etiology

Eosinophilic pustular folliculitis (Ofuji's disease) is an idiopathic disorder hypothesized to be infectious. This form of folliculitis is characterized by an eosinophilic inflammatory infiltrate within and surrounding hair follicles.

Clinical features

Three forms of Ofjui's disease exist. The classical form was originally described as a form of pruritic folliculitis of the scalp in Japanese men. More commonly in the United States is the immunosuppressed form most frequently occurring in individuals with human immunodeficiency virus infection. Finally, there also is a form occurring in children. In all types, follicular papules and pustules are seen. Unlike in bacterial folliculitis, urticarial papules are also present, and the pustules are frequently surrounded by a bright red urticarial halo. In the classical form, annular papules and pustules occur on the scalp and trunk. Although the diagnosis can be suspected in patients with acquired immunodeficiency syndrome, diagnosis ultimately depends on the histologic finding of an eosinophilic pustule within the follicular infundibulum. In the infantile form annular lesions are usually absent and there is a predilection for the scalp.

The differential diagnosis includes Grover's disease (transient acantholytic dermatosis) and miliaria pustulosa. Grover's disease primarily affects adult men and is characterized by pruritic nondescript papules that are not follicular based. A characteristic feature of Grover's disease is severe pruritus with minimal clinical findings. In miliaria, the lesions are smaller and not follicular based. They appear suddenly after severe sweating.

Treatment (Table 12.3)

Treatment is difficult. Topical or systemic steroids, Indomethacin, ultraviolet light therapy, itraconazole, topical permethrin, and oral metronidazole have been reported to help. HIV related cases improve with strong antiviral therapy.

Miliaria

Definition and etiology

Miliaria is an eruption due to obstruction of eccrine glands. It can be subdivided into miliaria crystallina, rubra, or profunda depending on the site of obstruction. The sites of obstruction are the stratum corneum in miliaria crystallina, the epidermis in miliaria rubra, and within the dermis in miliaria profunda.

Table 12.2 Treatment of bacterial folliculitis

Treatment	Precautions
Universal	
Consider culture to confirm diagnosis and determine sensitivities	
Treat any source of *Staphylococcus*	Pets can occasionally carry *Staphylococcus*
If chronic consider culture nasal nares	Nasal carriage often requires cocktail of antibiotics to clear
Avoid tight fitting clothes	
Women who shave legs with the grain	Frequent changing of razor blades may be helpful
Benzyl peroxide or Hibiclens wash	May be irritating
Severe cases	
Oral antibiotics as per culture	

Table 12.3 Treatment of eosinophilic pustular folliculitis

Treatment	Precautions
Universal	
Skin biopsy or scraping to confirm the diagnosis	
Oral antihistamines	May help with pruritus
Mild disease	
Topical corticosteroid bid	Atrophy, steroid-induced acne
Topical calcineurin inhibitor bid	May burn or sting
Permethrin 5% cream q day	Irritation
Moderate-to-severe disease	
Indomethacin 50–75mg q day	May be treatment of choice for classical variant. Gastrointestinal upset common. Risk of bleeding
UVB therapy	Risk of sunburn and skin cancer
Short course oral corticosteroids 1 mg/kg/day	Steroid side effects: hyperglycemia, insomnia, hypertension, fluid retention
Itraconazole 100–400 mg/day	Liver toxicity
Metronidazole 250 mg tid	Has Antabuse affect when taken with alcohol. May cause nausea, vomiting, metallic taste
Antiviral therapy	HIV associated cases may improve

Clinical features

Miliaria presents as an acute pruritic eruption after an episode of severe sweating. Covered sites such as the trunk or diaper are most commonly involved. In miliaria crystallina, small pinpoint-sized vesicles are seen. In miliaria rubra, small vesicles, papules, and pustules are present. In miliaria profunda, papular lesions predominate. The major differential diagnostic considerations are folliculitis and Grover's disease. The lesions of folliculitis are predominantly pustular and not vesicular, as in miliaria. Folliculitis is centered on hair follicles. Although sweating may have a pathogenic role in producing the lesions of Grover's disease, it is typically a chronic nonpruritic eruption in elderly men that requires a biopsy for definitive diagnosis.

Treatment (Table 12.4)

The eruption of miliaria is usually self-limited and does not require therapy. Wearing occlusive clothing and sweating should be minimized. Cool baths, compresses, and air conditioning may be helpful.

Acute generalized exanthematous pustulosis

Definition and etiology

Acute generalized exanthematous pustulosis is a severe exanthematous and pustular skin rash usually associated with high fevers, which is usually due to a variety of different medications.

Clinical features

Acute generalized exanthematous pustulosis is most commonly produced by a variety of different antibiotics and can be confused with pustular psoriasis or an exanthem if the pustules are obscured by the exanthematous portion of the rash. Occasionally a variety of infections have also been reported to be etiologic agent. The lesions are predominantly truncal; numerous pustules on an erythematous base are found; and the pustules are not follicular centered. As in pustular psoriasis, fever is frequently present. The onset of the rash 1–11 days after ingestion of a medication, the lack of a family history of psoriasis, and the lack of classic psoriatic lesions help distinguish pustular drug eruptions from pustular psoriasis. The differential could also include DRESS (drug reaction with eosinophilia and systemic symptoms). Patients with DRESS are very sick, have lymphadenopathy, evidence for hepatitis, and peripheral eosinophilia.

Treatment (Table 12.5)

Acute generalized exanthematous pustulosis may improve spontaneously after the medication is discontinued. Supportive skin care is frequently all that is needed, but some patients have been treated with oral prednisone.

Psoriasis

Definition and etiology

Psoriasis is an inflammatory disease characterized by increased epidermal proliferation. The cause of psoriasis is unknown, but abnormal epidermal kinetics, activation of the immune system within the skin, and genetic factors must be taken into account.

Clinical features

Approximately one-third of individuals with psoriasis have a positive family history. Psoriasis is a relatively common skin disease, affecting about 2% of the population of the United States. Asians are

Table 12.4 Treatment of miliaria rubra

Treatment
Avoid sweating
Avoid occlusive clothing
Cool baths
Compresses
Topical corticosteroids if pruritic

Table 12.5 Treatment of acute generalized exanthematous pustulosis

Treatment	Precautions
Universal	
Eliminate causative medication	Eruption is often self-limited and resolves in approximately 2 weeks, and no treatment may be necessary after medication eliminated
Consider biopsy to exclude pustular psoriasis	
Mild disease	
Topical corticosteroids such as triamcinolone 0.1% cream bid	May produce atrophy and steroid acne Avoid in intertriginous areas and on face
Moderate-to-severe disease	
Oral corticosteroids	Steroid side effects: hyperglycemia, insomnia, hypertension, fluid retention

less commonly affected. The most common age of onset is during the third decade, but psoriasis can present at any age. In most cases of psoriasis, examination reveals bright red erythematous plaques covered with white to silvery-colored scale. Areas of predilection include the elbows, knees, scalp, and sacrum. Extensor surface involvement predominates. Pitting of the nails and onychodystrophy occur frequently. Nails may appear to have an oil drop under them and small pits. Pustular psoriasis is a rare variant of psoriasis in which pustules are found. Pustular psoriasis can be further divided into four subtypes: palmoplantar acral pustular psoriasis (see Chapter 4), acute generalized pustular psoriasis of von Zumbusch, subacute annular psoriasis, and a mixed type. Recently, it has been discovered that some patients with pustular psoriasis have an Il-36 receptor antagonist deficiency or mutation.

Acute generalized pustular psoriasis of the von Zumbusch type occurs in patients with a history of classic psoriasis. The generalized pustular flare-up is precipitated by a variety of factors, such as corticosteroid withdrawal, pregnancy, infection, sunlight, or irritating topical therapy (e.g., coal tar or anthralin). Patients are seriously ill with fever and have an elevated erythrocyte sedimentation rate as well as leukocytosis and arthritis. Pre-existing lesions become bright red and develop pustules. Sheets of pustules spread to previously uninvolved skin to cover the entire integument. Isolated pustules, annular lesions, and plaques of pustules are found. In the subacute annular form of pustular psoriasis, the lesions start as annular areas of erythema that become raised and edematous and have a serpiginous appearance. Eventually, pustules appear at the advancing edge of the lesions. Unlike in the acute form, lesions develop slowly, and patients are not as sick. In the mixed form, features of both the acute and the subacute annular form are seen.

The major differential diagnostic considerations include acute generalized exanthematous pustulosis, subcorneal pustular dermatosis (Sneddon-Wilkinson, disease), IgA pemphigus, bacterial folliculitis, and acrodermatitis continua (Hallopeau's acrodermatitis). Acute generalized exanthematous pustulosis occurs 3 to 5 days after onset of administration of certain medications. Patients are usually not as sick as patients with pustular psoriasis, do not have high fever, have minimal leukocytosis, and do not have a history of preceding psoriatic lesions.

In subcorneal pustular dermatosis, the lesions are mostly localized to flexural areas such as the axilla and groin. A characteristic finding is pustules with a meniscus of clear overlying fluid. In acrodermatitis continua, which may also be a variant of pustular psoriasis, the pustules predominantly start around fingernails and cause confusion with paronychia infection.

Treatment (Table 12.6)

The treatment of choice for generalized pustular psoriasis is oral acitretin, cyclosporine, methotrexate, or infliximab. Alternative therapies include standard therapies for psoriasis such as TNF inhibitors, Il-17 inhibitors, Il-12, 23 inhibitors, apremilast, phototherapy, etc.

Table 12.6 Treatment of psoriasis

Universal	Precautions
Look and eliminate trigger factors such as streptoccocal infections and medications	
Mild-to-moderate disease	
Topical steroids bid	Atrophy, steroid induced acne
Topical calcipotriene bid	Slight irritation Overuse could cause hypercalcemia
Topical tar preparations such as liquor carbonis detergens 5% bid	Irritation
Topical tazarotene 0.05%, 0.1% cream or gel	Pregnancy category X Frequently irritating
Anthralin	Stains clothing, skin and irritation
Severe disease	
Acitretin 25–75 mg daily	Dry skin, hair loss, elevated serum lipids, birth defects Periodic liver function tests, and lipid profile Birth defects
Methotrexate 10–25 mg q week	Risk of liver toxicity, anemia, nausea, vomiting
Cyclosporine 5 mg/kg/day	Hypertension, renal insufficiency, immunosupression
TNF inhibitors Etanercept: start 50 mg SC 2×/week × 3 months than 50 mg SC q week Adalimumab: start 80 mg SC on day one then 40 mg sq day eight followed by 40 mg SC q 2 weeks Infliximab: 5 mg/kg IV week 0, 2 and 6 then q8 weeks	Risk of severe infection and increased risk of malignancies especially lymphoma
IL-12, 23 blocker Ustekinumab (weight dependent dosage) for less than 100 kg: 45 mg SC × 1 on week 0 and week 4 then q12 weeks	No black box warning, but still risk of severe infections and possibly malignancy
IL-17 blockers Secukinumab: start 300mg SC q week × 5 than 300 mg SC q4 weeks ixekizumab: start 160 mg SC × 1 then 80 mg SC q 2 weeks × 12 week. Then once a month Brodalumab: start 210 mg SC at weeks 0, 1 and 2, then 210 mg SC q 2 weeks	Black box warning only for brodalumab for suicidal ideation and risk Risk of severe infection especially candidal Risk of colitis
Ultraviolet light-narrow band UvB	Risk of burning and skin cancer
PUVA (psoralen plus UVA light)	Risk of burning and increased risk of skin cancer
Apremilast 30 mg orally bid	Risk of depression, diarrhea, nausea, headache, weight loss

Section 3

NEOPLASMS

Chapter 13 Epidermal growths

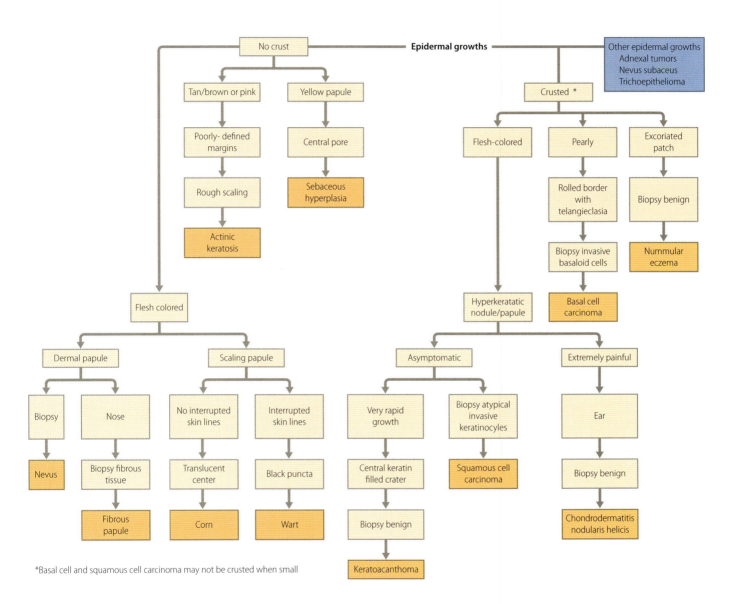

*Basal cell and squamous cell carcinoma may not be crusted when small

INTRODUCTION

Epidermal growths are caused by a proliferation of basal cells, or keratinocytes. They can be recognized by superficial thickening of the skin, which is often accompanied by increased production of keratin (manifested as scaling). It is important to differentiate scale (keratin) from crust (dried-up blood), since a crusting growth suggests a malignant process. For all growths that are crusted or ulcerated, a biopsy is mandatory unless there is a clear-cut history of preceding injury or irritation. A couple of the diseases discussed in this chapter are not epidermal growths. Sebaceous hyperplasia, flesh-colored nevi, and fibrous papule of the nose are included because they so closely resemble basal cell carcinoma. Likewise, nummular eczema, an inflammatory process, can mimic superficial basal cell carcinoma clinically.

1. PLANTAR WART VERSUS CORN

■ Features in common: scaling papule or plaque of the feet

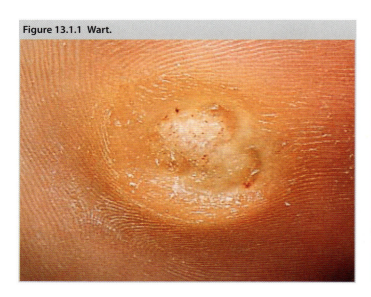

Figure 13.1.1 Wart.

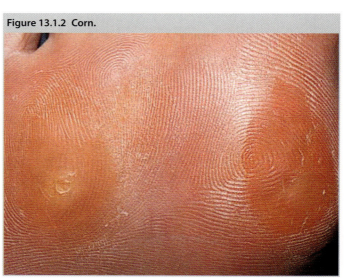

Figure 13.1.2 Corn.

■ Distinguishing features

		Plantar wart	Corn
Physical examination	Morphology	Interrupted skin lines Black puncta No translucent center Koebner's phenomenon present	No interrupted skin lines No black puncta Translucent center No Koebner's phenomenon
	Distribution	Feet, not related to pressure points Elsewhere	Feet sites of pressure Rarely hands
History	Symptoms	Usually not painful More painful upon pinching	Painful More pain upon pressure Ill-fitting shoes Bone projections
	Exacerbating factors	Immunosuppression	Not immunosuppressed
Associated findings		Rarely squamous cell carcinoma	None
Epidemiology		Children predominate	Adults predominate
Biopsy		Usually not done Epidermal papillomatosis and koilocytosis	Not done Keratin-filled epidermal invagination
Laboratory		None	None
Outcome		Resolves spontaneously or with destructive treatment	Resolves when pressure and friction removed

Differential diagnosis of scaling papules of feet

- Squamous cell carcinoma
- Adnexal tumor
- Seborrheic keratosis

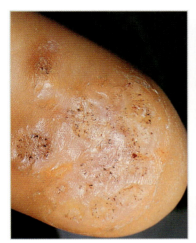

Figure 13.1.3 Wart. *Clue to diagnosis:* interrupted skin lines, black puncta.

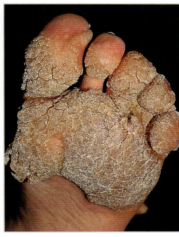

Figure 13.1.4 Warts in a cardiac transplant patient.

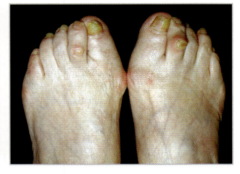

Figure 13.1.5 Corn.

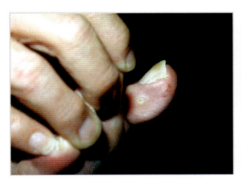

Figure 13.1.6 Corn.

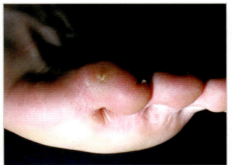

Figure 13.1.7 Corn.

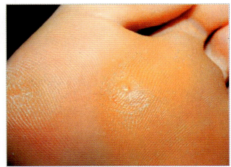

Figure 13.1.8 Corn. Note that when pared down, skin lines are intact.

2. SEBORRHEIC KERATOSIS VERSUS ACTINIC KERATOSIS

■ Features in common: scaling tan or brown papules

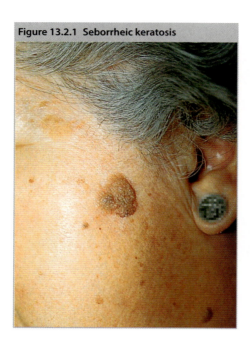

Figure 13.2.1 Seborrheic keratosis

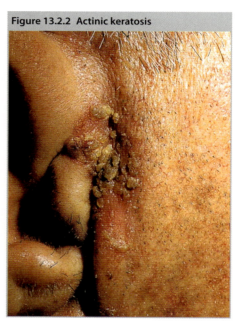

Figure 13.2.2 Actinic keratosis

■ Distinguishing features

	Seborrheic keratosis	Actinic keratosis
Physical examination Morphology	Well-demarcated Smooth greasy scale Pasted-on look	Poorly demarcated Rough scale Not pasted-on
Distribution	Generalized	Sun-exposed skin
History Symptoms	None	None
Exacerbating factors	None	Sunlight exposure Immunosuppression
Associated findings	None	Sun-damaged skin Skin cancer
Epidemiology	Common Middle-aged and elderly All skin types No relation to sun exposure	Common Adults Fair-complected skin A lot of sun exposure
Biopsy	Usually not necessary Biopsy required for irritated or atypical lesions Uniform benign keratinocytes, horn cysts	Usually not necessary Biopsy required for thick or indurated lesions Partial-thickness atypical keratinocytes, that spare adnexal structures
Laboratory	None	None
Outcome	Persistent No malignant potential	Spontaneously involute (20%) Malignant potential for squamous cell carcinoma (< 0.1%)

Seborrheic keratosis versus actinic keratosis   221

Differential diagnosis

- Wart
- Squamous cell carcinoma
- Melanoma
- Basal cell carcinoma

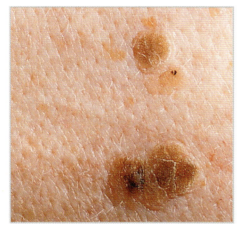

Figure 13.2.3 Seborrheic keratosis. *Clue to diagnosis:* well demarcated, pasted-on appearance.

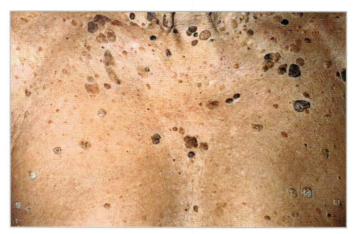

Figure 13.2.4 Seborrheic keratoses that are tan and brown.

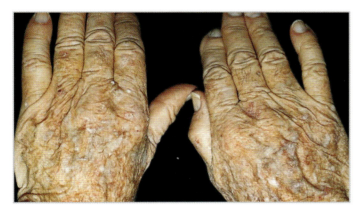

Figure 13.2.5 Actinic keratosis. *Clue to diagnosis:* ill-marginated, rough scale.

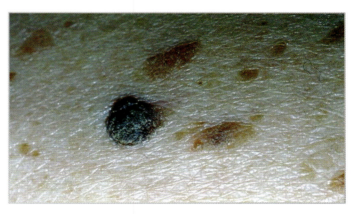

Figure 13.2.6 Seborrheic keratosis.

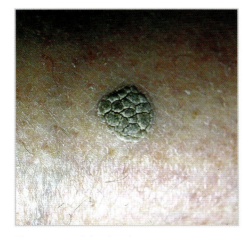

Figure 13.2.7 Seborrheic keratosis.

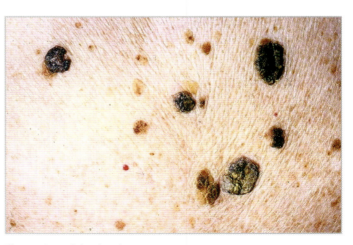

Figure 13.2.8 Seborrheic keratoses.

EPIDERMAL GROWTHS

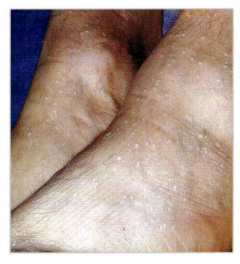

Figure 13.2.9 Stucco keratosis.

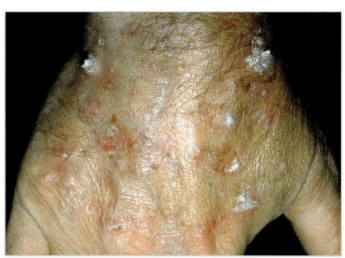

Figure 13.2.10 Actinic keratosis.

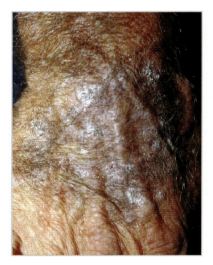

Figure 13.2.11 Actinic keratosis.

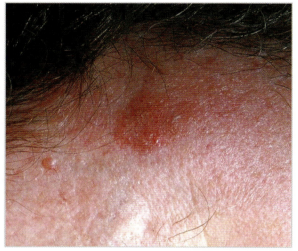

Figure 13.2.12 Actinic keratosis.

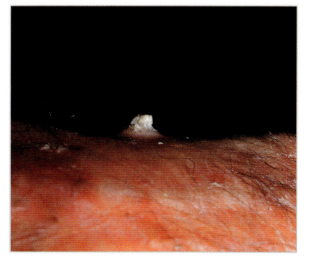

Figure 13.2.13 Actinic keratosis: cutaneous horn.

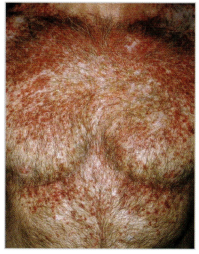

Figure 13.2.14 Actinic keratosis treated with 5-fluorouracil.

3. ACTINIC KERATOSIS VERSUS SQUAMOUS CELL CARCINOMA

Features in common: scaling papule or nodule

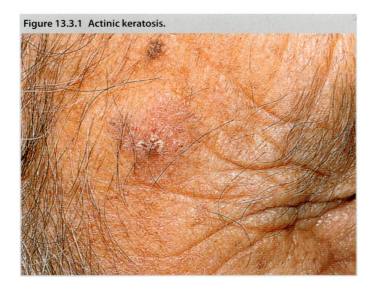

Figure 13.3.1 Actinic keratosis.

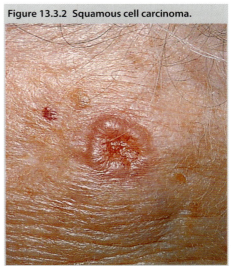

Figure 13.3.2 Squamous cell carcinoma.

Distinguishing features

	Actinic keratosis	Squamous cell carcinoma
Physical examination		
Morphology	Poorly demarcated Rough scale Not indurated No crust	Fairly well demarcated No rough scale Indurated May crust
Distribution	Sun-exposed skin	Usually sun-exposed
History		
Symptoms	No bleeding Sunlight exposure	May bleed Sunlight exposure
Exacerbating factors	Immunosuppression	Immunosuppression
Associated findings	Sun-damaged skin Skin cancer No chronic injury Cutaneous horn	Sun-damaged skin Actinic keratosis Chronic injury: burn scar, irradiation site, draining sinus, erosive discoid lupus erythematosus Cutaneous horn
Epidemiology	Common	Less common
Biopsy	Usually not necessary; biopsy for thick or indurated lesions Partial-thickness atypical keratinocytes that spare adnexal structures	Yes Full-thickness atypia and invasive atypical keratinocytes
Laboratory	None	None
Outcome	Spontaneously involute (20%) Do not metastasize Malignant potential for squamous cell cancer (<0.1%)	Do not involute Usually do not metastasize except for lesions in scars on lips and in chronic ulcers or long-neglected lesions

EPIDERMAL GROWTHS

Differential diagnosis of scaling isolated papules or nodules

- Basal cell carcinoma
- Chondrodermatitis nodularis helicis (ear)
- Keratoacanthoma
- Wart
- Adnexal tumor
- Seborrheic keratosis
- Epidermal nevus

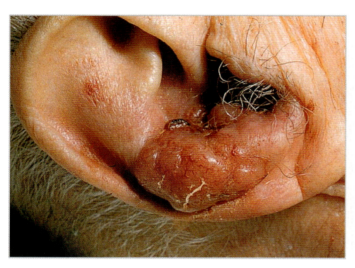

Figure 13.3.3 Squamous cell carcinoma. *Clue to diagnosis:* crusted indurated nodule.

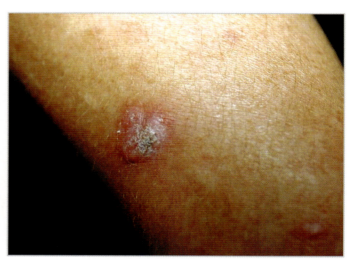

Figure 13.3.4 Squamous cell carcinoma.

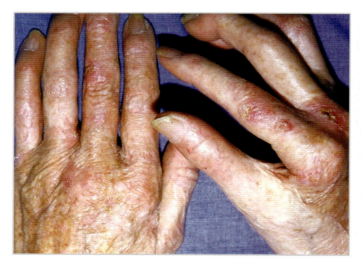

Figure 13.3.5 Squamous cell carcinoma in chronic radiation, induced dermatitis.

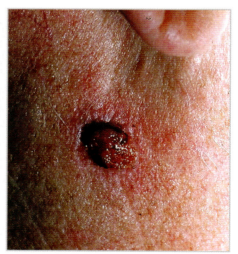

Figure 13.3.6 Squamous cell carcinoma.

Actinic keratosis versus squamous cell carcinoma

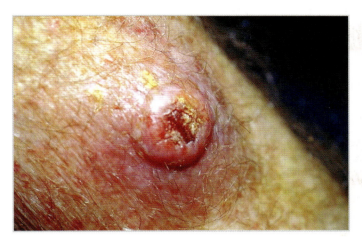

Figure 13.3.7 Squamous cell carcinoma.

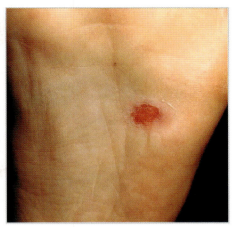

Figure 13.3.8 Squamous cell carcinoma *in situ* Bowen's disease.

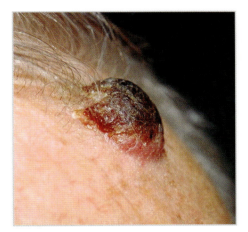

Figure 13.3.9 Squamous cell carcinoma.

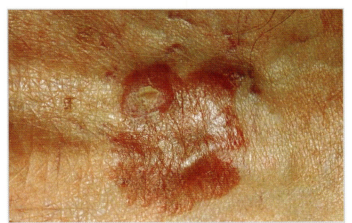

Figure 13.3.10 Squamous cell carcinoma.

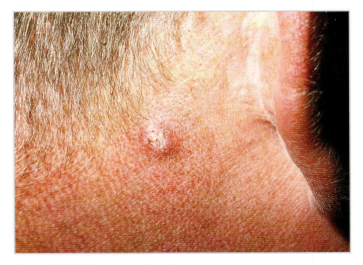

Figure 13.3.11 Squamous cell carcinoma.

4. SQUAMOUS CELL CARCINOMA VERSUS WART

■ Features in common: scaling papule or nodule

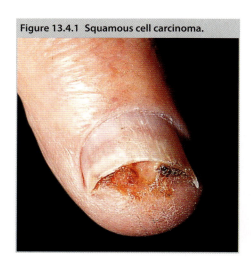

Figure 13.4.1 Squamous cell carcinoma.

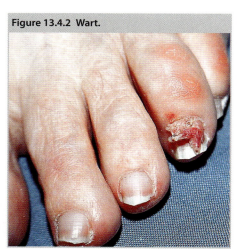

Figure 13.4.2 Wart.

■ Distinguishing features

	Squamous cell carcinoma	Wart
Physical examination Morphology Distribution	Not papillomatous May crust Endophytic No Koebner's phenomenon No black puncta Single lesion Usually sun-exposed skin	Papillomatous No crust Exophytic Koebner's phenomenon Black puncta Multiple lesions Predominantly hands, feet
History Symptoms Exacerbating factors	May bleed Sunlight exposure Immunosuppression	No bleeding Immunosuppression
Associated findings	Sun-damaged skin Actinic keratoses Chronic injury (burn scar, irradiation site, draining sinus, erosive discoid lupus erythematosus) Cutaneous horn	No sun-damaged skin No actinic keratoses No chronic injury Cutaneous horn
Epidemiology	Less common Adults Fair skin A lot of sun exposure	Common Children and adults All skin types No relation to sunlight
Biopsy	Yes Full-thickness atypia and invasive atypical keratinocytes	Usually not done Epidermal papillomatosis and koilocytosis
Laboratory	None	None
Outcome	Do not involute Usually do not metastasize except for lesions in scars, on lips, and in chronic ulcers or long-neglected lesions	Spontaneously involute Do not metastasize

Different types of squamous cell carcinoma

- Actinic-induced
- Chemical-induced
- Thermal-induced (Kangri cancer)
- Radiation-induced
- Chronic ulcer (Marjolin's ulcer)
- Squamous cell carcinoma in situ (Bowen's disease, erythroplasia of Queyrat)
- Verrucous carcinoma (erythroplasia of Queyrat, giant condyloma of Buschke–Löwenstein, epithelioma cuniculatum, and oral florid papillomatosis)

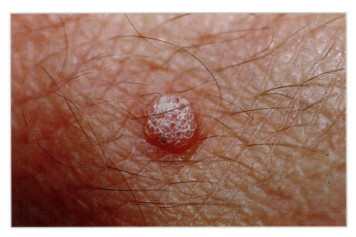

Figure 13.4.3 Wart.

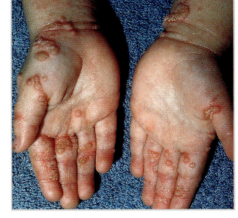

Figure 13.4.4 Warts.

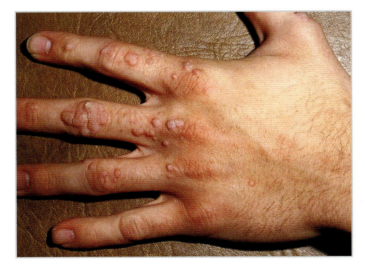

Figure 13.4.5 Warts.

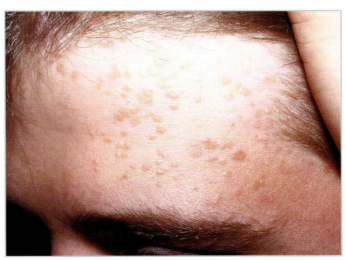

Figure 13.4.6 Flat warts.

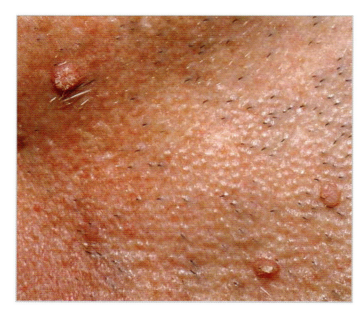

Figure 13.4.7 Filiform warts.

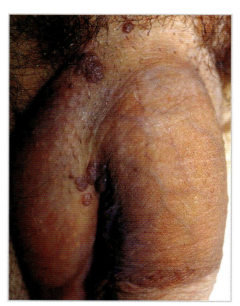

Figure 13.4.8 Genital warts.

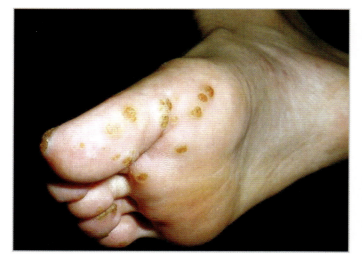

Figure 13.4.9 Plantar warts.

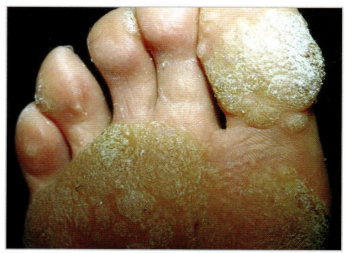

Figure 13.4.10 Plantar warts.

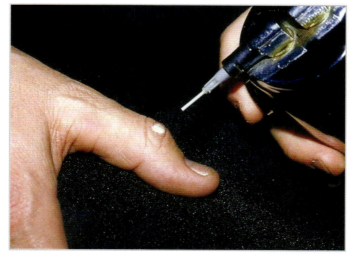

Figure 13.4.11 Warts: treatment with cryotherapy.

5. KERATOCANTHOMA VERSUS SQUAMOUS CELL CARCINOMA

■ Features in common: flesh-colored nodule

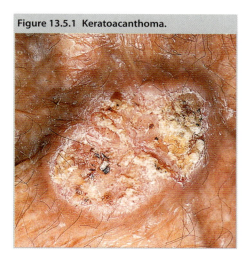

Figure 13.5.1 Keratoacanthoma.

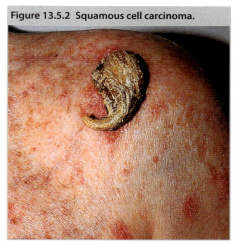

Figure 13.5.2 Squamous cell carcinoma.

■ Distinguishing features

	Keratocanthoma	Squamous cell carcinoma
Physical examination		
Morphology	Central keratin-filled crater No crust	Rare crater May crust
Distribution	Usually sun-exposed skin	Usually sun-exposed skin
History		
Symptoms	No bleeding Rapid growth	May bleed Not rapid growth
Exacerbating factors	None	Sunlight exposure Immunosuppression
Associated findings	Muir–Torre syndrome (sebaceous tumors, keratoacanthomas, low-grade internal malignancies) Sun-damaged skin Contact with tar Rarely acute injury	No syndrome Sun-damaged skin Actinic keratosis Chronic injury (burn scar, irradiation site, draining sinus, erosive discoid lupus erythematosus)
Epidemiology	Uncommon Familial multiple keratoacanthoma	Less common Not familial
Biopsy	Yes: keratin core, buttress of pseudoepitheliomatous hyperplasia, eosinophilic keratinocytes	Yes: full-thickness atypia and invasive atypical keratinocytes
Laboratory	None	None
Outcome	May spontaneously involute Rarely metastasizes	Does not involute Usually do not metastasize except for lesions in scars, on lip, and in chronic ulcers or long-neglected lesions

Types of keratoacanthoma

- Solitary
- Subungual
- Giant
- Multiple

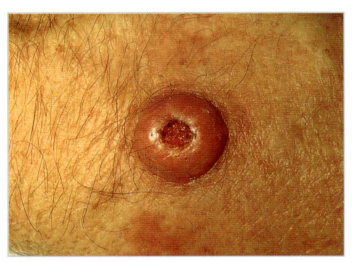

Figure 13.5.3 Keratoacanthoma. *Clue to diagnosis:* keratin-filled central crater.

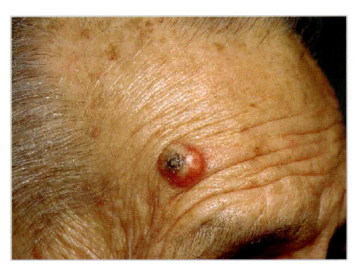

Figure 13.5.4 Keratoacanthoma.

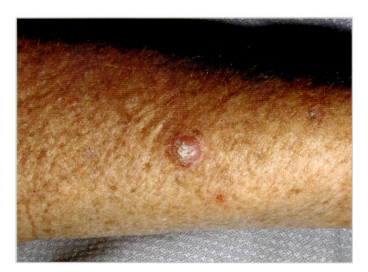

Figure 13.5.5 Keratoacanthoma.

6. CHONDRODERMATITIS NODULARIS HELICIS VERSUS SQUAMOUS CELL CARCINOMA

Features in common: flesh-colored nodule

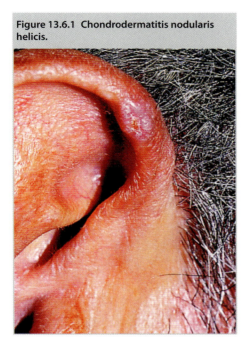

Figure 13.6.1 Chondrodermatitis nodularis helicis.

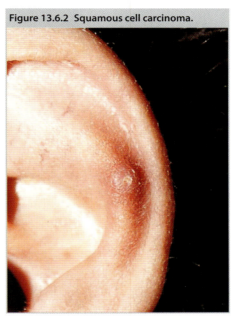

Figure 13.6.2 Squamous cell carcinoma.

Distinguishing features

	Chondrodermatitis nodularis helicis	Squamous cell carcinoma
Physical examination		
Morphology	Scale Crust	Scale May crust
Distribution	Ear (helix, anthelix)	Usually sun-exposed skin
History		
Symptoms	Painful	Not painful
Exacerbating factors	Sleeping on affected ear, trauma	Sunlight exposure, immunosuppression
Associated findings	No sun-damaged skin No actinic keratosis	Sun-damaged skin Actinic keratosis Chronic injury (burn scar, irradiation site, draining sinus, erosive discoid lupus erythematosus)
Epidemiology	Uncommon	Less common
Biopsy	Yes: ulcerated epidermis with adjacent acanthosis, degenerated collagen, inflammation, surrounding granulation tissue	Yes: full-thickness atypia and invasive atypical keratinocytes
Laboratory	None	None
Outcome	Does not involute Does not metastasize	Does not involute Usually do not metastasize except for lesions in scars, on lips, and in chronic ulcers or long-neglected lesions

Differential diagnosis of flesh-colored nodule

- Basal cell carcinoma
- Seborrheic keratosis
- Adnexal tumor
- Chondrodermatitis nodularis helicis
- Fibrous papule
- Nevus
- Neurofibroma
- Skin tag
- Dermatofibroma
- Leiomyoma
- Syringoma
- Sebaceous hyperplasia
- Squamous cell carcinoma

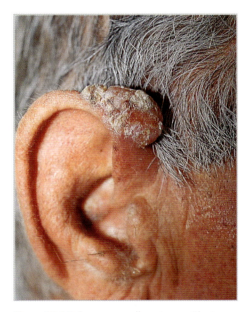

Figure 13.6.3 Squamous cell carcinoma. *Clue to diagnosis:* scaling and crusted nodule.

7. SQUAMOUS CELL CARCINOMA VERSUS BASAL CELL CARCINOMA (NODULAR)

■ Features in common: crusted nodule or plaque

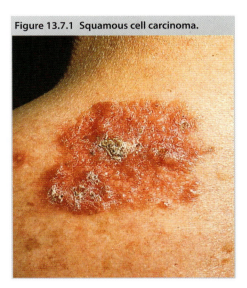

Figure 13.7.1 Squamous cell carcinoma.

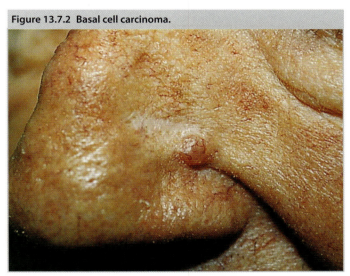

Figure 13.7.2 Basal cell carcinoma.

■ Distinguishing features

	Squamous cell carcinoma	Basal cell carcinoma (nodular)
Physical examination Morphology	Flesh-colored Scaling No central depression No telangiectasia No raised border	Pearly/translucent Usually no scaling Central depression Telangiectasia Raised rolled border
Distribution	Usually sun-exposed skin	Sun-exposed skin
History Symptoms Exacerbating factors	May bleed Sunlight exposure Immunosuppression	May bleed Sunlight exposure No immunosuppression
Associated findings	Sun-damaged skin Actinic keratosis Chronic injury (burn scar, irradiation site, draining sinus, erosive discoid lupus erythematosus)	Sun-damaged skin Actinic keratosis No injury
Epidemiology	Less common	Rarely inherited (basal cell nevus syndrome) Relatively common
Biopsy	Yes: full-thickness atypia and invasive keratinocytes	Yes: invasive basaloid cells with peripheral atypical palisading and clefts from stroma
Laboratory	None	None
Outcome	Usually do not metastasize except for lesions on lips and in chronic ulcers or long-neglected lesions	Metastasis very uncommon, usually in very long neglected lesions

Differential diagnosis of crusted nodule

- Basal cell carcinoma
- Chondrodermatitis nodularis helicis
- Keratoacanthoma
- Wart
- Adnexal tumor
- Seborrheic keratosis
- Squamous cell carcinoma
- Melanoma
- Metastatic carcinoma

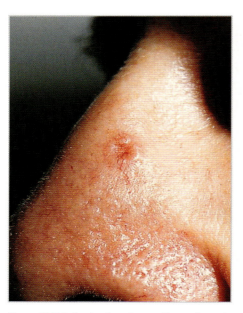

Figure 13.7.3 Basal cell carcinoma. *Clue to diagnosis:* pearly nodule with central crust and rolled border with telangiectasia.

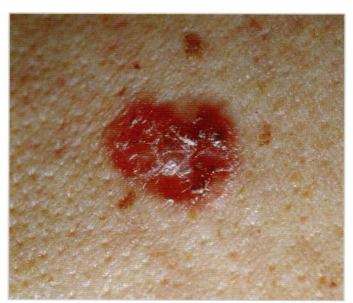

Figure 13.7.4 Basal cell carcinoma.

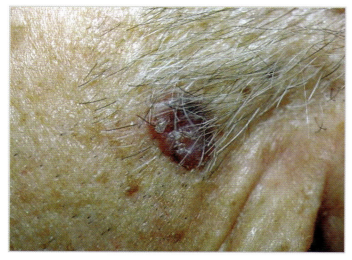

Figure 13.7.5 Basal cell carcinoma.

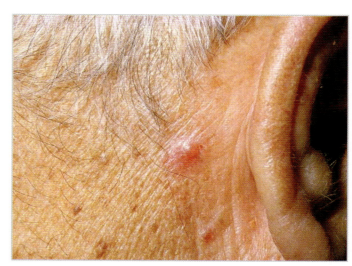

Figure 13.7.6 Basal cell carcinoma.

Squamous cell carcinoma versus basal cell carcinoma (nodular)

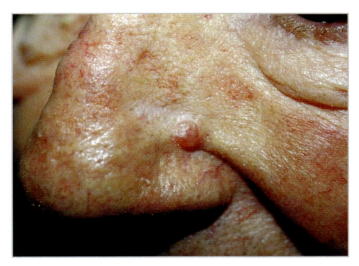

Figure 13.7.7 Basal cell carcinoma.

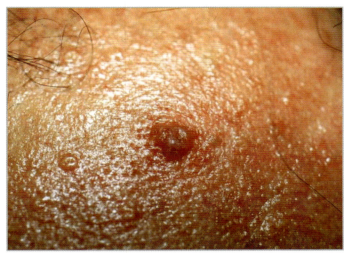

Figure 13.7.8 Basal cell carcinoma.

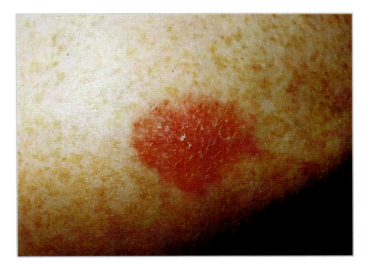

Figure 13.7.9 Basal cell carcinoma.

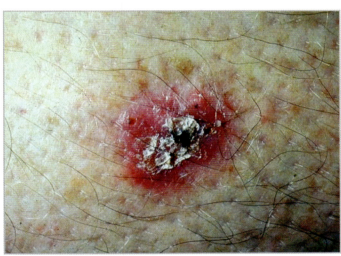

Figure 13.7.10 Basal cell carcinoma: superficial type.

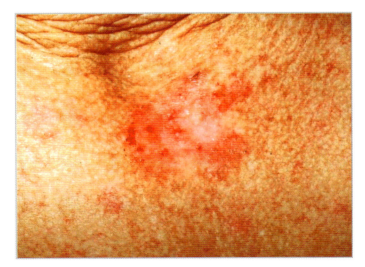

Figure 13.7.11 Basal cell carcinoma: scarring type.

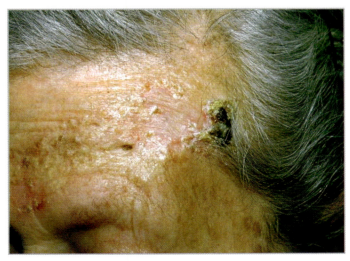

Figure 13.7.12 Basal cell carcinoma.

EPIDERMAL GROWTHS

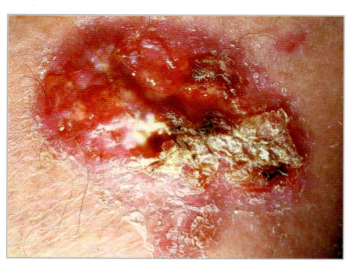

Figure 13.7.13 Basal cell carcinoma.

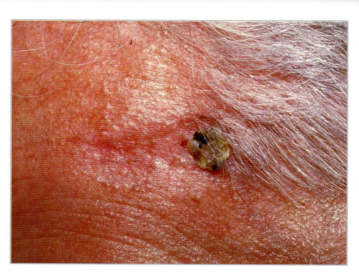

Figure 13.7.14 Basal cell carcinoma.

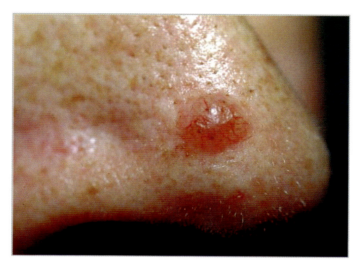

Figure 13.7.15 Basal cell carcinoma: nodular type.

8. BASAL CELL CARCINOMA (NODULAR) VERSUS INTRADERMAL NEVUS

Features in common: flesh-colored to pearly nodule

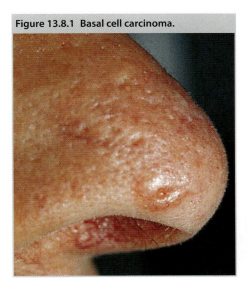

Figure 13.8.1 Basal cell carcinoma.

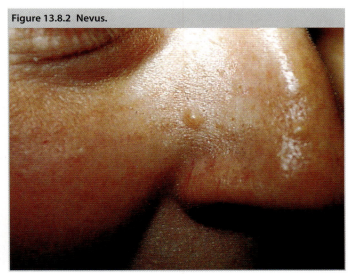

Figure 13.8.2 Nevus.

Distinguishing features

	Basal cell carcinoma (nodular)	Intradermal nevus
Physical examination Morphology	Pearly/translucent May scale Central depression May crust Telangiectasia Raised rolled border	Flesh-colored, flecks of brown may be present No scale No central depression No crust No telangiectasia No raised border
Distribution	Sun-exposed skin	Anywhere
History Symptoms	May bleed Present months to a few years	Does not bleed Present for decades
Exacerbating factors	Sunlight exposure	None
Associated findings	Sun-damaged skin Actinic keratosis	None
Epidemiology	Adults Common Rarely inherited (Basal cell nevus syndrome)	Children and adults Common
Biopsy	Yes: invasive basaloid cells with peripheral palisading and clefts from stroma	If uncertain: nests of nevus cells
Laboratory	None	None
Outcome	Gradually enlarges if not treated	Stable

Clinical types of basal cell carcinoma

- Nodular
- Superficial
- Cystic
- Pigmented
- Fibroepitheliomatous
- Keratoid/follicular
- Morpheaform

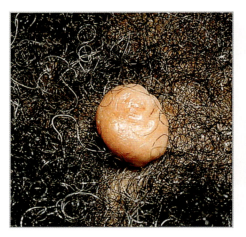

Figure 13.8.3 Nevus. *Clue to diagnosis:* flesh-colored, stable, smooth nodule.

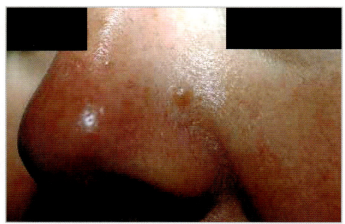

Figure 13.8.4 Nevus.

9. SEBACEOUS HYPERPLASIA VERSUS BASAL CELL CARCINOMA

■ Features in common: pearly to yellow papule

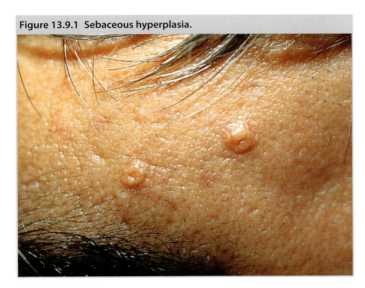

Figure 13.9.1 Sebaceous hyperplasia.

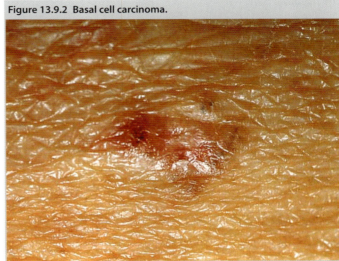

Figure 13.9.2 Basal cell carcinoma.

■ Distinguishing features

	Sebaceous hyperplasia	Basal cell carcinoma
Physical examination Morphology	Yellow No scale Central pore No crust No telangiectasia	Pearly/translucent May scale Central depression May crust Telangiectasia
Distribution	Sun-exposed skin on face	Sun-exposed skin
History Symptoms	Does not bleed	May bleed
Exacerbating factors	Sunlight exposure Medications (cyclosporine, anabolic steroids)	Sunlight exposure No medications
Associated findings	Sun-damaged skin Actinic keratosis	Sun-damaged skin Actinic keratosis
Epidemiology	Common Adults	Common Adults Rarely inherited (basal cell nevus syndrome)
Biopsy	If uncertain: hyperplasia of sebaceous glands	Yes: invasive basaloid cells with peripheral palisading and clefts from stroma
Laboratory	None	None
Outcome	Stable	Gradually enlarges if not treated

Differential diagnosis of pearly to yellow papule or nodule

- Trichoepithelioma
- Syringoma
- Fibrous papule
- Neurofibroma
- Xanthoma
- Juvenile xanthogranuloma
- Basal cell carcinoma
- Sebaceous hyperplasia

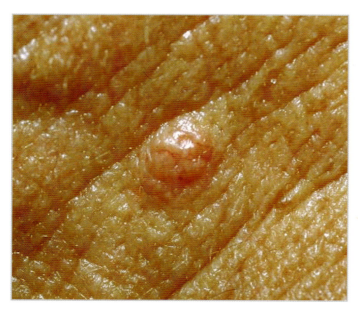

Figure 13.9.3 Sebaceous hyperplasia.

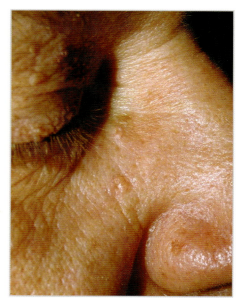

Figure 13.9.4 Sebaceous hyperplasia.

10. FIBROUS PAPULE OF NOSE VERSUS BASAL CELL CARCINOMA

■ Features in common: flesh-colored to pearly papule on nose

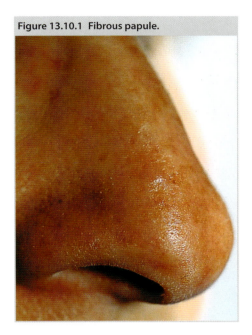

Figure 13.10.1 Fibrous papule.

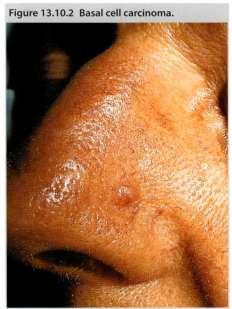

Figure 13.10.2 Basal cell carcinoma.

■ Distinguishing features

	Fibrous papule of nose	Basal cell carcinoma
Physical examination Morphology	Flesh colored No scale No depression No telangiectasia No rolled border Small size	Pearly/translucent May scale Central depression Telangiectasia Raised rolled border Small or large size
Distribution	Nose, nasolabial fold	Sun-exposed skin
History Symptoms	Does not bleed	May bleed
Exacerbating factors	None	Sunlight exposure
Associated findings	No sun-damaged skin No actinic keratoses	Sun-damaged skin Actinic keratoses
Epidemiology	Common Adults	Common Adults Rarely inherited (basal cell nevus syndrome)
Biopsy	If uncertain: benign spindle-shaped cells	Yes: invasive basaloid cells with peripheral palisading and clefts from stroma
Laboratory	None	None
Outcome	Stable	Gradually enlarges if not treated

11. BASAL CELL CARCINOMA (SUPERFICIAL) VERSUS NUMMULAR ECZEMA

Features in common: solitary scaling patch

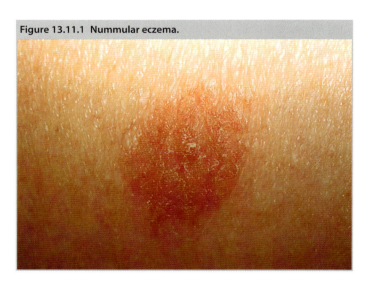

Figure 13.11.1 Nummular eczema.

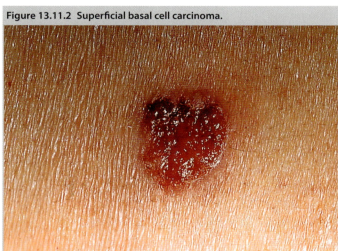

Figure 13.11.2 Superficial basal cell carcinoma.

Distinguishing features

	Nummular eczema	Basal cell carcinoma (superficial)
Physical examination		
Morphology	No crust No pearly border Vesicles may be present Round	May be crusted Pearly rolled border No vesicles May be irregularly shaped
Distribution	Generalized	Sun-exposed
History		
Symptoms	Itchy Does not bleed	Not itchy May bleed
Exacerbating factors	Dry skin	Sunlight exposure
Associated findings	None	Sun-damaged skin Actinic keratosis
Epidemiology	Common	Common
Biopsy	If uncertain: spongiosis	Yes: invasive basaloid cells
Laboratory	None	None
Outcome	Resolves with treatment	Gradually enlarges if not treated

Differential diagnosis of solitary scaling patch

- Nummular eczema
- Basal cell carcinoma
- Squamous cell carcinoma in situ (Bowen's disease)
- Psoriasis
- Actinic keratoses
- Fixed drug eruption
- Tinea

12. EPIDERMAL GROWTHS

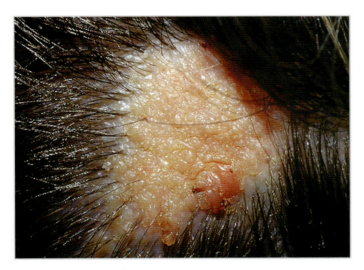

Figure 13.12.1 Nevus sebaceus.

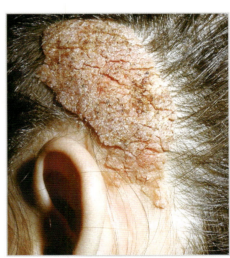

Figure 13.12.2 Epidermal nevus.

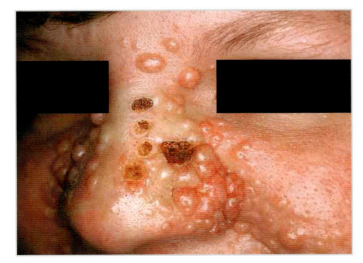

Figure 13.12.3 Trichoepithelioma.

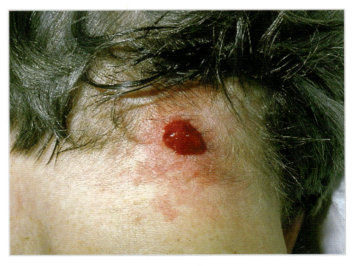

Figure 13.12.4 Syringocystadenoma papilliferum.

244　EPIDERMAL GROWTHS

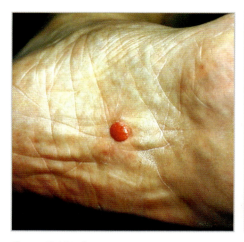
Figure 13.12.5 Eccrine poroma.

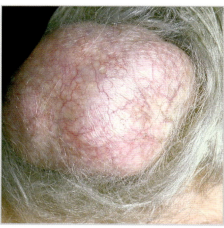
Figure 13.12.6 Cylindroma.

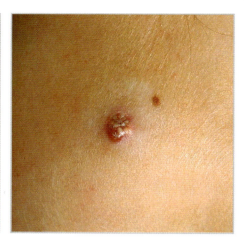
Figure 13.12.7 Pilomatrixoma.

13. OTHER EXAMPLES

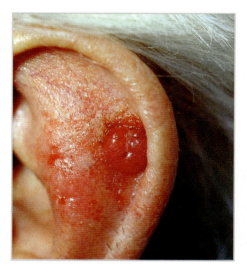
Figure 13.13.1 Merkel cell carcinoma.

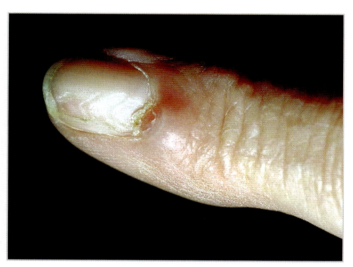
Figure 13.13.2 Digital mucous cyst.

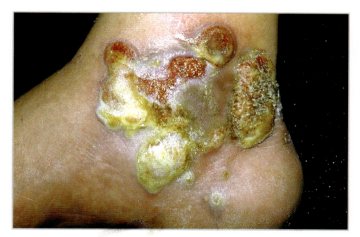
Figure 13.13.3 Lymphoma.

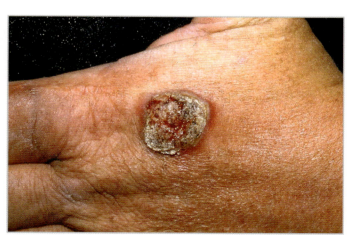
Figure 13.13.4 Lymphoma.

Other examples 245

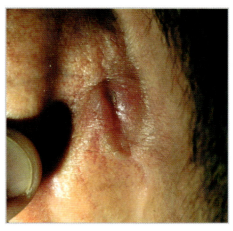

Figure 13.13.5 Granuloma fissuratum.

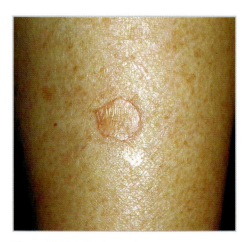

Figure 13.13.6 Porokeratosis.

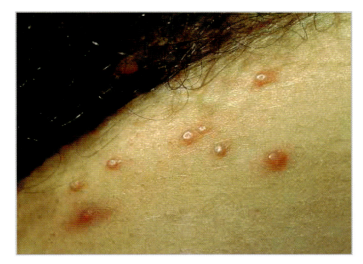

Figure 13.13.7 Molluscum contagiosum.

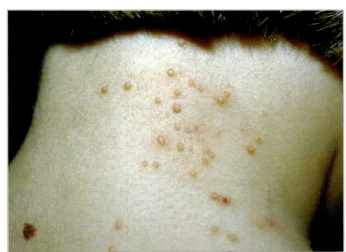

Figure 13.13.8 Molluscum contagiosum.

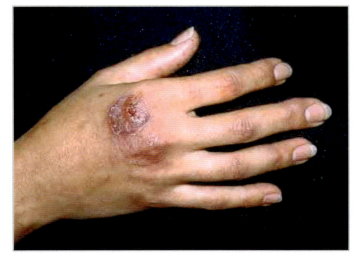

Figure 13.13.9 Fibroma.

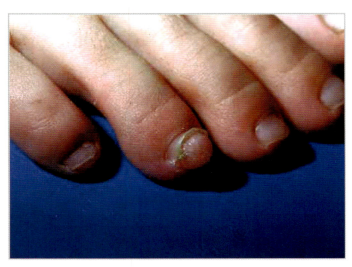

Figure 13.13.10 Blastomycosis-like pyoderma.

246 EPIDERMAL GROWTHS

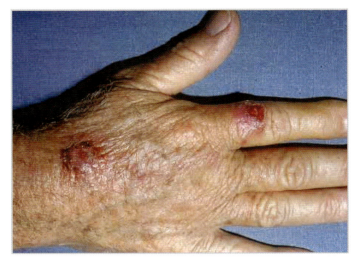

Figure 13.13.11 Sporotrichosis.

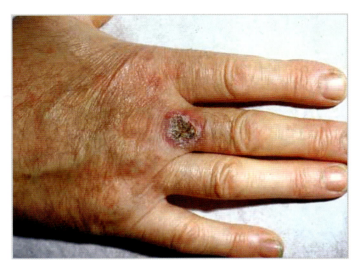

Figure 13.13.12 Sporotrichosis.

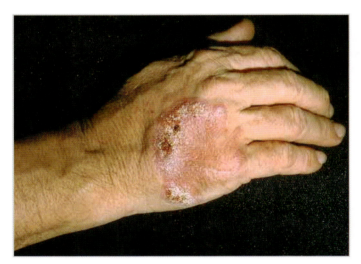

Figure 13.13.13 Sporotrichosis.

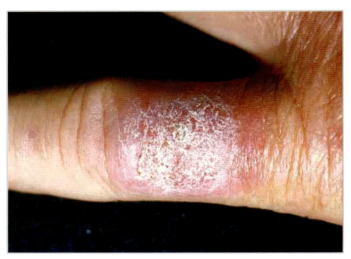

Figure 13.13.14 Sporotrichosis.

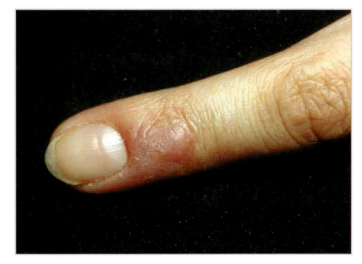

Figure 13.13.15 Mycobacterium marinum.

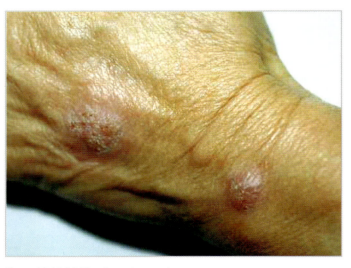

Figure 13.13.16 Mycobacterium marinum.

Other examples

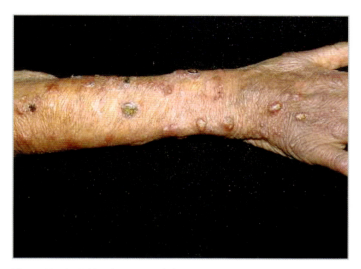

Figure 13.13.17 Mycobacterium chelonae.

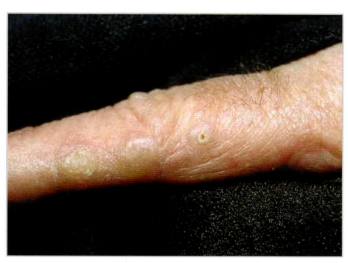

Figure 13.13.18 Arsenical keratosis.

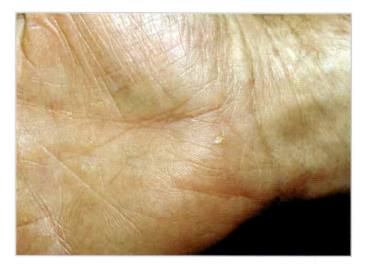

Figure 13.13.19 Arsenical keratosis.

DISEASE DISCUSSION

Actinic keratosis

Definition and etiology
Actinic keratosis is a potentially premalignant epidermal neoplasm that is caused by ultraviolet-radiation-induced damage to the keratinocyte.

Clinical features
Lightly pigmented skin and abundant sunlight predispose individuals to actinic keratoses. Fair-complected whites, particularly of Irish or Anglo-Saxon heritage (who have the least amount of protective pigment), are at greatest risk of developing cutaneous photodamage and actinic keratoses. Individuals who live close to the Equator, where there is an abundance of natural sunlight, and those who engage in large amounts of outdoor activity either recreationally or occupationally are more prone to develop actinic keratoses.

On examination, actinic keratoses are rough, scaling, ill-marginated papules and patches that are sometimes easier to feel than see. They occur on the sun-damaged skin of the face, posterior neck, upper trunk, and dorsum of the hands and forearms. They may appear flesh-colored, tan, or reddish.

The usual differential diagnosis of actinic keratosis includes seborrheic keratosis, squamous cell carcinoma, wart, and basal cell carcinoma. Unlike seborrheic keratoses, actinic keratoses have indistinct borders, have a red color rather than brown, and do not have a pasted-on appearance. Squamous cell carcinoma looks like actinic keratosis except that squamous cell carcinoma is larger and usually indurated. Basal cell carcinomas are pearly colored, not red; have telangiectasias; and usually do not scale. Warts are more papillomatous, skin-colored exophytic lesions. The biopsy of actinic keratosis reveals partial-thickness dysplasia of the epidermis that spares adnexal structures.

Treatment (Table 13.1)
Not all actinic keratoses need to be treated. Although there is a potential for developing into squamous cell carcinoma, this possibility appears to be quite small. Additionally, a number of actinic keratoses, up to 20%, spontaneously disappear. It is therefore only the more prominent actinic keratoses and ones irritating to the patient that need to be treated. This can be done by freezing the lesion with liquid nitrogen or by administering topical chemotherapy with 5-fluorouracil (Efudex cream 5%) applied twice a day until marked inflammation occurs, usually in 2 to 3 weeks. Alternative topical chemotherapy includes diclofenac, imiquimod, and ingenol. Treatment-resistant or thick and indurated actinic keratoses should undergo biopsy to rule out squamous cell carcinoma. Measures should be taken to prevent further ultraviolet light damage by reducing sunlight exposure with protective clothing and sunscreens (sun protection factor of 30 or greater), and by avoiding outdoor exposure during the midday (10:00 am to 2:00 pm), the time of most intense ultraviolet radiation.

Basal cell carcinoma

Definition and etiology
Basal cell carcinoma is a malignant neoplasm arising from the basal cells of the epidermis. Most basal cell carcinomas are caused by sunlight-induced damage to the skin.

Table 13.1 Treatment of actinic keratosis

Treatment	Precautions
Sun protection: broad spectrum sunscreen with SPF 30 or greater and repeat every 2 hours if in the sun, protective clothing , avoid midday sun	Vitamin D deficiency, rare allergic contact dermatitis
Cryotherapy with liquid nitrogen	Painful, scars, hypopigmentation
5-Fluorouracil 5% cream bid for 2–3 weeks	Painful, crusting and weeping, allergic contact dermatitis
Alternatives: diclofenac, imiquimod, ingenol mebutate	Pain, crusting and weeping Expensive
Photodynamic therapy	Pain, crusting and weeping
None: small, non-indurated	Do not miss a squamous cell carcinoma

Clinical features
Basal cell carcinoma is the most frequent malignancy in the United States, with more than 800,000 new cases reported annually. Although basal cell carcinoma almost never metastasizes, its malignant nature is emphasized by the local destruction that it can cause. As with other sun-induced neoplasms of the skin, fair-complected individuals and those with a lot of sunlight exposure are most likely to develop basal cell carcinoma.

Clinically, there are four major types of basal cell carcinomas: nodular, superficial, morpheaform, and pigmented. They are, of course, found most commonly on sun-exposed skin. *Nodular basal cell carcinomas*, the most common type, appears as a pearly semi-translucent papule or nodule that has a depressed center, telangiectasia, and rolled waxy border. Crusting and ulceration frequently occur.

The most common location is on the face, particularly the nose. *Superficial basal cell carcinomas* look quite different. They are red, slightly scaling, slightly crusted, well demarcated eczematous-appearing patches that most commonly occur on the trunk.

Infiltrative or morpheaform basal cell carcinoma appears as an atrophic, whiteish, scar-like eroded or crusted plaque. *Pigmented basal cell carcinoma* is a shiny brown, blue, or black papule or nodule.

The differential diagnosis of basal cell carcinoma depends on the type. For nodular basal cell carcinoma, the differential diagnosis includes sebaceous hyperplasia, fibrous papule of the nose, nonpigmented nevus, and squamous cell carcinoma. Dermatitis, psoriasis, and Bowen's disease (squamous cell carcinoma in situ) appear similar to superficial basal cell carcinomas. Seborrheic keratosis, pigmented nevus, and, most important, malignant melanoma must be ruled out in the case of pigmented basal cell carcinoma. For crusted nonhealing scar like lesions, the differential diagnosis is mainly between basal cell and squamous cell carcinoma.

A skin biopsy, either shave, punch, or excision, should be accomplished to confirm the diagnosis of basal cell carcinoma. The tumor is composed of a thickened epidermis with invasive buds and lobules of basaloid cells.

Treatment (Table 13.2)
Curettage and electrodesiccation of the lesion or excision are the most common surgical modalities used to treat basal cell carcinoma. Because of the locally destructive nature and potential for recurrence

Table 13.2 Treatment of basal cell carcinoma

Treatment	Precaution
Excision	Bleeding, infection, scar
Curettage and electrodessication	Experience needed, infection, scar
Mohs micrographic surgery	Mostly head and neck or recurrent tumor
Alternatives: radiation, cryotherapy, 5-fluorouracil, imiquimod, vismodegib	Use cautiously and in very selected cases

of the disease, treatment should be done by an experienced clinician who can individualize the therapeutic modality based on location of the lesion, histopathologic type, size of the basal cell carcinoma, and its primary or recurrent status. Less commonly used treatments are radiation therapy, cryosurgery, and topical chemotherapy. A specialized surgical technique, Mohs' surgery, is indicated for most basal cell carcinomas of the head and neck, for recurrent basal cell carcinoma, and for primary tumors with a high risk of recurrence. Vismodegib is indicated for metastatic, very difficult surgical basal cell carcinomas, and basal cell nevus syndrome patients.

Chondrodermatitis nodularis chronica helicis

Definition and etiology

Chondrodermatitis nodularis chronica helicis is a localized reaction of the skin in the helix of the ear related to chronic trauma and possibly poor circulation, producing a nonhealing nodule.

Clinical features

Tenderness and pain are the most common reasons the patient seeks medical care. Sleeping on the affected ear is often impossible. There may be a history of antecedent trauma.

The examination reveals a tender, pink, crusted, scaling papule or nodule on the superior rim of the helix or the antihelix. Because the surface is usually eroded, the differential diagnosis always includes basal cell or squamous cell carcinoma. Therefore, these lesions should always undergo biopsy. In the case of chondrodermatitis nodularis chronica helicis, biopsy findings reveal degenerative changes of the collagen, chronic inflammation, thin epidermis, and ulcer.

Treatment (Table 13.3)

Use of topical or intralesional steroids or cryotherapy frequently results in healing. Special pillows containing a hole are also available, which help minimize trauma to the ear while sleeping. For stubborn lesions, surgical excision of the involved cartilage is necessary.

Table 13.3 Treatment of chondrodermatitis nodularis helicis

Treatment	Precautions
Universal	
Avoid pressure on ear – use foam padding or special pillow	Biopsy to rule out skin cancer
Clobetasol ointment 0.5% bid	Atrophy with chronic use
Intralesional triamcinolone 40 mg/mL	Atrophy
Cryotherapy with liquid nitrogen	Painful, scar, hypopigmentation
Excision	Bleeding, infection, scar

Corn

Definition and etiology

Corns are localized thickening of the epidermis with a central keratin core secondary to chronic pressure or friction over bony prominences. They most commonly occur on the toes or feet.

Clinical features

Pain is the reason that patients with corns seek medical care. There is often a history of ill-fitting shoes or foot injury. The examination reveals a flesh-colored to yellow, well-circumscribed, hyperkeratotic papule or nodule over a bony prominence. The center has a hyperkeratotic plug that on paring with a scalpel reveals a translucent core and preservation of the skin lines.

The differential diagnosis is usually straightforward, although confusion with a plantar wart may occur. The presence of skin lines, translucent core, and lack of black puncta identify the lesion as a corn.

Treatment (Table 13.4)

Pain due to the corn can be relieved by reducing friction and pressure. Paring down the hyperkeratotic surface provides immediate relief. Changing shoes, shielding the site with orthotic devices, and surgically removing a bony exostosis are therapeutic options.

Nummular eczema

Definition and etiology

Nummular eczema is idiopathic inflammation of the skin characteristically occurring in oval or coin-shaped patches.

Clinical features

The hallmark of nummular eczema is an oval pruritic patch. The individual patches are discrete, well-marginated, erythematous, scaling, edematous, slightly weeping, and crusted. Vesicles may also be present. There may be a few or many lesions on the trunk and extremities.

The differential diagnosis of a single patch of nummular eczema includes superficial basal cell carcinoma and squamous cell carcinoma in situ (Bowen's disease).

Lesions of nummular dermatitis are round, whereas lesions of basal cell carcinoma or squamous cell carcinoma may be shaped irregularly. Skin biopsy findings reveal spongiosis typical of dermatitis. Any eczematous-appearing patch that is chronic and unresponsive to topical steroids should undergo biopsy to rule out carcinoma.

Treatment (Table 13.5)

Treatment of nummular eczema is similar to other eczemas. However, it can often be difficult control with weeping and crusting. Harsh soaps

Table 13.4 Treatment of corn

Treatment	Precaution
Remove friction and pressure: change shoes, protective pads/rings	None
Salicylic acid plaster 40%	Maceration
Pair down with scalpel	Too vigorous paring causing pain and bleeding
Surgery	Pain, infection, scar, temporary disability
Cryotherapy	Pain, blister, hypopigmentation

EPIDERMAL GROWTHS

Table 13.5 Treatment of nummular eczema

Treatment	Precautions
Universal	
Avoid irritants Moisturizers Mild cleansing agents like Dove or Aveeno	None
Mild disease	
Hydrocortisone cream/ointment 1% bid	Rarely causes allergic contact dermatitis
Pimecrolimus cream 1% bid	Burning sensation
Moderate disease	
Triamcinolone cream/ointment 0.1% bid	Atrophy with chronic application; especially intertriginous areas
	Steroid acne of face
	Glaucoma and cataracts if apply on eyelids
Tacrolimus ointment 0.1% bid	Burning sensation
Cetirizine 10 mg bid, Diphenhydramine 25–50 mg qid Gabapentin 100–300 mg qid	Sedation
Oatmeal or tar baths Bleach bathes for skin infections: 1/4 cup in half full bathtub	None
Severe disease	
Clobetasol cream/ointment 0.5% bid	Atrophy with chronic application; especially intertriginous areas
	Steroid acne of face
	Glaucoma and cataracts if apply on eyelids
Prednisone 40–60 mg daily tapered over 2–3 weeks	Hyperglycemia, hypertension, insomnia, mood change, weight gain, infection, osteoporosis
Mycophenolate mofetil 1000–1500 mg bid	Nausea, diarrhea, bone marrow suppression, infection, birth defects
Ultraviolet light: nUVB	Burn, skin cancer
Antipruritics and baths as for moderate	

and irritants should be avoided. Topical steroids and emollients for dry skin are the treatments of choice to start. Often, systemic medications are necessary.

Fibrous papule
Definition and etiology
Fibrous papule is an idiopathic flesh-colored papule that occurs on the nose of middle-aged individuals.

Clinical features
Fibrous papule is asymptomatic. Its onset in adults and history of gradual growth cause concern that this lesion may represent a basal cell carcinoma. A biopsy reveals spindle-shaped, stellate, and multinucleated fibroblasts surrounded by telangiectatic vessels as well as sclerotic collagen bundles in the superficial dermis.

Treatment (Table 13.6)
Other than for cosmetic reasons, no therapy is needed. A shave biopsy to differentiate a fibrous papule from basal cell carcinoma usually gives excellent cosmetic results.

Keratoacanthoma
Definition and etiology
Keratoacanthoma is a rapidly growing epidermal neoplasm with a propensity for spontaneous involution. The relationship between keratoacanthoma and squamous cell carcinoma continues to be debated. Some argue that keratoacanthoma is squamous cell carcinoma, whereas others believe that keratoacanthoma is a unique tumor.

Clinical features
Solitary acanthomas are the most common form of this neoplasm. They grow quite rapidly and usually occur on the sun-exposed skin of older individuals. Multiple familial and sporadic eruptive keratoacanthomas rarely occur. Keratoacanthomas, sebaceous tumors, and multiple low-grade visceral malignancies occur in Muir-Torre syndrome. In addition to ultraviolet light damage of the skin, pitch, tar, and human papillomavirus have been reported as possible cofactors in the development of keratoacanthoma.

Keratoacanthoma is a dome-shaped flesh-colored nodule that has rolled borders and a central crater filled with a keratin plug.

The differential diagnosis of keratoacanthoma includes other epidermal tumors, particularly squamous cell carcinoma. A skin biopsy is necessary. The pathologic changes, however, may make it difficult to differentiate keratoacanthoma from low-grade squamous cell carcinoma. Typically, keratoacanthoma has a keratin-filled central crater surrounded by pseudoepitheliomatous hyperplasia of the epidermis, which contains benign keratinocytes with an eosinophilic, glassy cytoplasm.

Treatment (Table 13.7)
Management can be guided by the results of the biopsy. Since the biologic behaviour is not always predictable, awaiting spontaneous regression of the lesion over a 4- to 12-month period is usually not recommended. A complete surgical excision should be accomplished.

Table 13.6 Treatment of fibrous papule

Treatment	Precautions
None necessary	Do not miss a basal cell carcinoma
Shave biopsy to confirm diagnosis	Scar

Table 13.7 Treatment of keratoacanthoma

Treatment	Precautions
Excision	Bleeding, infection, scar,
Curettage and electrodessication	Experience needed, infection, scar
Mohs micrographic surgery	Mostly head and neck, recurrent tumor
Alternatives: radiation, cryotherapy, intralesional 5-fluorouracil or bleomycin	Use cautiously and in very selected cases
None if completely regressed	Do not leave residual tumor

Other treatments for keratoacanthoma include radiotherapy, electrodesiccation and curettage, and intralesional 5-fluorouracil or bleomycin.

■ Melanocytic nevus

Definition and etiology
A melanocytic nevus (mole) is a congenital or acquired benign neoplasm of melanocytes.

Clinical features
Nevi should be considered a normal skin finding. They vary in number from an average of a couple of dozen in whites to less than a dozen in blacks. Most nevi develop between the ages of 6 months and 35 years. Pregnancy and adolescence particularly influence nevi; during these times they enlarge, darken in color, and itch. Otherwise, nevi are asymptomatic and are usually brought to the attention of a physician because of irritation, change in appearance, or cosmetic reasons.

Nevi should be relatively uniform in color, surface, and border. They may be flesh-colored to darkly pigmented, non-scaling, dome-shaped papules or nodules.

The main disease in the differential diagnosis of a flesh-colored nevus, particularly on the nose or face, is nodular basal cell carcinoma. A history of the lesion having been present since childhood strongly suggests a nevus. Early nodular basal cell carcinomas may lack the typical central depression, the pearly rolled border, telangiectasia, and crusting. A skin biopsy easily differentiates these two neoplasms: a nevus reveals nests of benign nevus cells. Most important, is to differentiate a nevus from a malignant melanoma. A regular brown color, surface, and border are characteristic features of a nevus. For a pigmented lesion that appears much different than the individual's other nevi, be concerned that this 'ugly duckling' may represent a malignant melanoma.

Treatment (Table 13.8)
Unless the nevus is irritated, cosmetically unattractive, or changing, no therapy is necessary. Depending on the situation, a punch, shave, or excisional biopsy will provide adequate tissue for pathologic examination and will also remove the lesion.

■ Sebaceous hyperplasia

Definition and etiology
Sebaceous hyperplasia is a benign neoplasm of sebaceous glands.

Clinical features
Sebaceous hyperplasia is an asymptomatic growth that occurs most commonly on the sun-damaged skin of the face. It appears as a yellowish papule or a small nodule with a central pore or umbilication. It has no scale or crusting. Other than aesthetics, its only importance is its differentiation from basal cell carcinoma. When diagnosis is uncertain, biopsy findings reveal typical hypertrophied multilobulate sebaceous glands.

Treatment (Table 13.9)
No therapy is necessary. Local electrodesiccation can be used cautiously to destroy these benign growths.

■ Seborrheic keratosis

Definition and etiology
Seborrheic keratosis is a benign neoplasm of the epidermis that usually appears during middle age.

Clinical features
Unless irritated, seborrheic keratoses are asymptomatic. Most patients seek medical care when these benign tumors become irritated or displeasing cosmetically or when they are concerned that they may represent skin cancer.

Seborrheic keratoses typically are well-demarcated, slightly scaling, greasy appearing, tan to dark brown *pasted-on* papules and plaques. Their surface is often verrucous or crumbly in appearance with small keratin-filled pits. They occur anywhere on the body with the exception of the palms and soles.

The well-marginated, pasted-on appearance and the finding of multiple similar appearing papules and plaques make the diagnosis of seborrheic keratosis generally straightforward. On occasion, though, they can mimic warts, actinic keratosis, nevus, pigmented basal cell carcinoma, and malignant melanoma. When the diagnosis is uncertain, biopsy findings reveal the typical uniform, well-demarcated intraepithelial proliferation of small benign squamous cells.

Treatment (Table 13.10)
No treatment is necessary for seborrheic keratoses unless they are irritated or cosmetically unacceptable. Freezing with liquid nitrogen is generally most efficient and most effective. Curettage or shave can be done for thicker lesions. A biopsy is not done unless there is concern about malignancy.

Table 13.9 Treatment of sebaceous hyperplasia

Treatment	Precautions
None	Do not miss a basal cell carcinoma
Electrodessication	Scar
Trichloroacetic or bichloroacetic acid	Scar

Table 13.8 Treatment of melanocytic nevus

Treatment	Precautions
None if not worrisome	Do not miss a melanoma
Shave biopsy	Scar
Deep shave excision, punch biopsy, or excision for suspicious lesion	Scar, infection, bleeding
Serial photographs	If change, biopsy

Table 13.10 Treatment of seborrheic keratoses

Treatment	Precautions
None	Do not miss a melanoma
Cryotherapy with liquid nitrogen	Painful, hypopigmentation
Curettage	Scar
Shave biopsy/excision	Scar, infection

Squamous cell carcinoma

Definition and etiology

Squamous cell carcinoma is a malignant neoplasm of keratinocytes that is locally invasive and has the potential to metastasize. Ultraviolet radiation, x-rays, papillomavirus infection, and chemical carcinogens such as soot and arsenic cause squamous cell carcinoma.

Clinical features

Squamous cell carcinoma is the second most common skin cancer in the United States, with more than 100,000 new cases diagnosed annually. As with other sunlight induced skin cancers, the frequency of squamous cell carcinoma is increased in those who are fair complected or engage in many outdoor activities. The history of a bleeding growth or ulcer should arouse suspicion of squamous cell carcinoma. Squamous cell carcinoma most often arises in sun-damaged skin. It also develops on the mucous membranes and in areas of chronic injury such as burn scars, chronic radio-dermatitic lesions, chronic draining sinuses, and areas of erosive discoid lupus erythematosus. The examination reveals a hard papule or nodule that is erythematous to flesh-colored, smooth, scaling, and crusted. Squamous cell carcinoma in situ (Bowen's disease) has a different appearance, being a well-demarcated, slightly scaling, slightly crusted, eczematous-appearing patch.

The differential diagnosis of squamous cell carcinoma includes keratoacanthoma (which some consider a subset of squamous cell carcinoma), hypertrophic actinic keratosis, wart, basal cell carcinoma, and seborrheic keratosis. Any lesion that is crusted or ulcerated should be suspected of being squamous cell carcinoma, and biopsy must be done. This reveals a hyperkeratotic thickened epidermis containing atypical keratinocytes that invade the dermis.

Treatment (Table 13.11)

Squamous cell carcinoma should be totally excised. Follow-up to monitor for local recurrence as well as metastases is required. The squamous cell carcinomas most likely to metastasize in immunosuppressed patients and are lesions that are large, histologically poorly differentiated, have deep invasion, perineural invasion, or occur in damaged skin or the mucous membranes of the lips, glans penis, and vulva. Metastasis is generally to the regional lymph nodes, and careful attention should be given to examining the patient for lymphadenopathy.

Wart

Definition and etiology

Warts (verruca vulgaris) are benign neoplasms of the epidermis that are caused by the papillomavirus.

Clinical features

Warts affect people of all ages but are most common in children and young adults. Anogenital warts are usually sexually transmitted by adults and are probably the most common sexually transmitted disease. In children, genital warts should raise the suspicion of sexual abuse, but is not conclusive evidence of abuse. In immunosuppressed patients, particularly transplant recipients, warts can be a difficult problem. Warts have a somewhat different appearance depending on their type.

Common and plantar warts, which occur on the hands and feet, have a flesh-colored, scaling, and corrugated surface that characteristically interrupts skin lines and contains black puncta. Flat warts usually occur on the head and hand, are subtle, flesh-colored or reddish, slightly raised, flat-topped papules 2–5 mm in size. Venereal or genital warts (condyloma acuminatum) are soft, moist, often cauliflower-like, flesh and brown-colored papules and plaques in the perineum. A linear arrangement (Koebner phenomenon) of warts occurs from autoinoculation.

The diagnosis of warts is usually straightforward from their typical clinical appearance. In adults who have a persistent lesion that crusts and is unresponsive to usual wart therapies, squamous cell carcinoma should be considered. A skin biopsy of a wart will reveal benign epidermal papillomatoses and large keratinocytes with small pyknotic nuclei (koilocytes). Plantar warts sometimes can be confused with corns or calluses. Pairing off the thick hyperkeratotic surface reveals the interruption of skin lines and black puncta of a wart. Flat warts may be confused with comedones when on the face and lichen planus when on the hands. Genital warts can appear similar to seborrheic keratoses and also the lesions of secondary syphilis, condyloma latum.

Treatment (Table 13.12)

The treatment of warts is destructive and usually painful. The goal is to eliminate the skin that is infected with the virus. The two most common methods are topical acids available over the counter and liquid nitrogen cryotherapy in the office. Overzealous treatment that results in unbearable discomfort and scarring should be avoided. Untreated, many warts, perhaps half, will spontaneously resolve in 1 or 2 years. Other treatment modalities include podophyllin, imiquimod and sinecatechins (especially for genital warts), intralesionally bleomycin, cantharidin, surgical excision, electrodesiccation, and laser therapy.

Table 13.11 Treatment of squamous cell carcinoma

Treatment	Precautions
Excision	Bleeding, infection, scar
Curettage and electrodessication	Experience needed, infection, scar
Mohs micrographic surgery	Mostly head and neck, recurrent tumor
Alternatives: radiation, cryotherapy, intralesional 5-fluorouracil, or bleomycin	Use cautiously and in very selected cases

Table 13.12 Treatment of wart

Treatment	Precautions
None: await spontaneous involution	May spread and enlarge
Cryotherapy with liquid nitrogen	Pain, scar, hypopigmentation
Salicylic acid 17–40% under occlusion	Maceration
Alternatives: cantharidin, tretinoin (flat warts), podophyllin (genital warts) podofilox (genital warts), sinecatechins (genital warts) imiquimod (genital warts)	Local irritation/blistering
Surgical destruction	Scar

Chapter 14 Pigmented growths

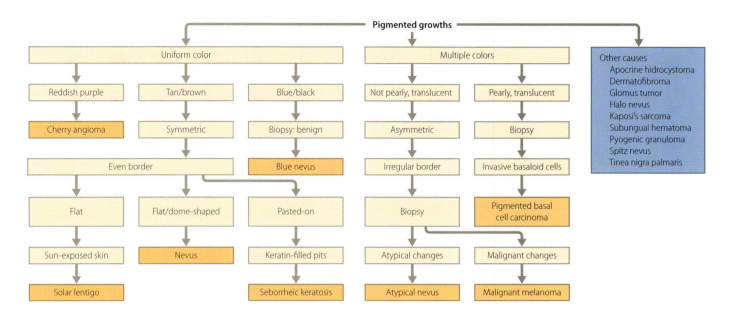

INTRODUCTION

Pigmented growths are an important group of neoplasms because their differential diagnosis includes malignant melanoma, which if recognized early is curable but if untreated is deadly. The neoplasms in this chapter are characterized by an increased amount of pigment or pigment-forming cells. For any pigmented growth in which the diagnosis is uncertain or in which malignant melanoma is a possibility, a biopsy is mandatory. Common pigmented lesions other than melanocytic nevus or melanoma include seborrheic keratosis, pigmented basal cell carcinoma, solar lentigines, and cherry angiomas. In seborrhoeic keratosis, pigmented basal cell carcinoma, and solar lentigines, the increased pigment is in keratinocytes, in contrast to cherry angiomas which only appear pigmented because of blood-filled vessels in the dermis.

1. MELANOCYTIC NEVUS VERSUS MALIGNANT MELANOMA

■ Features in common: pigmented papule

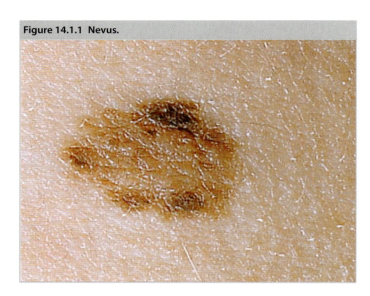

Figure 14.1.1 Nevus.

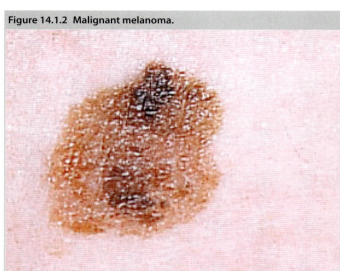

Figure 14.1.2 Malignant melanoma.

■ Distinguishing features

	Melanocytic nevus	Malignant melanoma*
Physical examination Morphology	Uniform color: tan, brown Symmetric Regular border < 6 mm in size (usually)	Multiple colors: black, blue, pink, white, tan, brown Asymmetric Irregular border > 6 mm in size
Distribution	Generalized	Generalized
History Symptoms	No change in size or color No bleeding	Change in size and color Bleeds
Exacerbating factors	Sunlight	Sunlight
Associated findings	None	Sun-damaged skin Lymphadenopathy
Epidemiology	Common	Uncommon Rarely familial
Biopsy	Yes, if worrisome lesion; shows melanocytes in nests No atypia	Yes; malignant melanocytes arranged in single cells and nests Atypia present
Laboratory	None	None initially
Outcome	Does not metastasize	May metastasize
* Large melanomas may bleed and have loss of hair follicles, but if one waits for these features to appear, the lesions will be deep and the patient's prognosis very poor.		

Differential diagnosis of pigmented papules

- Melanoma
- Pigmented basal cell carcinoma
- Seborrheic keratosis
- Hemangioma, angiokeratoma
- Nevi: atypical, Spitz, halo, blue
- Kaposi's sarcoma
- Lentigo
- Tattoo
- Hemorrhage (talon noir)

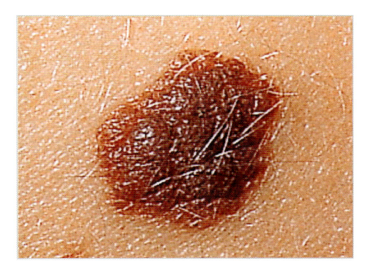

Figure 14.1.3 Nevus. *Clue to diagnosis:* even brown color, border, surface.

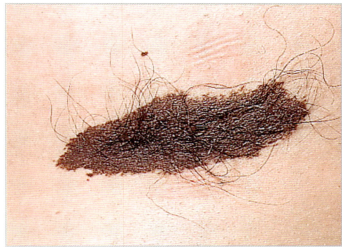

Figure 14.1.4 Congenital nevus.

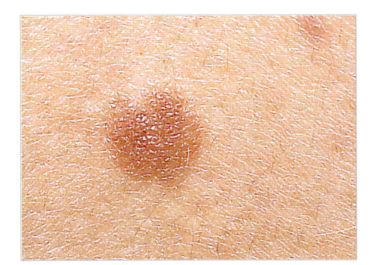

Figure 14.1.5 Compound nevus.

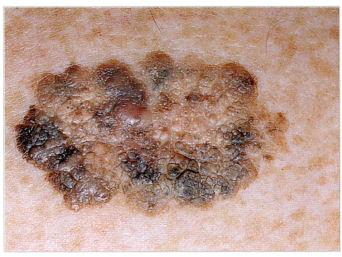

Figure 14.1.6 Malignant melanoma. *Clue to diagnosis:* multiple colors (red, white, blue).

256 PIGMENTED GROWTHS

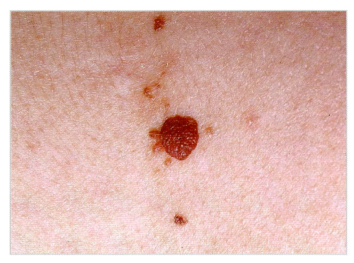

Figure 14.1.7 Nevus.

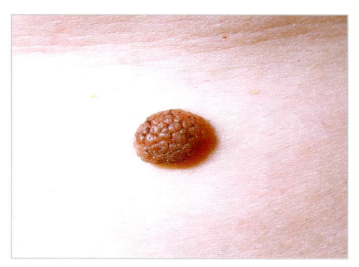

Figure 14.1.8 Nevus.

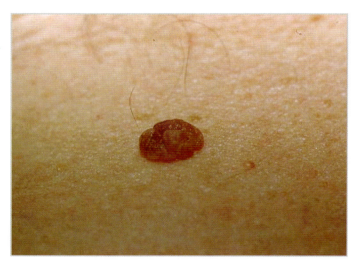

Figure 14.1.9 Nevus.

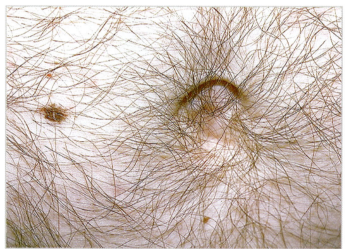

Figure 14.1.10 Nevus.

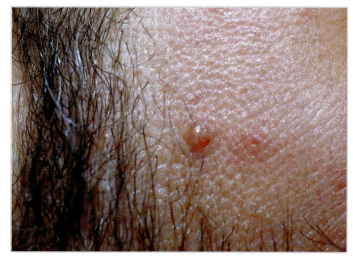

Figure 14.1.11 Nevus.

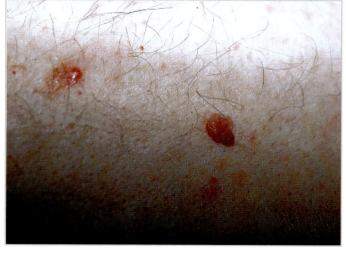

Figure 14.1.12 Nevus.

Melanocytic nevus versus malignant melanoma

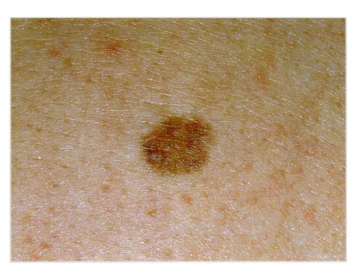

Figure 14.1.13 Nevus.

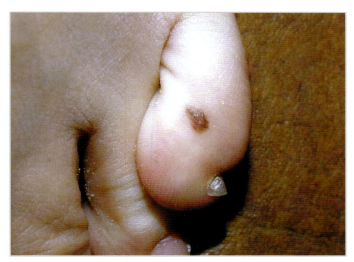

Figure 14.1.14 Nevus.

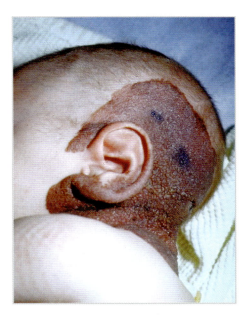

Figure 14.1.15 Nevus: congenital.

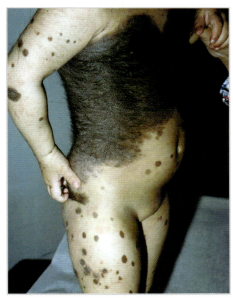

Figure 14.1.16 Nevus: congenital.

PIGMENTED GROWTHS

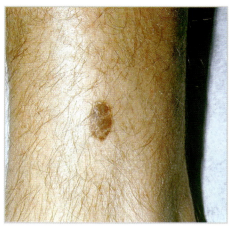

Figure 14.1.17 Nevus: congenital.

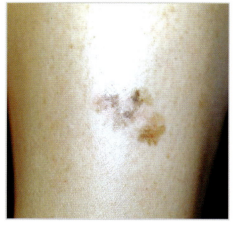

Figure 14.1.18 Malignant melanoma.

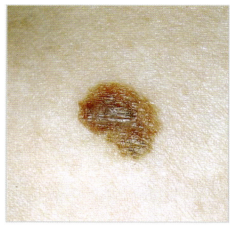

Figure 14.1.19 Malignant melanoma.

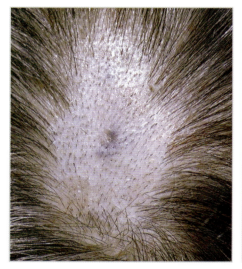

Figure 14.1.20 Malignant melanoma.

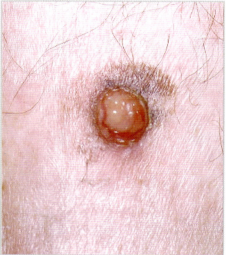

Figure 14.1.21 Malignant melanoma.

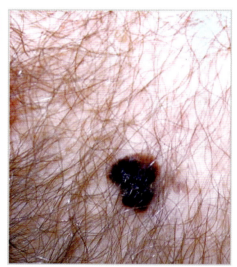

Figure 14.1.22 Malignant melanoma.

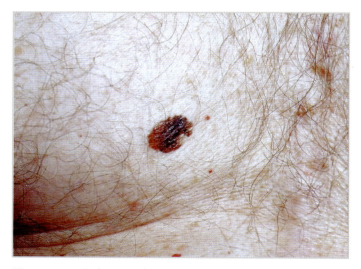

Figure 14.1.23 Malignant melanoma.

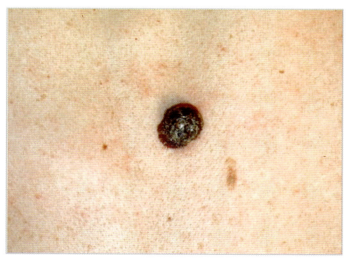

Figure 14.1.24 Malignant melanoma.

Melanocytic nevus versus malignant melanoma

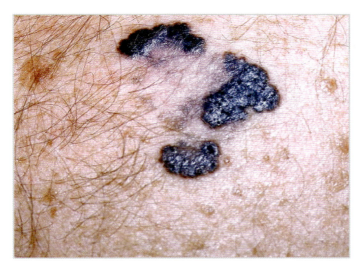

Figure 14.1.25 Malignant melanoma.

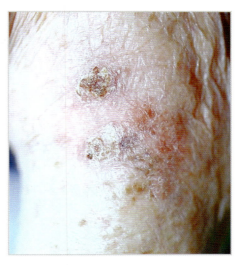

Figure 14.1.26 Malignant melanoma.

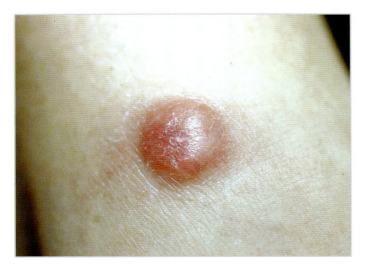

Figure 14.1.27 Malignant melanoma: metastatic.

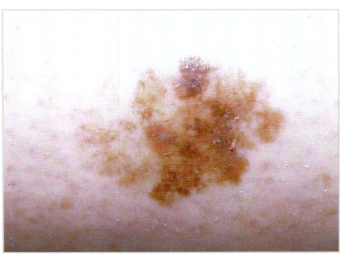

Figure 14.1.28 Malignant melanoma in a patient with familial atypical mole and melanoma syndrome.

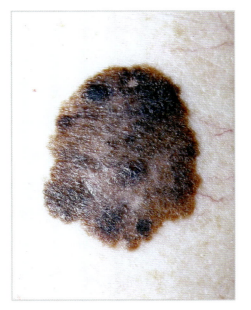

Figure 14.1.29 Malignant melanoma.

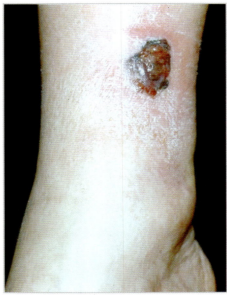

Figure 14.1.30 Malignant melanoma.

PIGMENTED GROWTHS

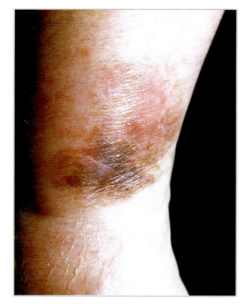

Figure 14.1.31 Malignant melanoma.

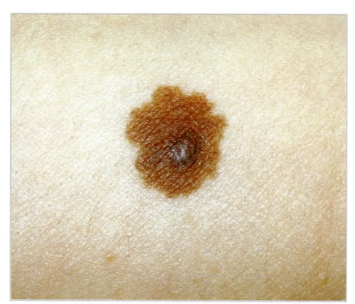

Figure 14.1.32 Malignant melanoma.

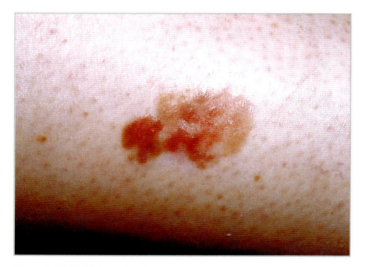

Figure 14.1.33 Malignant melanoma.

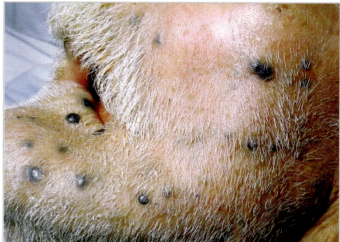

Figure 14.1.34 Malignant melanoma: metastatic.

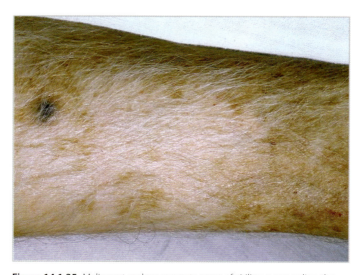

Figure 14.1.35 Malignant melanoma: note areas of vitiligo surrounding the melanoma.

2. ATYPICAL NEVUS VERSUS MALIGNANT MELANOMA

■ Features in common: pigmented papules

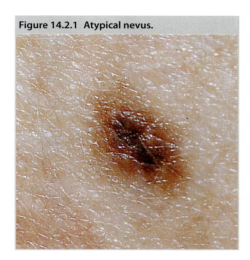

Figure 14.2.1 Atypical nevus.

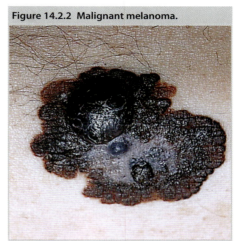

Figure 14.2.2 Malignant melanoma.

■ Distinguishing features

	Atypical nevus	Malignant melanoma*
Physical examination Morphology	Multiple colors: black, blue, pink, white, tan, brown Asymmetric Irregular border < 6 mm in size	Multiple colors: black, blue, pink, white, tan, brown Asymmetric Irregular border > 6 mm in size
Distribution	Generalized	Generalized
History Symptoms Exacerbating factors	Change in size or color Sunlight	Change in size and color Sunlight
Associated findings	None	Sun-damaged skin Lymphadenopathy
Epidemiology	Common Rarely familial	Uncommon Rarely familial
Biopsy	Yes; melanocytes not atypical, architectural disorder	Yes; malignant melanocytes arranged in single cells and nests
Laboratory	None	None initially
Outcome	Does not metastasize	May metastasize

*Large melanomas may bleed and have loss of hair follicles, but if one waits for these features to appear, the lesions will be deep and the patient's prognosis very poor.

3. SEBORRHEIC KERATOSIS VERSUS MELANOCYTIC NEVUS

■ Features in common: tan or brown papule or plaque

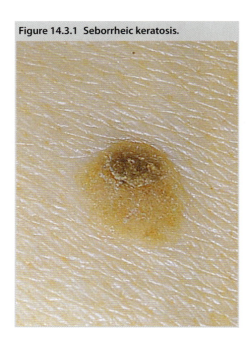

Figure 14.3.1 Seborrheic keratosis.

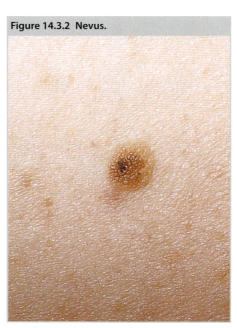

Figure 14.3.2 Nevus.

■ Distinguishing features

	Seborrheic keratosis	Melanocytic nevus
Physical examination Morphology	Pasted-on appearance Keratin-filled pits Greasy	Not pasted-on No pits Not greasy
Distribution	Generalized	Generalized
History Symptoms	None	None
Exacerbating factors	None	Sunlight
Associated findings	None	None
Epidemiology	Common Middle-aged and elderly	Common More common in young adults
Biopsy	No, unless worrisome or irritated	No, unless worrisome or irritated; shows nested melanocytes
Laboratory	None	None
Outcome	Chronic	Chronic

Differential diagnosis of brown papule or plaque

- Basal cell carcinoma
- Blue nevus
- Hemangioma
- Malignant melanoma
- Seborrheic keratosis

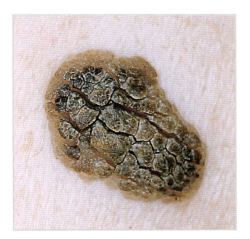

Figure 14.3.3 Seborrheic keratosis. *Clue to diagnosis:* pasted-on well-demarcated plaque.

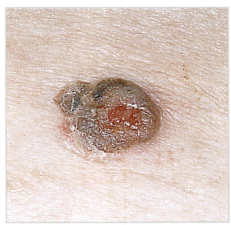

Figure 14.3.4 Irritated seborrheic keratosis.

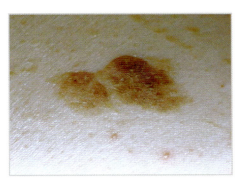

Figure 14.3.5 Seborrheic keratosis.

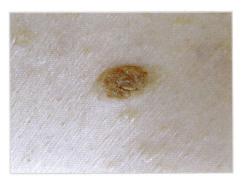

Figure 14.3.6 Seborrheic keratosis.

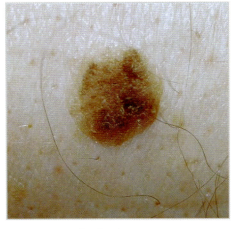

Figure 14.3.7 Seborrheic keratosis.

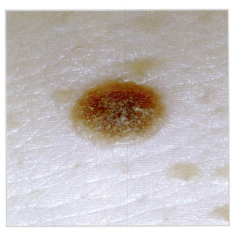

Figure 14.3.8 Seborrheic keratosis.

264 PIGMENTED GROWTHS

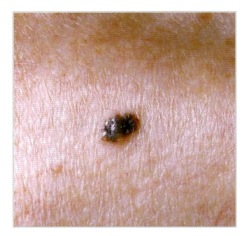

Figure 14.3.9 Seborrheic keratosis.

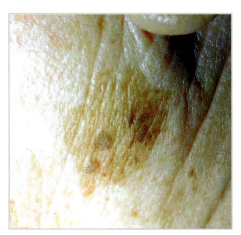

Figure 14.3.10 Seborrheic keratosis.

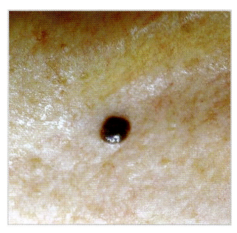

Figure 14.3.11 Seborrheic keratosis.

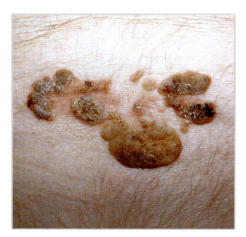

Figure 14.3.12 Seborrheic keratosis.

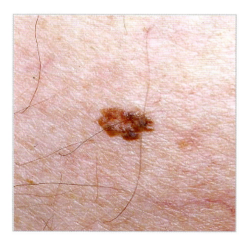

Figure 14.3.13 Seborrheic keratosis.

4. MALIGNANT MELANOMA VERSUS PIGMENTED BASAL CELL CARCINOMA

■ Features in common: pigmented papule

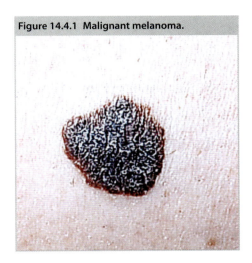

Figure 14.4.1 Malignant melanoma.

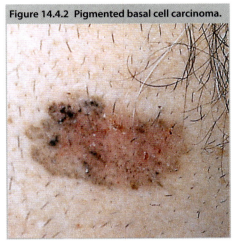

Figure 14.4.2 Pigmented basal cell carcinoma.

■ Distinguishing features

	Malignant melanoma*	Pigmented basal cell carcinoma
Physical examination Morphology	No telangiectasias Not pearly or translucent Multiple colors: black, blue, pink, white, tan, brown No crust Asymmetric Irregular border	Telangiectasias Pearly or translucent Multiple colors: black, blue Crust may be present Asymmetric Irregular border
Distribution	Generalized	Generalized
History Symptoms	Change in size and color	Change in size and color
Exacerbating factors	Sunlight	Sunlight
Associated findings	Sun-damaged skin Lymphadenopathy	Sun-damaged skin No lymphadenopathy
Epidemiology	Less common Rarely familial	Common Not familial
Biopsy	Yes; malignant melanocytes arranged in single cells and nests	Yes; invasive buds and lobules of basaloid cells
Laboratory	None initially	None
Outcome	May metastasize	Does not metastasize

*Large melanomas may bleed and have loss of hair follicles, but if one waits for these features to appear, the lesions will be deep and the patient's prognosis very poor.

Differential diagnosis of pigmented papules

- Nevus
- Seborrheic keratosis
- Hemangioma
- Malignant melanoma
- Pigmented basal cell carcinoma

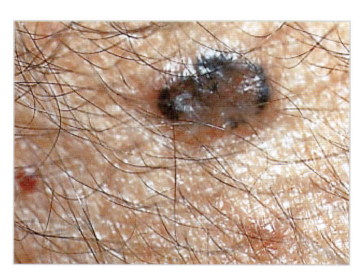

Figure 14.4.3 Pigmented basal cell carcinoma. *Clue to diagnosis:* pearly or translucent color.

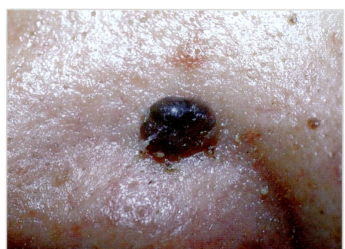

Figure 14.4.4 Pigmented basal cell carcinoma.

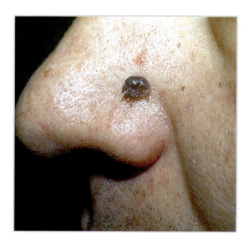

Figure 14.4.5 Pigmented basal cell carcinoma.

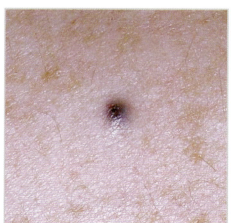

Figure 14.4.6 Pigmented basal cell carcinoma.

5. BLUE NEVUS VERSUS MALIGNANT MELANOMA

■ Features in common: blue or black papule or nodule

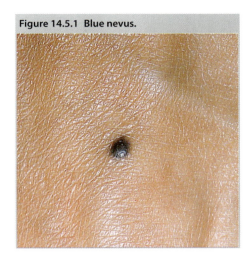

Figure 14.5.1 Blue nevus.

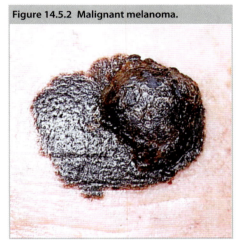

Figure 14.5.2 Malignant melanoma.

■ Distinguishing features

	Blue nevus	Malignant melanoma*
Physical examination Morphology	Uniform color: blue/black Symmetric Regular border	Multiple colors: black, blue, pink, white, tan, brown Asymmetric Irregular border
Distribution	Generalized	Generalized
History Symptoms	No itching No change in size or color No bleeding	Itches Change in size and color Bleeds
Exacerbating factors	None	Sunlight
Associated findings	None	Sun-damaged skin Lymphadenopathy
Epidemiology	Common Not familial	Uncommon Rarely familial
Biopsy	Yes; if worrisome lesion; shows melanocytes in nests No atypia	Yes; malignant melanocytes arranged in single cells and nests Atypia present
Laboratory	None	Chest X-ray
Outcome	Does not metastasize	May metastasize

*Large melanomas may bleed and have loss of hair follicles, but if one waits for these features to appear, the lesions will be deep and the patient's prognosis very poor.

Differential diagnosis of blue or black papule or nodule

- Pigmented basal cell carcinoma
- Seborrheic keratosis
- Hemangioma
- Angiokeratoma
- Atypical nevus
- Nevus
- Tattoo
- Hemorrhage (talon noir)
- Malignant melanoma

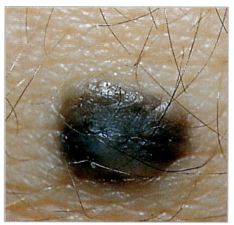

Figure 14.5.3 Blue nevus. *Clue to diagnosis:* even color, border, surface.

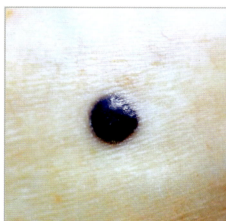

Figure 14.5.4 Blue nevus.

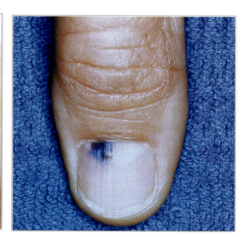

Figure 14.5.5 Blue nevus.

6. SOLAR LENTIGO VERSUS LENTIGO MALIGNA MELANOMA

Features in common: pigmented macule

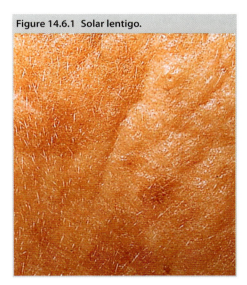

Figure 14.6.1 Solar lentigo.

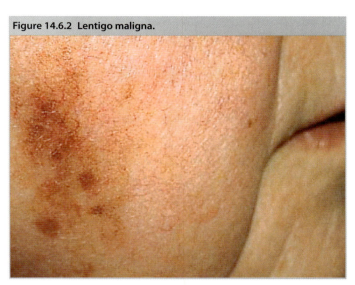

Figure 14.6.2 Lentigo maligna.

Distinguishing features

	Solar lentigo	Lentigo maligna melanoma*
Physical examination Morphology	Uniform color: tan, brown Symmetric Regular border	Multiple colors: black, blue, pink, white, tan, brown Asymmetric Irregular border
Distribution	Sun-exposed areas	Sun-exposed and non-sun-exposed areas
History Symptoms	No change in size or color	Change in size and color
Exacerbating factors	Sunlight	Sunlight
Associated findings	Sun-damaged skin No lymphadenopathy	Sun-damaged skin Lymphadenopathy
Epidemiology	Common	Uncommon
Biopsy	Yes, if worrisome lesion; shows uniform pigmentation along basal layers of elongated rete ridges	Yes; malignant melanocytes arranged in single cells and nests
Laboratory	None	Chest X-ray
Outcome	Does not metastasize	May metastasize

*Large melanomas may bleed and have loss of hair follicles, but if one waits for these features to appear, the lesions will be deep and the patient's prognosis very poor.

Differential diagnosis of pigmented macules

- Common causes
  - Freckle
  - Simple lentigo
  - Solar lentigo
  - Café au lait spot
  - Becker's nevus
  - Mongolian spot
  - Congenital nevus
  - Seborrheic keratosis
  - Postinflammatory hyperpigmentation
- Rarer causes
  - Syndromes: LEOPARD, NAME, Peutz–Jeghers
  - Degos' disease
  - Confluent and reticulate papillomatosis
  - Ochronosis
  - Granuloma faciale
  - Lichen planus
  - Nevi of Ota and Ito
  - Lentigo maligna melanoma

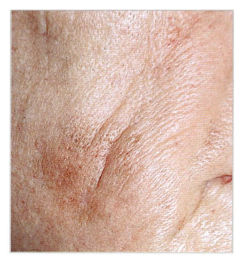

Figure 14.6.3 Solar lentigo. *Clue to diagnosis:* Even brown or tan color.

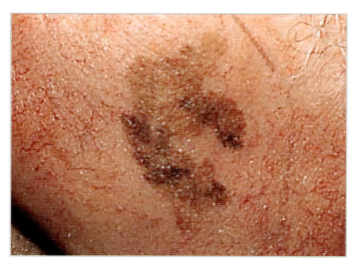

Figure 14.6.4 Lentigo maligna. *Clue to diagnosis:* Uneven blue, black, brown color.

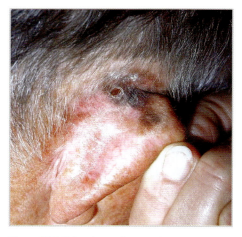

Figure 14.6.5 Lentigo maligna melanoma.

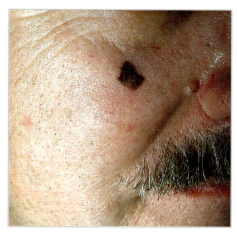

Figure 14.6.6 Lentigo maligna melanoma.

7. CHERRY ANGIOMA VERSUS MALIGNANT MELANOMA

Features in common: reddish papule or nodule

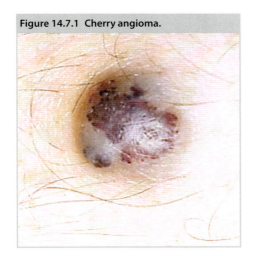

Figure 14.7.1 Cherry angioma.

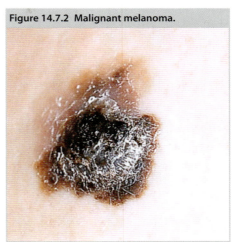

Figure 14.7.2 Malignant melanoma.

Distinguishing features

	Cherry angioma	Malignant melanoma*
Physical examination		
Morphology	Uniform color: red, violet May blanch Symmetric Regular border	Multiple colors: black, blue, pink, white, tan, brown Does not blanch Asymmetric Irregular border
Distribution	Generalized	Generalized
History		
Symptoms	No change in size or color	Change in size and color
Exacerbating factors	None	Sunlight
Associated findings	None	Sun-damaged skin Lymphadenopathy
Epidemiology	Common Not familial	Uncommon Rarely familial
Biopsy	Yes; if worrisome lesion; shows blood vessels	Yes; malignant melanocytes arranged in single cells and nests
Laboratory	None	None initially
Outcome	Does not metastasize	May metastasize

*Large melanomas may bleed and have loss of hair follicles, but if one waits for these features to appear, the lesions will be deep and the patient's prognosis very poor.

Differential diagnosis of reddish papule or nodule

- Angiokeratoma
- Pyogenic granuloma
- Kaposi's sarcoma
- Dermatofibroma
- Angiolymphoid hyperplasia
- Tattoo
- Metastatic cancer, especially renal cell cancer
- Cherry angioma
- Malignant melanoma

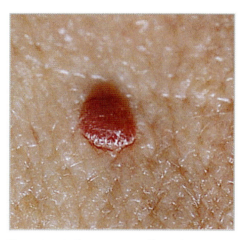

Figure 14.7.3 Cherry angioma. *Clue to diagnosis:* Red vascular appearance.

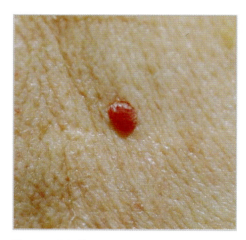

Figure 14.7.4 Cherry angioma.

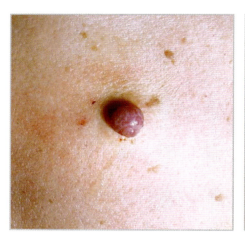

Figure 14.7.5 Cherry angioma.

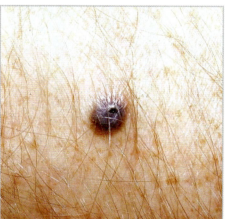

Figure 14.7.6 Cherry angioma.

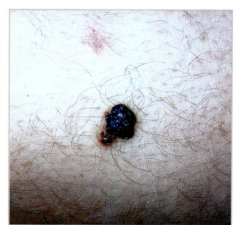

Figure 14.7.7 Cherry angioma.

8. PIGMENTED GROWTHS

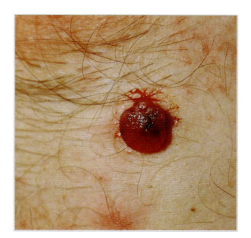

Figure 14.8.1 Pyogenic granuloma.

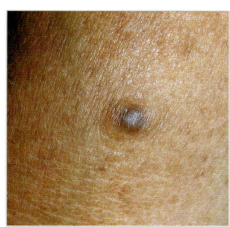

Figure 14.8.2 Dermatofibroma.

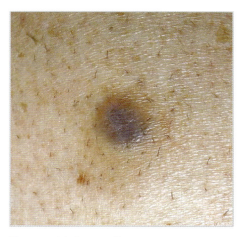

Figure 14.8.3 Dermatofibroma.

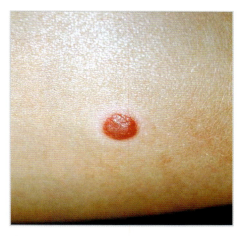

Figure 14.8.4 Spitz nevus.

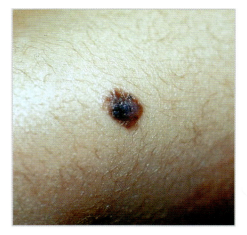

Figure 14.8.5 Spitz nevus.

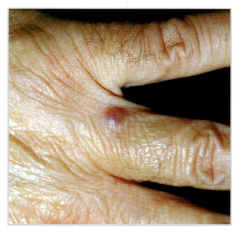

Figure 14.8.6 Kaposi's sarcoma.

274 PIGMENTED GROWTHS

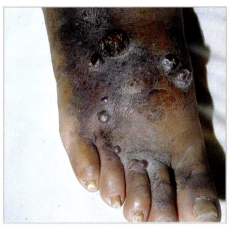

Figure 14.8.7 Kaposi's sarcoma.

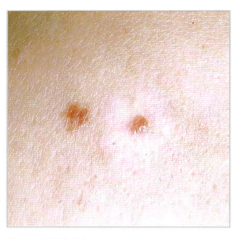

Figure 14.8.8 Halo nevus.

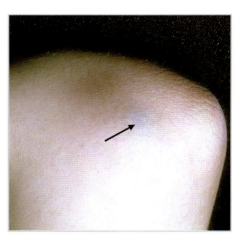

Figure 14.8.9 Glomus (arrow).

9. OTHER EXAMPLES

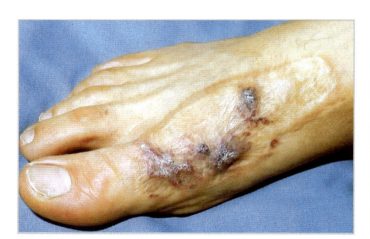

Figure 14.9.1 Verrucous hemangioma.

Figure 14.9.2 Nevus spilus.

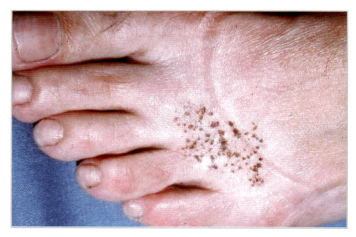

Figure 14.9.3 Nevus spilus.

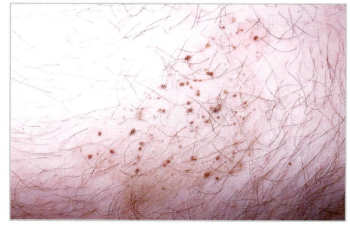

Figure 14.9.4 Nevus spilus.

Other examples

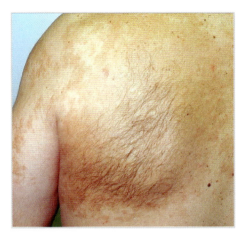
Figure 14.9.5 Becker's nevus.

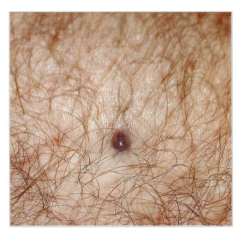
Figure 14.9.6 Lymphangioma.

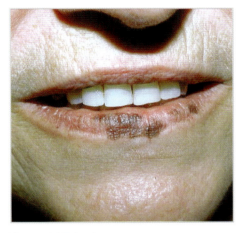
Figure 14.9.7 Lentigo.

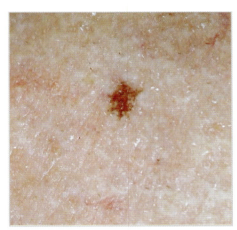
Figure 14.9.8 Ink-spot lentigo.

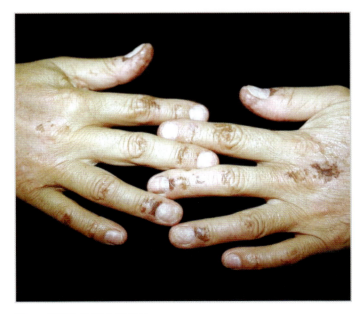
Figure 14.9.9 PUVA lentigines.

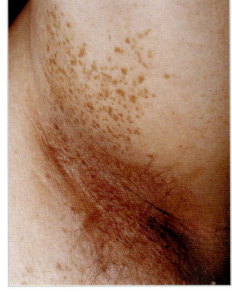
Figure 14.9.10 Lentigo: Crowe's sign found in neurofibromatosis (axilla).

PIGMENTED GROWTHS

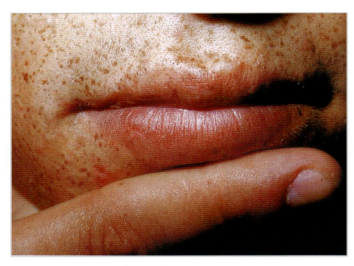

Figure 14.9.11 Peutz–Jeghers syndrome.

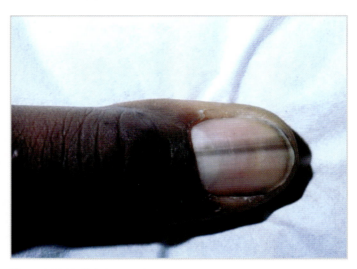

Figure 14.9.12 Nail pigmentation.

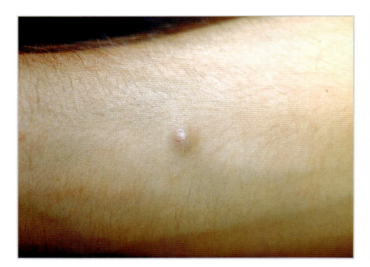

Figure 14.9.13 Eccrine spiradenoma.

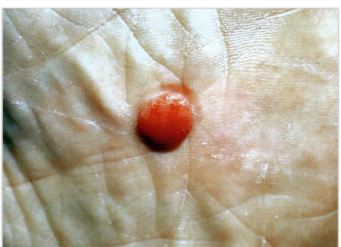

Figure 14.9.14 Eccrine poroma.

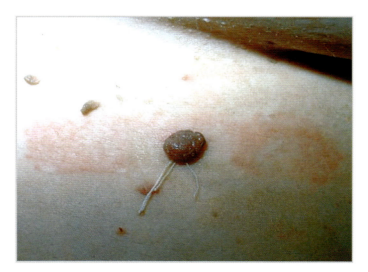

Figure 14.9.15 Skin tag.

DISEASE DISCUSSION

■ Cherry angioma

Definition and etiology
Cherry angioma is a benign neoplasm of blood vessels.

Clinical features
The most common form of hemangioma is the superficial cherry hemangioma that occurs in adults. Its appearance varies from a pinpoint-sized, red petechial appearing macule to a red, blue, or purple smooth dome-shaped papule or nodule.

Hemangiomas most commonly occur on the trunk, begin in early adulthood, and increase in number with age. When they are blue to purple, the differential diagnosis includes blue nevus and malignant melanoma. Blanching with pressure is a diagnostic feature of cherry angioma but may not always be found. When the diagnosis is in doubt, a biopsy should be performed and will reveal benign proliferation of small dilated blood vessels.

Treatment (Table 14.1)
Treatment of cherry angioma is usually not necessary. If removal is desired, it can be destroyed with light electrodesiccation, scalpel or scissors excision, or a laser.

■ Malignant melanoma

Definition and etiology
Malignant melanoma is a cancerous proliferation of melanocytes. Although the precise cause of malignant melanoma is unknown, sunlight and heredity appear to be the most important risk factors.

Clinical features
The incidence of malignant melanoma is increasing, with more than 35,000 new cases diagnosed yearly in the United States. It is estimated that 1% of individuals in the United States will develop malignant melanoma in their lifetimes. The highest incidence of malignant melanoma in the world is in Queensland, Australia, where there is abundant equatorial sunlight and a predominantly fair-skinned population.

Occasionally, there is a family history of malignant melanoma. Most individuals notice a change in the malignant melanoma prior to diagnosis, such as development of a new growth, increase in size, change in color, and rarely bleeding or itching.

The characteristic signs of a majority of malignant melanomas are referred to as the ABCDs: (1) *asymmetry*, (2) *border irregularity* (notched border), (3) *color variation* (red, white, blue), and (4) *diameter* greater than 6 mm. Four clinical types of malignant melanoma have been described: (1) superficial spreading malignant melanoma, (2) lentigo maligna melanoma, (3) nodular melanoma, and (4) acral lentiginous melanoma. These clinical subtypes are somewhat arbitrary, since they exhibit similar features. The superficial spreading melanoma is the most common type and demonstrates all the characteristic ABCD signs. It occurs most frequently in young and middle-aged white adults on all skin surfaces, with preference for the back and legs. Superficial spreading malignant melanoma may be present a couple of years before it metastasizes. Lentigo maligna melanoma occurs in elderly whites on sun-exposed skin, especially the head and neck. It also has the ABCD signs and can reach a diameter of 5 to 7 cm before becoming invasive and metastatic. Nodular melanoma is a rapidly growing blue, black, red, or, occasionally, flesh-colored nodule affecting young to middle-aged whites. Unfortunately, nodular melanoma often metastasizes before clinical attention is sought and the diagnosis is made. The ABCD signs do not work for nodular melanoma. Therefore, any growing or changing melanocytic neoplasm should undergo biopsy. Acral-lentiginous melanoma occurs on the palms, the soles, and the distal portion of the toes and fingers. It demonstrates the ABCD signs but unfortunately often has already metastasized before diagnosis.

In contrast to other malignant melanomas, blacks and Asians most commonly have acral-lentiginous melanoma. Atypical or suspicious pigmented lesions should undergo biopsy to rule out malignant melanoma. Watching and waiting before a diagnosis is made may result in death. The preferable method of biopsy is by excision with narrow 2–3 mm margins of normal skin. The biopsy findings reveal malignant melanocytes within the epidermis and dermis scattered individually and in various-sized nests, usually associated with inflammation. The differential diagnosis of malignant melanoma includes nevus, atypical nevus, blue nevus, seborrheic keratosis, cherry angioma, pigmented basal cell carcinoma, actinic lentigo, pyogenic granuloma, and dermatofibroma.

Early melanomas cannot always be distinguished from atypical nevi, since the latter can also have multiple colors and asymmetry and will be larger than 6 mm. Dermatoscopic examination may help in some lesions; however, any questionable borderline or changing lesions should undergo biopsy.

Treatment (Table 14.2)
Surgical excision is the treatment of choice and, if done early, is curative. Superficial spreading and lentigo maligna melanoma characteristically have an initial horizontal growth phase that is premetastatic and allows for early diagnosis and surgical cure.

Acral-lentiginous and nodular melanoma, unfortunately, are usually already in a vertical growth phase and therefore are often metastatic before diagnosis. The prognosis for malignant melanoma is best predicted by tumor thickness, with greater depth of invasion correlated with poor 5-year survival. Patients with malignant melanoma with a thickness of less than 0.75 mm have a 5-year survival rate of 99%, whereas those with disease of more than 3 mm in thickness have a poor prognosis, with less than 50% surviving 5 years. Beliefs about the extent of surgery necessary for malignant melanoma have evolved and are still somewhat controversial. A 1-cm margin of normal skin around the melanoma is certainly adequate for thin lesions less than 1.0 mm thick, and it is probably adequate for all melanomas, no matter how deeply invasive. Elective regional lymph node dissection is not usually recommended in thin melanomas. If metastases develop,

Table 14.1 Treatment of cherry angioma

Treatment	Precautions
None	Do not miss a melanoma for dark lesions
Electrodesiccation	Scar
Shave with scalpel or snip with scissors	Scar
Laser	Eye protection, scar

Table 14.2 Treatment of malignant melanoma

Treatment	Precautions
Wide excision with margins determined by melanoma thickness In situ: 0.5 cm margin, <2 mm to 1 cm margin, >2 mm to 2 cm margin	Infection, bleeding, scar
Staging sentinel lymph node biopsy for >1 mm thickness	Infection, bleeding, scar, lymphedema
Chemotherapy (dacarbazine, etc.)	Numerous
Immunotherapy (interferon, interleukin, ipilimumab, nivolumab)	Numerous
Kinase inhibitors (dabrafenib, vemurafenib, trametinib)	Numerous
Radiation	Burn, chronic radiodermatitis

chemotherapy, immunotherapy, and kinase inhibitors are usually palliative and not curative.

Periodic follow-up of patients is recommended. The history and physical examination of the skin, lymph nodes, liver, and spleen are the most important parameters in detecting recurrence or metastasis. Certainly, extensive laboratory tests such as brain, bone, liver, and spleen scans are not indicated unless the history or physical examination suggests metastasis to these organs.

■ Melanocytic nevus

Definition and etiology
A nevus or mole is a benign neoplasm of melanocytes. Nevi are so common that they can be considered a normal skin finding.

Clinical features
Nevi are congenital (occurring in 1% of newborns) or are acquired in childhood, adolescence, or early adulthood. Whites have an average of 15–40 nevi per person, whereas blacks have 11. Symptomatic nevi should be regarded suspiciously at any time other than during pregnancy or adolescence, when darkening in color, itching, and development of new nevi are not uncommon.

Nevi can be subdivided histologically and clinically. Junctional nevi are macular, with nevus cells confined to the basal layer of the epidermis. Intradermal nevi are papular, with nevus cells within the dermis, and compound nevi are also papular, with nevus cells in the epidermis and dermis. These different types of nevi vary in appearance and coloration but individually have a fairly symmetric configuration, a regular border, a uniform flesh to brown color, and a relatively small diameter. They may have a smooth or varicoid surface and may be sessile or polypoid. The absence or presence of skin lines or hair has no diagnostic significance.

The most important disease in the differential diagnosis of a nevus is malignant melanoma. For all suspicious lesions, a biopsy is mandatory. The histologic examination of a nevus reveals uniform cells with an epithelioid, a lymphoid, or a spindle-cell appearance; cells are arranged in nests in the basal layer of the epidermis and papillary dermis. When nevus cells extend deeper into the dermis, cord or sheetlike formations occur. Usually, melanin pigment can be found in some of the cells.

A *blue nevu*s appears as a steel-blue papule or nodule. It usually appears in childhood, and its significance lies in its differentiation from nodular melanoma.

The biopsy findings reveal benign cells, generally with a lot of melanin pigment.

Atypical nevus (Clark's or dysplastic nevus) is important because it resembles malignant melanoma clinically, may be a precursor of malignant melanoma in some cases, and is the characteristic finding in individuals with the rare familial atypical mole and malignant melanoma syndrome. Atypical moles can be very difficult to differentiate from malignant melanoma, since they have similar clinical features.

The atypical nevus is often asymmetric, has an irregular border that blends into the normal surrounding skin, and varies in color from tan, brown, and pink to (sometimes) black. The surface is often irregular, having macular and papular portions. Atypical moles are common, with 5% of normal whites in the United States having these lesions. The risk of malignant melanoma in individuals with one or two atypical nevi is controversial but appears to be quite small. Individuals who have the familial atypical mole and melanoma syndrome will develop malignant melanoma in their lifetime, and they require close follow-up. Fortunately, this syndrome is rare. The biopsy findings in an atypical mole reveal architectural disorder of the melanocytes, dermal fibrotic response, and varying amounts of cytologic atypia.

Treatment (Table 14.3)
For a common nevus, no therapy is required unless there has been a worrisome change in color, shape, size, or amount of bleeding or itching. For suspicious lesions, a deep shave or an excisional biopsy with narrow margins is recommended. For clinically benign and cosmetically unsightly nevi, a shave excision with a scalpel is acceptable. However, this leaves some residual nevus cells at the biopsy site that may become darkly pigmented. All removed nevi should be examined by a pathologist to confirm their benign nature. For congenital nevi, only those that are large (greater than 20 cm in diameter) have a definitely increased potential to become malignant melanoma.

Otherwise, congenital nevi can be treated similarly to acquired nevi. For an individual with atypical moles, it should be decided whether this individual has familial atypical mole and melanoma syndrome, in which case close clinical follow-up is required with periodic full-skin examinations by the physician as well as monthly patient self-examinations. Sun protection is particularly prudent for these individuals.

■ Pigmented basal cell carcinoma

Definition and etiology
Basal cell carcinoma is a malignant neoplasm arising from the basal cells of the epidermis. Most basal cell carcinomas are caused by sunlight-induced damage to the skin. A pigmented basal cell carcinoma, as the name implies, contains blue and black pigment.

Clinical features
Basal cell carcinoma is the most frequent malignancy in the United States, with more than 750,000 new cases reported annually. Although basal cell carcinoma almost never metastasizes, its malignant nature is emphasized by the local destruction that it can cause. As with other

Table 14.3 Treatment of nevus

Treatment	Precautions
None if not worrisome	Do not miss a melanoma
Shave biopsy	Scar
Deep shave excision, punch biopsy, or excision for suspicious lesion	Scar, infection, bleeding
Serial photographs	If change, biopsy

sun-induced neoplasms of the skin, fair-complected individuals and those with a lot of sunlight exposure are most likely to develop basal cell carcinoma. Pigmented basal cell carcinoma is a pearly, translucent, blue or black papule or nodule. Seborrheic keratosis, pigmented nevus, and, most important, malignant melanoma must be ruled out in the case of pigmented basal cell carcinoma. A skin biopsy, which reveals a thickened epidermis with invasive buds and lobules of malignant basal cells, should be accomplished to confirm the diagnosis. Seborrheic keratosis has a rough, stuck-on appearance. Nevi and malignant melanomas do not contain telangiectasias or have a pearly appearance.

Treatment (Table 14.4)

Curettage and electrodesiccation of the lesion or excision is the most common surgical modality used to treat basal cell carcinoma. Less commonly used treatments are radiation therapy, cryosurgery, and topical chemotherapy. A specialized surgical technique, Mohs' surgery, is indicated for recurrent basal cell carcinoma and for primary tumors with a high risk of recurrence.

■ Seborrheic keratosis

Definition and etiology

Seborrheic keratosis is a benign neoplasm of the epidermis that usually appears during middle age.

Clinical features

Unless irritated, seborrheic keratoses are asymptomatic. Most patients seek medical care when these benign tumors become irritated or displeasing cosmetically or when they are concerned that they may represent skin cancer, particularly malignant melanoma.

Seborrheic keratoses typically are well-demarcated, slightly scaling, greasy appearing, tan to dark brown, pasted-on symmetric papules and plaques. Their surface is often verrucous or crumbly in appearance and has small keratin-filled pits. They occur anywhere on the body with the exception of the palms and soles. The well-marginated (even bordered), symmetric, pasted-on appearance and the finding of multiple similar-appearing papules and plaques make the diagnosis of seborrheic keratosis generally straightforward. On occasion, though, they can mimic a wart, actinic keratosis, nevus, pigmented basal cell carcinoma, or malignant melanoma. When diagnosis is uncertain, biopsy findings reveal typical uniform well demarcated intraepithelial proliferation of small, benign squamous cells.

Treatment (Table 14.5)

No treatment is necessary for seborrheic keratoses unless they are irritated or cosmetically unacceptable. Freezing with liquid nitrogen is generally the most efficient and most effective method of treatment. Curettage or shave can be done for thicker lesions. Excisional surgery is not done unless there is concern about malignancy.

■ Solar lentigo

Definition and etiology

Solar lentigo is a brown macule induced by sunlight exposure and represents a proliferation of both keratinocytes and pigment.

Clinical features

Solar (actinic) lentigines arise in middle age and are numerous in sun-exposed skin. They are tan to brown macules ranging in size from a couple of millimeters to several centimeters. They occur on exposed areas of the body, dorsum of the hands, neck, head, and shoulders.

The main diseases in the differential diagnosis of solar lentigo are lentigo maligna melanoma and a thin seborrheic keratosis. A biopsy is mandatory for any lesion that develops an irregular border and color, particularly very dark brown or black hues. The biopsy findings in solar lentigo are characterized by hyperplastic epidermal rete ridges that contain increased amounts of melanin.

Treatment (Table 14.6)

No treatment is necessary, since solar lentigo is not a premalignant lesion. For cosmetic purposes, it may be treated with cryotherapy or laser.

Table 14.5 Treatment of seborrheic keratosis

Treatment	Precautions
None	Do not miss a melanoma
Cryotherapy with liquid nitrogen	Painful, scar, hypopigmentation
Curettage	Scar
Shave	Scar

Table 14.4 Treatment of pigmented basal cell carcinoma

Treatment	Precautions
Excision	Bleeding, infection, scar
Curettage and electrodessication	Experience needed, infection, scar
Mohs micrographic surgery	Mostly head and neck, recurrent tumor
Alternatives: radiation, cryotherapy, 5-fluorouracil, imiquimod, vismodegib	Use cautiously and in very selected cases

Table 14.6 Treatment of solar lentigo

Treatment	Precautions
None	Do not miss a melanoma
Sun protection	None
Cryotherapy	Scar, hypopigmentation
Laser	Eye protection, scar

Chapter 15   Benign dermal neoplasms

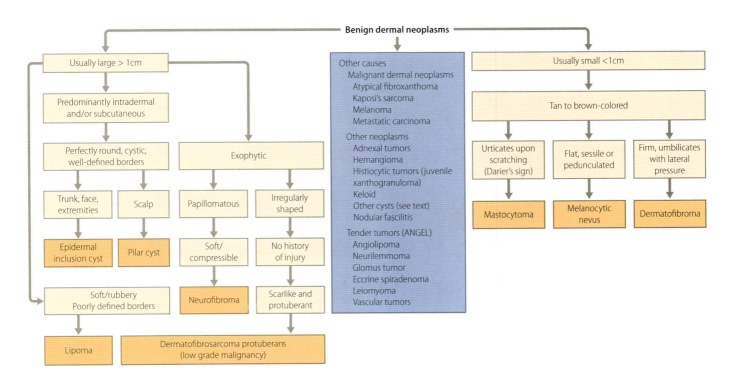

INTRODUCTION

The dermis and subcutaneous tissue contain a wide variety of cell types from which neoplasms may develop. Fibroblasts, sebocytes, hair follicles, smooth muscle cells, and nerves all may give rise to a variety of both benign and malignant neoplasms. Despite this broad and complex spectrum of dermal tumors, the vast majority of neoplasms encountered in clinical practice are limited to a subset of common and readily identified growths. Recognition of the different types of neoplasms is often possible based on color, size, location, and tactile properties. The most common tan-brown growths are nevi and dermatofibromas. Dermatofibromas can be distinguished from nevi by their 'center of gravity' in the mid to upper dermis and by the presence of puckering on lateral pressure.

Mastocytomas are benign growths arising from mast cells, most commonly seen in children. Usually they are red-brown or tan, are larger than nevi, and develop a surrounding wheal when stroked. Neurofibromas typically present as large exophytic pedunculated growths that can be pushed back into the skin to produce a dimple. Cysts are mobile well-demarcated deep dermal nodules that sometimes have an overlying dilated pore. Lipomas are softer and less demarcated and often have lobulated borders. Despite clinical clues, biopsy needs to be performed for some dermal neoplasms to allow for accurate diagnosis.

History of rapid growth, pain, or hemorrhage should prompt a close evaluation of any dermal neoplasm. This chapter helps clinicians develop a paradigm for deciding whether a neoplasm can simply be followed or whether it warrants biopsy or excision.

1. DERMATOFIBROMA VERSUS MELANOCYTIC NEVUS (INTRADERMAL)

■ Features in common: tan to brown-colored dermal papules or nodules

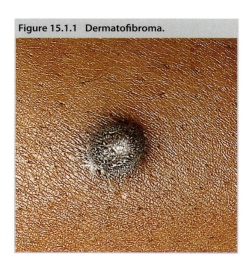

Figure 15.1.1 Dermatofibroma.

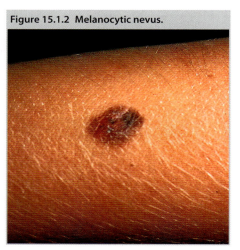

Figure 15.1.2 Melanocytic nevus.

■ Distinguishing features

	Dermatofibroma	Melanocytic nevus (intradermal)
Physical examination		
Morphology	Color: varies from yellow and reddish to dark brown Slight scale Not protuberant	Color: less varied, various shades of brown to skin-colored No scale Protuberant
Distribution	Dimples on lateral pressure (Fitzpatrick's dimple sign) Most frequently on extremities	No dimple sign Anywhere
History		
Symptoms	Antecedent history of an insect bite, folliculitis, or cyst occasionally pruritic	No antecedent history of bite, folliculitis, or cyst Rarely pruritic
Exacerbating factors	None	None
Associated findings	None	Family history of multiple moles
Epidemiology	Adults	Children and adults
Biopsy	No Epidermal hyperplasia, within dermis increased number of haphazardly distributed fibroblasts surrounding and entrapping collagen bundles	Sometimes Collection of melanocytes in nests; melanocytes 'mature' and become more spindle-shaped in the deeper dermis
Laboratory	None	None
Outcome	May involute over many years	May involute over many years

Dermatofibroma versus melanocytic nevus (intradermal)

Differential diagnosis of brown lesions

- Melanocytic nevus
- Dermatofibroma
- Lentigo: solar or simplex
- Café au lait spot
- Becker's nevus
- Mongolian spot
- Nevus of Ota
- Nevus of Ito
- Urticaria pigmentosa
- Juvenile xanthogranuloma
- Seborrheic keratosis
- Pigmented basal cell carcinoma

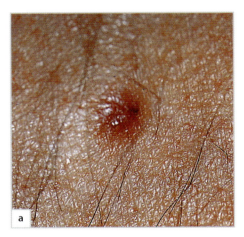 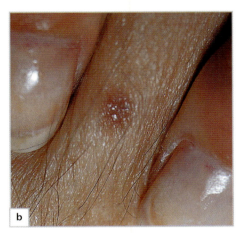

Figure 15.1.3 Dermatofibroma. *Clue to diagnosis:* (a) central pucker; (b) upon pressure.

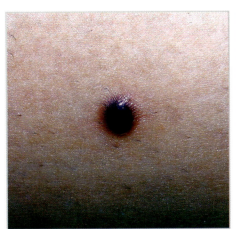 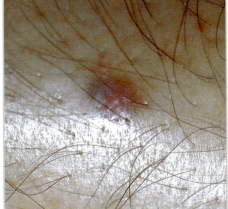 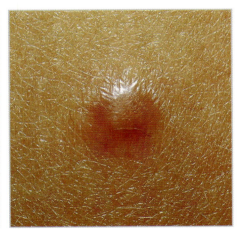

Figure 15.1.4 Dermatofibroma.   **Figure 15.1.5** Dermatofibroma.   **Figure 15.1.6** Dermatofibroma.

2. DERMATOFIBROMA VERSUS DERMATOFIBROSARCOMA PROTUBERANS

Features in common: dermal plaques or papules

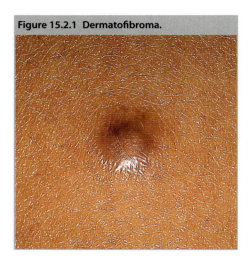

Figure 15.2.1 Dermatofibroma.

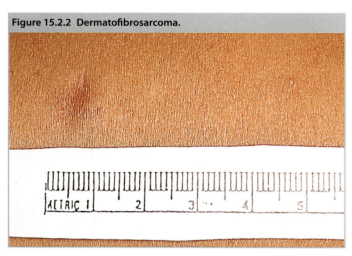

Figure 15.2.2 Dermatofibrosarcoma.

Distinguishing features

	Dermatofibroma	Dermatofibrosarcoma protuberans
Physical examination		
Morphology	Small < 1 cm (symmetric) Dimples on lateral pressure (Fitzpatrick's, dimple sign) Not protuberant Epidermis acanthotic and does not ulcerate Slight scale	Large > 1 cm (asymmetric) No dimple sign Protuberant tumor Epidermis atrophic and shiny and may ulcerate No scale
Distribution	Most frequently on extremities	Most common on back
History		
Symptoms	No growth Occasionally antecedent history of an insect bite, "pimple," or antecedent cyst No history of recurrence Occasionally pruritic	Slow growth No history of bite, 'pimple,' or antecedent cyst History of recurrence after prior removal in many cases Asymptomatic
Exacerbating factors	None	None
Associated findings	None	None
Epidemiology	Young adults Slightly more common in women	Adults Male predominance
Biopsy	No Epidermal hyperplasia; increased number of haphazardly distributed fibroblasts surrounding and entrapping collagen bundle Immunohistochemistry: factor XIIIa positive	Yes No epidermal hyperplasia; dense collection of fibroblast-like cells that form cartwheels and extend into subcutaneous tissue, forming fenestrated septae Immunohistochemistry: CD34 positive Fluorescent in situ hybridization studies show T(17, 22) translocation
Laboratory	None	None
Outcome	May resolve or involute over many years	Continued growth: frequently recurrent; rarely metastatic

Synonyms for variants of dermatofibroma

- Dermatofibroma with monster giant cells
- Epithelioid cell histiocytoma
- Fibroma durum
- Fibrous histiocytoma
- Granular cell dermatofibroma
- Nodular subepidermal fibrosis
- Sclerosing hemangioma

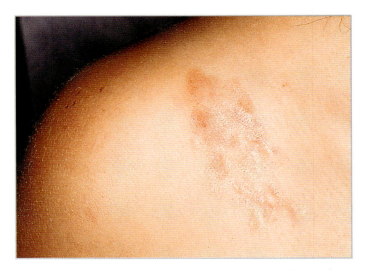

Figure 15.2.3 Dermatofibrosarcoma. *Clue to diagnosis:* irregular shape with protuberant nodules.

3. NEUROFIBROMA VERSUS MELANOCYTIC NEVUS (INTRADERMAL)

■ Features in common: exophytic tumor

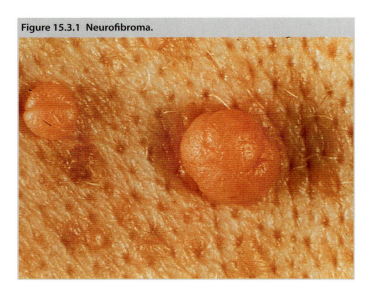

Figure 15.3.1 Neurofibroma.

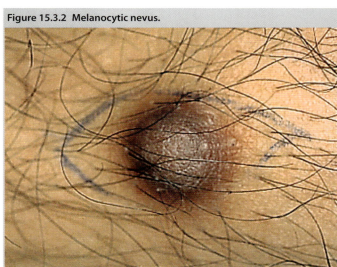

Figure 15.3.2 Melanocytic nevus.

■ Distinguishing features

	Neurofibroma	Melanocytic nevus (intradermal)
Physical examination Morphology	Skin colored Lesions polypoid or pedunculated "Button hole sign": invagination of lesion into skin with pressure	Various shades of brown to skin-colored Lesions flat or sessile: no invagination with pressure
Distribution	Any cutaneous surface	Any cutaneous surface
History Symptoms	None	None
Exacerbating factors	None	None
Associated findings	All ages No family history of multiple moles If multiple may be associated with neurofibromatosis: café au lait spots, axillary freckling, acoustic neuroma	All ages Family history of multiple moles No café au lait spots or axillary freckling
Epidemiology	Usually sporadic Neurofibromatosis: autosomal dominant inheritance	Young adults No sex predilection
Biopsy	No Small wavy spindle cells surrounded by a pale eosinophilic, slightly myxoid stroma containing mast cells	Sometimes Collection of melanocytes in nests Melanocytes "mature" and become more lymphoid and fibroblast-like in the deeper dermis
Laboratory	None	None
Outcome	Persists; rarely may evolve into neurofibro-sarcoma in patients with neurofibromatosis	May involute over many years

Riccardi's classification of neurofibromatosis

Type A: Congenital onset with total body involvement; neurofibromas present
1. Neurofibromatosis 1 (NF-1, von Recklinghausen's neurofibromatosis): most common form
2. Neurofibromatosis 2 (NF-2, acoustic neurofibromatosis)
3. Neurofibromatosis 3 (NF-3, mixed neurofibromatosis)
4. Neurofibromatosis 4 (NF-4, variant neurofibromatosis)

Type B: Limited in distribution or late onset; neurofibromas not always found
5. Neurofibromatosis 5 (NF-5, segmental neurofibromatosis)
6. Neurofibromatosis 6 (NF-6, café au lait neurofibromatosis)
7. Neurofibromatosis 7 (NF-7, late-onset neurofibromatosis)

Type C: Neurofibromatosis 8 (NF-8, unclassifiable)

Diagnostic criteria for von Recklinghausen's neurofibromatosis

Two of following seven criteria required:
1. Six or more café au lait spots over 5 mm in diameter in children or over 1.5 cm in diameter in adults
2. Two or more neurofibromas or a single plexiform neurofibroma (histologic diagnosis)
3. Crowe's sign: freckling in axillary or inguinal areas
4. Optic glioma
5. Lisch nodules on iris
6. Osseous lesions: sphenoid dysplasia, thinning of long-bone cortex
7. First-degree relative with neurofibromatosis

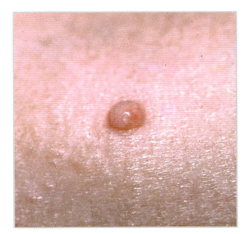

Figure 15.3.3 Neurofibroma: *Clue to diagnosis:* skin tag like lesion in non-intertriginous skin.

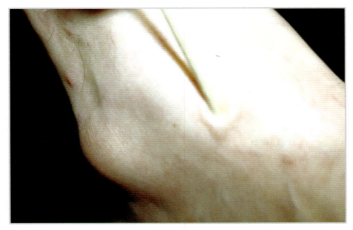

Figure 15.3.4 Neurofibroma: *Clue to diagnosis:* 'button hole' sign. Neurofibromas will form a 'hole' upon pressure.

BENIGN DERMAL NEOPLASMS

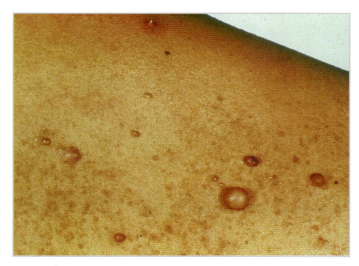

Figure 15.3.5 Multiple neurofibromas in patient with neurofibromatosis.

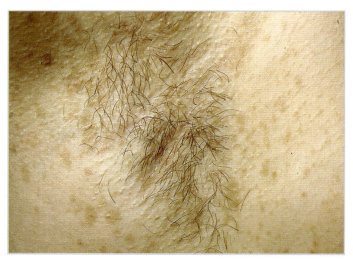

Figure 15.3.6 Crow's sign: axillary freckling in patient with neurofibromatosis.

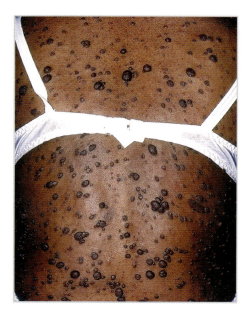

Figure 15.3.7 Multiple neurofibromas in patient with neurofibromatosis.

4. MASTOCYTOMA VERSUS MELANOCYTIC NEVUS (INTRADERMAL OR COMPOUND)

Features in common: brown macules, papules, and nodules

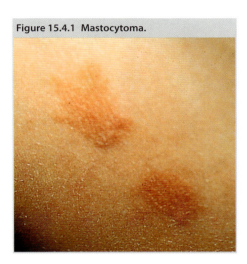

Figure 15.4.1 Mastocytoma.

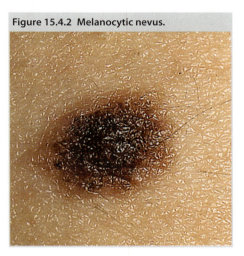

Figure 15.4.2 Melanocytic nevus.

Distinguishing features

	Mastocytoma	Melanocytic nevus (intradermal)
Physical examination Morphology	Brown to red Indistinct borders Positive Darier's sign: production of a wheal upon rubbing the lesion Occasionally bullous lesions	Various shades of brown to skin-colored Sharp borders No Darier's sign No bullous lesions
Distribution	Predominantly truncal	Any cutaneous surface
History Symptoms	Intense pruritus	No pruritus
Exacerbating factors	Rubbing or scratching Medications: aspirin, codeine, morphine, alcohol, polymyxin B	None
Associated findings	Flushing attacks with headaches, dyspnea, wheezing, diarrhea, and syncope may be seen	Family history of multiple moles
Epidemiology	Predominantly babies, infants, and children	All ages
Biopsy	Yes Proliferation of mast cells in dermis	Sometimes Collection of melanocytes in nests Melanocytes 'mature' and become more lymphoid and fibroblast-like in the deeper dermis
Laboratory	Usually none necessary Increased urine 5-hydroxyindoleacetic acid (5-HIAA) widespread and/or systemic lesions	None
Outcome	Spontaneous resolution over several years	May resolve over many years

Differential diagnosis of cutaneous dermal growths in infants and young children

- Dermatofibroma
- Dermoid cyst
- Hemangioma
- Infantile myofibroma
- Juvenile xanthogranuloma or other histiocytic tumors
- Leiomyoma and smooth muscle hamartoma
- Mastocytoma (urticaria pigmentosa)
- Melanocytic lesions
  - Blue nevus
  - Café au lait spot
  - Congenital nevus
  - Mongolian spot
  - Nevi of Ito and Ota
  - Spitz nevus
- Molluscum contagiosum (mimicker of growth)
- Neurofibroma
- Pilomatrixoma

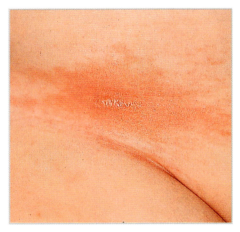

Figure 15.4.3 Mastocytoma. *Clue to diagnosis:* Darier's sign (i.e. an urticarial flare develops upon rubbing the lesion).

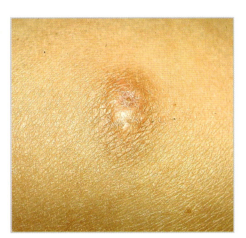

Figure 15.4.4 Mastocytoma.

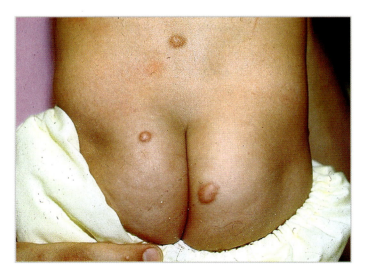

Figure 15.4.5 Urticaria pigmentosa (multiple mastocytomas).

5. LIPOMA VERSUS EPIDERMAL INCLUSION CYST

Features in common: mobile subcutaneous nodules

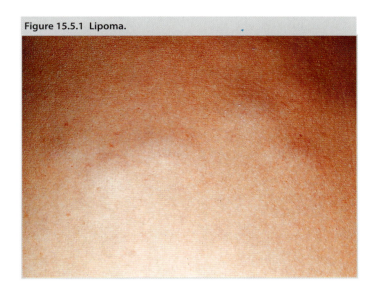

Figure 15.5.1 Lipoma.

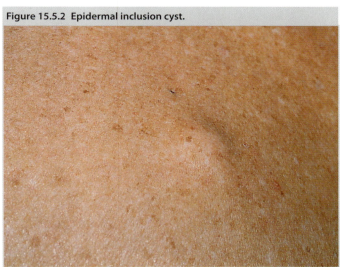

Figure 15.5.2 Epidermal inclusion cyst.

Distinguishing features

	Lipoma	Epidermal inclusion cyst
Physical examination		
Morphology	Lobulated subcutaneous nodule with indistinct borders Indistinct borders Soft, rubbery, and compressible No central punctum No surrounding erythema	Smooth dermal and subcutaneous nodule Well-demarcated borders Firm but not soft Central punctum frequently present in overlying epidermis Erythema if ruptured or secondarily infected
Distribution	Trunk, neck, and forearms	Trunk, face, and scalp
History		
Symptoms	None (angiolipomas may be painful) No history of drainage	None Tender if ruptured or infected Drainage of yellow cheesy material occasionally Can form in hands after trauma
Exacerbating factors	None	Secondary infection
Associated findings	Obesity Rarely Gardner's syndrome Rarely inherited as autosomal dominant trait	Acne Rarely Gardner's syndrome
Epidemiology	Adults	Adults
Biopsy	No Lobular aggregate of mature-appearing fat	No Keratin-filled cyst lined with epithelium resembling normal epidermis
Laboratory	None	None
Outcome	Stable	Stable unless ruptures or becomes infected

BENIGN DERMAL NEOPLASMS

Differential diagnosis of benign subcutaneous nodules

- Adnexal tumors
- Cysts
  - Bronchogenic
  - Cutaneous ciliated
  - Dermoid
  - Epidermal inclusion
  - Hidrocystoma (apocrine and eccrine)
  - Median raphe
  - Mucous/ganglion
  - Pilar
  - Steatocystoma
  - Thyroglossal duct
  - Vellus
- Lipomas
  - Angiolipoma
  - Hibernoma
  - Spindle cell lipoma/pleomorphic lipoma
- Painful tumors (ANGEL)
  - Angiolipoma
  - Neurilemmoma
  - Glomus
  - Eccrine spiradenoma
  - Leiomyoma
- Miscellaneous
  - Dermatofibroma
  - Foreign body granuloma
  - Gouty tophus
  - Osteoma/calcinosis cutis
  - Pilomatrixoma
  - Rheumatoid nodule
  - Subcutaneous granuloma annulare
- Vascular tumors
  - Capillary hemangioma
  - Cavernous hemangioma
  - Lymphangioma

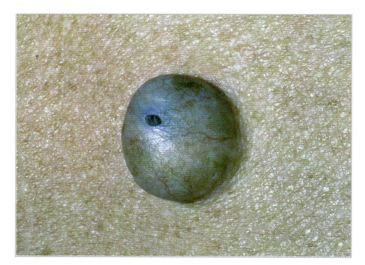

Figure 15.5.3 Epidermal inclusion cyst.

6. EPIDERMAL INCLUSION CYST VERSUS PILAR CYST

■ Features in common: subcutaneous and dermal cysts

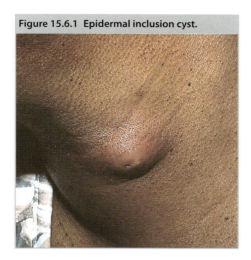

Figure 15.6.1 Epidermal inclusion cyst.

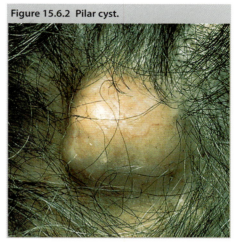

Figure 15.6.2 Pilar cyst.

■ Distinguishing features

	Epidermal inclusion cyst	Pilar cyst
Physical examination		
Morphology	Compressible Central punctum frequently in overlying epidermis Erythema if ruptured or infected	Noncompressible No central punctum No erythema
Distribution	Trunk, face, and scalp	Scalp
History		
Symptoms	Tender if ruptures Drainage of yellow cheesy material occasionally Can form in hands after trauma	None No history of drainage
Exacerbating factors	Secondary infection	None
Associated findings	Acne Rarely Gardner's syndrome Not inherited	No acne Not associated with Gardner's syndrome Autosomal dominant inheritance occasionally
Epidemiology	Adults	Adults
Biopsy	No Loose keratin-filled cyst lined with epithelium resembling normal epidermis	No Compact keratin-filled cyst lined with epithelium resembling follicular isthmus
Laboratory	None	None
Outcome	Stable; only of cosmetic concern unless ruptures	Stable; only of cosmetic concern

Miscellaneous dermal tumors (see algorithm)

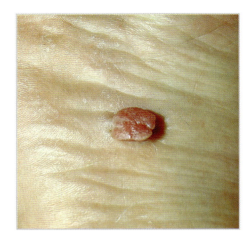

Figure 15.7.1 Poroma.

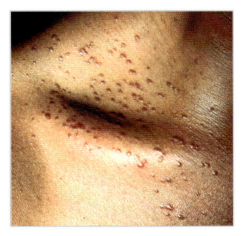

Figure 15.7.2 Syringoma. *Clue to diagnosis:* multiple papules around eye.

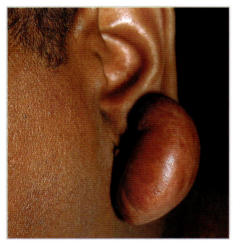

Figure 15.7.3 Keloid. *Clue to diagnosis:* history of injury or surgery.

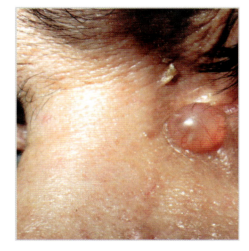

Figure 15.7.4 Hidrocystoma.

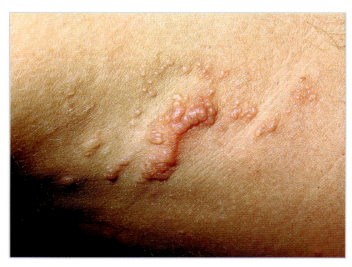

Figure 15.7.5 Lymphangioma. *Clue to diagnosis:* 'Frog spawn' appearance.

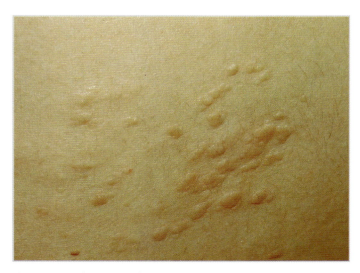

Figure 15.7.6 Shagreen patch in patient with tuberous sclerosus (collagenoma).

DISEASE DISCUSSION

▪ Dermatofibroma

Definition and etiology
A dermatofibroma is a nodular benign proliferation of fibroblasts, histiocytes, blood vessels, and lymphocytes. Although historically classified as a neoplasm, a dermatofibroma is a reactive scar like proliferation that may be caused by a wide variety of stimuli. Sometimes the lesions can be attributed to a ruptured cyst, an insect bite, folliculitis, or trauma.

Clinical features
Dermatofibromas are most commonly found on the lower extremities of young adults. Clinical examination reveals a firm, tan to light-brown dermal nodule. Slight epidermal lichenification due to rubbing and scaling may be present. Upon squeezing, the nodule puckers in from the side to the center; this phenomenon has been called Fitzpatrick's or dimple sign. Dermatofibromas are frequently confused with intradermal nevi because of their brown color. Fitzpatrick's sign is not present in nevi, however. Nevi are usually more exophytic and soft and frequently are not round. If a dermatofibroma has a prominent vascular component, such as in the sclerosing hemangioma variant, it can also be confused with a hemangioma. Hemangiomas are bright red and have a lobular appearance. Early developing lesions of dermatofibrosarcoma protuberans may be mistaken for scars or dermatofibromas. The clue to correct diagnosis of dermatofibrosarcoma protuberans is the typically larger size (greater than 1 cm), the irregular shape and borders, and the areas of protrusion from the skin.

Dermatofibrosarcoma protuberans will also recur if not completely excised, and multiple recurrences are common because of subclinical extension of the tumor.

Usually biopsies are not necessary to make a diagnosis of dermatofibroma. For worrisome or indeterminate lesions, biopsy results will reveal a nodular collection of haphazardly distributed fibroblasts that surround and entrap thick collagen bundles. A sparse inflammatory infiltrate, increased number of blood vessels, and lentiginous hyperplasia of the epidermis are also found.

Treatment (Table 15.1)
Since dermatofibromas are benign, no treatment is necessary; they gradually involute over many years. If they are bothersome, excision is the treatment of choice. Liquid nitrogen therapy can help flatten and soften the lesions.

Table 15.1 Treatment of dermatofibromas

Treatment	Precautions
Universal	
If diagnostic uncertainty or lesion growing and changing confirm diagnosis with biopsy	Occasionally other neoplasms such as basal cell carcinoma can arise in association with dermatofibromas
If symptomatic	
Excision is treatment of choice	Risk of scarring and infection
Cryotherapy	May soften lesion

▪ Dermatofibrosarcoma protuberans

Definition and etiology
Dermatofibrosarcoma protuberans (DFSP) is a low-grade sarcoma. Biopsy results reveal a spindle cell tumor arising within the dermis from fibroblast-like cells. DFSP recurs after incomplete removal and rarely metastasizes. Ninety per cent of cases involve a translocation between 17q22 and 22q13, the Col1A1 and PDFG beta genes.

Clinical features
Dermatofibrosarcoma occurs most commonly on the upper back of adult men.

A higher incidence is seen in blacks. Clinical examination reveals an irregularly shaped, asymmetric, firm, skin- to red-colored keloidal nodule or plaque on the skin that is several centimeters in size. The overlying epidermis is usually atrophic. Telangiectatic blood vessels are seen, and ulceration may be present. A characteristic feature of DFSP is single or multiple protuberant nodules.

The major diseases in the differential diagnosis are keloid and dermatofibroma.

Dermatofibromas are smaller, symmetric, and brown and exhibit dimpling upon squeezing. Unlike in DFSP, keloids occur after an injury and are frequently multiple.

They may also be symmetric exophytic masses. In all questionable cases or when dermatofibrosarcoma is suspected, the diagnosis should be confirmed with a biopsy. In some cases, when the biopsy results are equivocal the diagnosis can be confirmed by molecular studies looking for characteristic translocation.

Treatment (Table 15.2)
Since DFSP recurs very frequently and ultimately after numerous recurrences can metastasize, excision with wide margins is the treatment of choice. Mohs' surgery with microscopically controlled margins has been used successfully by a number of surgeons. Recently imatinib, a tyrosine kinase inhibitor, has been shown to shrink tumor size, and has been used preoperatively in some tumors, or in unresectable tumors. Radiation therapy has also been used as an adjunctive therapy in recurrent, unresectable, or metastatic tumors.

Table 15.2 Treatment of dermatofibrosarcoma protuberans

Treatment	Precautions
Wide local excision	Dermatofibrosarcoma protuberans frequently occurs so good margin control is essential
Mohs surgery	Adjective use of CD34 immunostaining may help with margin control
Imatinib	Helps shrink unresectable tumors. Numerous side effects- nausea vomiting, diarrhea, myalgias, fluid retention
Radiation therapy	Another adjunctive therapy if tumor is unresectable

Epidermal inclusion cyst

Definition and etiology
A cyst is a sac lined with epithelium. In an epidermal inclusion cyst, the lining epithelium resembles normal epidermis.

Clinical features
Cysts are easily recognized as mobile, well-circumscribed subcutaneous or dermal nodules. Accurate diagnosis of a cyst requires histologic confirmation because the majority of the neoplasm cannot be seen clinically. Epidermal inclusion cysts are the most common type of cyst seen in adults. They occur on the trunk, face, and sometimes the scalp. A central punctum in the overlying epidermis may be present.

Associated diseases include acne and uncommon entities such as Gardner's syndrome. Epidermal inclusion cysts on the hands can be produced by traumatic inoculation of epidermis into dermis in a puncture wound. The major differential diagnostic considerations are other cysts. Pilar cysts are more firm and are commonly found on the scalp because they are derived from hair follicles. Dermoid cysts are a type of hamartoma and most commonly occur lateral to the eyebrows. They usually present in infancy or early childhood.

Thyroglossal duct and bronchogenic duct cysts should be suspected with cystic lesions occurring in the midline area of the neck in babies and infants. Meningomyelocele should be suspected with centrally located cysts on the scalp in babies, infants, and young children. In adults, the sudden onset of multiple firm 'cystic' nodules should raise the suspicion of metastatic tumor (see Chapter 16). If the lesions are firm and tender, the differential diagnosis includes so-called ANGEL tumors: angiolipoma, neurilemmoma, glomus tumor, spiradenoma, and leiomyoma.

Treatment (Table 15.3)
Since epidermal inclusion cysts are benign, no treatment is necessary. For larger or cosmetically bothersome lesions, complete removal of the cyst and epithelial lining is the treatment of choice. If cyst wall remains, the cyst is likely to recur. Other therapies include incision and drainage with curettage of the cyst wall or intralesional corticosteroids if the cyst is inflamed.

Lipoma

Definition and etiology
A lipoma is a benign tumor composed of mature adipocytes.

Table 15.3 Treatment of epidermal inclusion cysts

Treatment	Precautions
Universal	
If unusual or sudden onset confirm diagnosis since adnexal tumors and metastatic tumors can present as cyst like lesions	
Asymptomatic	
No treatment necessary	
Symptomatic	
Excision	Treatment of choices
Incision and drainage	Frequently recurs
Intralesional steroids (Kenalog 10 mg/ml)	Helps with inflamed cysts May produce atrophy
Oral antibiotics	Helps if cyst infected

Clinical features
Lipomas are well-circumscribed, mobile, subcutaneous nodules most commonly found on the trunk, neck, and proximal extremities. The tumors are usually asymptomatic, but if they contain a large number of blood vessels (e.g. angiolipoma), they can be painful. Upon palpation, tumors have a soft spongy texture. A higher incidence of lipoma occurs in obese people, and a female predominance has been reported.

The major differential diagnostic consideration is a cyst. Epidermal inclusion cysts are usually not quite as deep, are better circumscribed, and are firmer and often have a punctum in the overlying epidermis. Cysts may have surrounding erythema if they rupture or become secondarily infected. Drainage from epidermal inclusion cysts is often a cheesy material or pus. Other entities to be considered include metastatic carcinoma and adnexal tumors (ANGEL tumors). Metastatic tumors should be suspected when numerous subcutaneous lesions develop suddenly. The sudden development of numerous lipomas would be extremely unlikely. Metastases are firm and occur in elderly individuals who usually have a history of prior cancer (see Chapter 16). Adnexal tumors, like cysts, usually are firmer than lipomas.

Treatment (Table 15.4)
Since lipomas are benign, no therapy is necessary. Lipomas do not develop into liposarcomas. If they are bothersome clinically, the treatment of choice is resection. Liposuction can also be performed if numerous biopsy-proven lipomas are present.

Mastocytoma

Definition and etiology
A mastocytoma is a benign tumor of mast cells.

Clinical features
Mastocytomas are tan to light brown macules, papules, and nodules most commonly found in children from birth to 2 years of age. A characteristic finding is Darier's sign (e.g., urtication upon rubbing). Usually the tumors are localized to the skin, but involvement of internal organs (bone, liver, and gastrointestinal tract) can produce flushing, headaches, diarrhea, dyspnea, and syncopal episodes. Because of their brown color, mastocytomas can be mistaken for nevi. Small acquired nevi more commonly develop in older children, adolescents, and young adults. Congenital nevi are larger than mastocytomas and may contain hair. Nevi are also darker brown and do not exhibit Darier's sign. Other lesions to be considered in the differential diagnosis include non-X histiocytoses (such as juvenile xanthogranuloma) and adnexal tumors. Lesions of juvenile xanthogranuloma are usually more yellow. In clinically indeterminate lesions, a biopsy should readily lead to a correct diagnosis. The biopsy findings reveal a collection

Table 15.4 Treatment of lipomas

Treatment	Precautions
If clinically unusual confirm diagnosis with biopsy	Lipomas are mobile so biopsying can be difficult
Asymptomatic	
No treatment necessary	
Symptomatic	
Surgical excision	Risk of scarring and infection
Liposuction	May be useful if multiple or very large tumors are present

Disease discussion

Table 15.5 Treatment of mastocytoma

Treatment	Comment
Universal	
Confirm diagnosis either clinically with Darier's sign or via biopsy	
Asymptomatic	
No treatment necessary	Reassure parents, and give list of mast cell degranulating agents
Symptomatic	
Antihistamines	May cause drowsiness or hyperactivity in children
Excision	Only helpful if one or two lesions are present
Topical corticosteroids bid	Risk of atrophy, and acne on the face.
Topical light or PUVA therapy	Risk of sun burn reaction, and increased risk of skin cancer
Supply epinephrine kit	Rare cases of anaphylaxis

Table 15.6 Treatment of nevi

Treatment	Precautions
Universal	
Biopsy if unsure of diagnosis to exclude possibility of melanoma	Since nevi and melanoma may exhibit histological overlapping features examination by a dermatopathologist is preferred
Council patients on following nevi for changes	
Ask about family history of atypical nevi and melanoma	Patients with family history of nevi and melanomas are much more likely to develop a melanoma during their lifetime
Sun screen and sun avoidance	Nevi more commonly found in sun exposed skin
Asymptomatic nevi	
No treatment necessary	There is no evidence that removing nevi will prevent a patient from developing a melanoma
Symptomatic nevi	
Excision	A margin of normal skin should be taken to prevent reoccurrence since recurrent nevi can resemble melanomas

of uniform-appearing mast cells that stain blue on Giemsa staining, interspersed eosinophils, and slight hyperpigmentation of the basal cell epidermal layer.

Treatment (Table 15.5)

Lesions may spontaneously regress over 5 to 6 years. Mast-cell-degranulating agents such as aspirin, alcohol, polymyxin B, morphine, and codeine should be avoided. Parents of patients with multiple mastocytomas (urticaria pigmentosa) should be given a prescription for an epinephrine kit (e.g. Ana-Kit, epi-pen) to prepare for the possibility of anaphylactic shock. Single lesions can be treated with a high-strength topical steroid under occlusion or with excision.

▇ Melanocytic nevus

Definition and etiology

A nevus or mole is a benign neoplasm of melanocytes. The major etiologic factors are sun exposure and familial inheritance.

Clinical features

Nevi can be acquired or congenital. The most common acquired nevus has been given various eponyms such as dysplastic nevus, atypical nevus, Clark's nevus, and nevus with architectural disorder. Nevi vary in appearance and coloration but most often have a fairly symmetric configuration, regular border, uniform flesh to brown color, and relatively small diameter. The most important mimicker of a nevus is a melanoma. Early melanomas frequently can be mistaken clinically for nevi, but unlike nevi melanomas will continue to grow and change. Nevi on the face and occasionally elsewhere are slightly raised soft papules that can be confused with basal cell carcinoma, but telangiectasias are usually absent. Nevi can be confused with dermatofibromas because of their brown color and intradermal location. Dimpling upon squeezing (Fitzpatrick's sign) is not seen in nevi. Nevi also usually have a darker brown color. Juvenile xanthogranulomas, xanthomas, mastocytomas, can be confused with intradermal nevi.

Epiluminescent microscopy (dermatoscopy, skin-surface microscopy) can accentuate an underlying pigment network and aid in accurate diagnosis. If the diagnosis is in question, the lesion should be biopsied.

Treatment (Table 15.6)

For common nevi, no therapy is required unless there has been a change in color, shape, or size or if bleeding or symptoms have occurred. For clinically indeterminate lesions, an excisional biopsy is mandated, especially to exclude a diagnosis of malignant melanoma.

▇ Neurofibroma

Definition and etiology

A neurofibroma is a common tumor of nerve sheath origin. Solitary neurofibromas are idiopathic, but the tendency for multiple neurofibromas can be inherited as an autosomal dominant trait in von Recklinghausen's disease (neurofibromatosis).

Clinical features: Cutaneous neurofibromas are soft, sessile or pedunculated, skin-colored to light pink tumors most commonly found on the trunk. Tumors can be partially pushed back into the skin. This finding is known as the 'buttonhole sign'. Rarer uncommonly encountered variants of neurofibromas such as plexiform, diffuse, and nodular types present as deep subcutaneous nodules and masses. In patients with neurofibromatosis, other associated findings include café au lait spots, axillary freckling, and Lisch nodules on the iris of the eye. The major differential diagnostic considerations are intradermal nevi (which usually retain some brown color) and skin tags, which usually are smaller and occur around the neck or axilla. A biopsy is usually not required but reveals a collection of small wavy spindle cells surrounded by a loose myxoid-appearing stroma.

Treatment (Table 15.7)

Neurofibroma is a benign tumor, and therefore treatment is not necessary.

Surgical excision is the treatment of choice for lesions that are irritated by clothing, cosmetically disfiguring, or painful or that require confirmation to make the diagnosis. Lesions in patients with von

Table 15.7 Treatment of neurofibroma

Treatment	Precautions
No treatment necessary unless symptomatic or growing and changing	Neurofibrosarcomas can develop within neurofibromas in patients with neurofibromatosis
Symptomatic	
Excision	Risk of scarring and infection

Recklinghausen's disease need to be followed closely because of the risk for sarcomatous change.

Pilar cyst

Definition and etiology
A pilar cyst (trichilemmal cyst) contains compact hair-type keratin with a cyst wall resembling the isthmus portion of a hair follicle. Pilar cysts can be idiopathic or can be inherited as an autosomal dominant trait.

Clinical features
Pilar cysts are most commonly found on the scalp of middle-aged adults. Pilar cysts are slightly more predominant in women. Examination reveals a firm flesh-colored mobile dermal nodule. The major differential diagnostic consideration is an epidermal inclusion cyst. Epidermal inclusion cysts occur most commonly on the trunk, are not as firm, and contain a central umbilication in the overlying epidermis.

Epidermal cysts more frequently rupture or become secondarily infected, producing surrounding erythema; they frequently may have a drainage of white cheesy material. The differential diagnosis also includes other cysts, metastatic tumors, and adnexal neoplasms. Dermoid cyst, a form of hamartoma, most commonly occurs lateral to the eyebrows in newborn babies. Thyroglossal duct and bronchogenic duct cysts should be suspected with cystic lesions in the midline area of the neck in babies and infants. In adults with the sudden onset of multiple firm 'cystic' nodules, metastatic disease should be excluded (see Chapter 16). If the lesions are firm and tender, the differential diagnosis would also include ANGEL tumors (angiolipoma, neurilemmoma, glomus tumor, eccrine spiradenoma and leiomyoma.

Table 15.8 Treatment of pilar cysts

Treatment	Precautions
Universal	
If unusual or sudden onset confirm diagnosis with biopsy or excision	Adnexal tumors and metastatic tumors can present as cyst like lesions
Asymptomatic	
No treatment necessary	
Symptomatic	
Excision	Treatment of choice
Incision and drainage	Frequently recurs
Intralesional steroids: triamcinolone (Kenalog) 10 mg/mL	Helps with inflamed cysts May produce atrophy
Oral antibiotics	Helps if cyst infected

Treatment (Table 15.8)
Pilar cysts are benign and need only be excised for cosmetic reasons or if symptomatic.

Chapter 16 Malignant dermal neoplasms

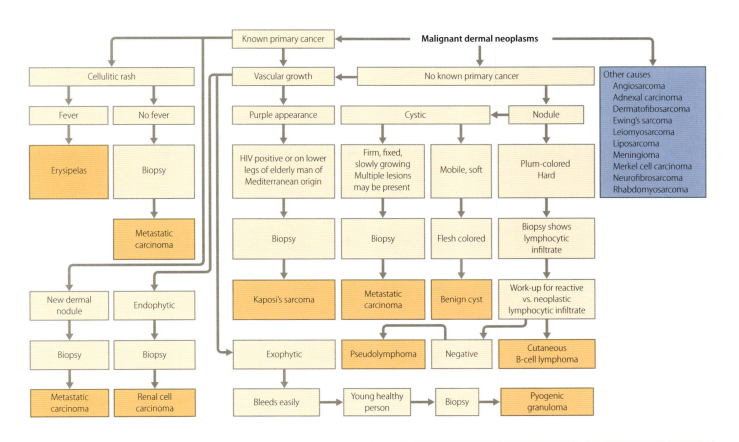

INTRODUCTION

This chapter reviews the differential diagnosis of common malignant tumors and their benign simulators. Prompt recognition of malignant tumors is necessary to prevent morbidity and mortality. Cutaneous metastases are especially important to diagnose because they can assume a variety of different morphologies that can be mistaken for benign entities. Metastatic nodules are often misdiagnosed as cysts. Lesions of metastatic renal cell carcinoma are often red colored in appearance and can be mistaken for hemangioma or pyogenic granuloma. Inflammatory metastases, so-called *carcinoma erysipeloids*, have a cellulitic or erysipelas-like appearance; it is inappropriate to treat them with intravenous antibiotics. Occasionally metastases can also have zosteriform morphology and be confused with herpes zoster. Metastases to the scalp can produce hair loss also known as alopecia neoplastica. Finally, some tumors like breast cancer can produce indurated skin mimicking morphea or scleroderma (metastasis en cuirasse).

Another malignant tumor that can be extremely difficult to diagnose is cutaneous B-cell lymphoma, especially since both the histologic and the clinical features of lymphomas and pseudolymphomas can be practically identical.

Kaposi's sarcoma related to human herpes virus type 8 infection, has several morphological expressions. The classical type seen on the lower legs of elderly men of Mediterranean descent can be mistaken for stasis dermatitis. The variant associated with immunosuppression or HIV disease can occur anywhere on the body and can be mistaken for a variety of different hemangiomas.

1. NODULAR METASTATIC DISEASE VERSUS CUTANEOUS CYST

■ Features in common: dermal nodules

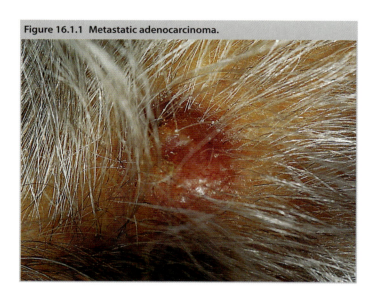

Figure 16.1.1 Metastatic adenocarcinoma.

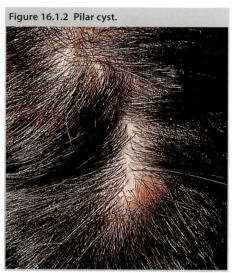

Figure 16.1.2 Pilar cyst.

■ Distinguishing features

	Nodular metastatic disease	Cutaneous cyst
Physical examination Morphology	Firm May be fixed to overlying skin No central punctum May ulcerate	Soft Not fixed to overlying skin Central punctum in epidermal inclusion cyst No ulceration
Distribution	Usually in vicinity of or body region near underlying cancer	Trunk, scalp, proximal extremities
History Symptoms	Sudden onset Often prior history of cancer Malaise, weight loss	Gradual onset No prior history of cancer No malaise or weight loss
Exacerbating factors	None	Secondary infection, rupture
Associated findings	Occasionally lymphadenopathy Hair loss if metastatic to scalp (overlying metastasis)	No lymphadenopathy unless infected No hair loss with scalp cysts
Epidemiology	Elderly Familial history of cancer	Adults No familial history of cancer
Biopsy	Yes Malignant tumor cells Special stains can be performed	No, unless diagnosis is uncertain Cavity lined with epithelium
Laboratory	Depending on primary tumor	None
Outcome	Poor	Excellent

Differential diagnosis of dermal nodules

- Adnexal tumors
- Calcinosis/osteoma cutis
- Cysts
- Dermatofibromas
- If tender, consider ANGEL tumors: angiolipoma, neurilemmoma, glomus tumor, eccrine spiradenoma, leiomyoma
- Lipomas
- Metastatic tumors

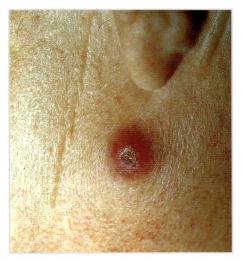

Figure 16.1.3 Metastatic adenocarcinomas.

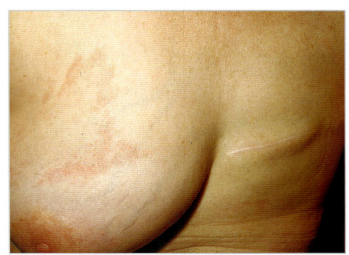

Figure 16.1.3 Metastatic adenocarcinomas.

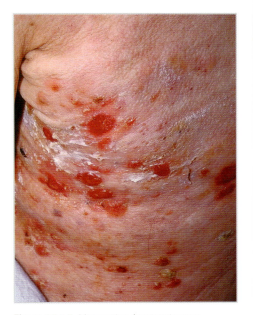

Figure 16.1.5 Metastatic adenocarcinomas.

2. CARCINOMA ERYSIPELOIDES VERSUS ERYSIPELAS

Features in common: large red macule

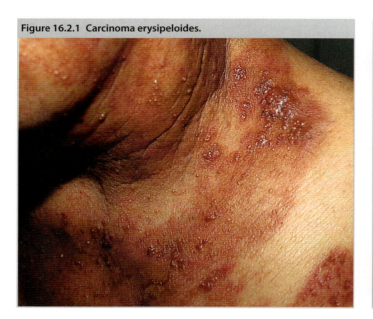

Figure 16.2.1 Carcinoma erysipeloides.

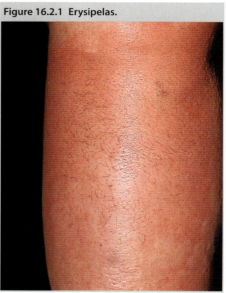

Figure 16.2.1 Erysipelas.

Distinguishing features

	Carcinoma erysipeloides	Erysipelas
Physical examination		
Morphology	Dusky red–maroon color Skin is firm indurated Telangiectasias may be present Gradual spread over days to weeks Nodular component may be present On chest may be associated with nipple retraction, edema, and breast enlargement	Bright red color Skin not indurated No telangiectasia Rapid spread over hours Nodules rarely present No nipple retraction, edema, and breast enlargement
Distribution	Most common on chest	Usually on face or lower legs
History		
Symptoms	Prior history of cancer No prior history of cellulitis Weight loss, malaise	No prior history of cancer Sometimes prior history of cellulitis No weight loss or malaise
Exacerbating factors	Neglect or inappropriate treatment	Immunosuppression
Associated findings	No fever Underlying malignancy No baseline lymphedema No prior history of thrombophlebitis	Fever No underlying malignancy Lymphedema: congenital, postsurgical, or stasis-related A prior history of thrombophlebitis or tinea pedis may be present with lesions on legs
Epidemiology	Adults Most often due to breast cancer	Adults Male and female
Biopsy	Yes Tumor cells within dilated lymphatic vessels	Not necessary Diffuse edema with neutrophilic infiltrate
Laboratory	Metastatic work-up	Leukocytosis, culture of skin biopsy or blood
Outcome	Poor	Resolves with treatment

3. METASTATIC RENAL CELL CARCINOMA VERSUS PYOGENIC GRANULOMA

Features in common: red vascular-appearing nodules

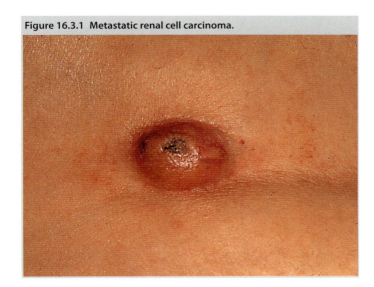

Figure 16.3.1 Metastatic renal cell carcinoma.

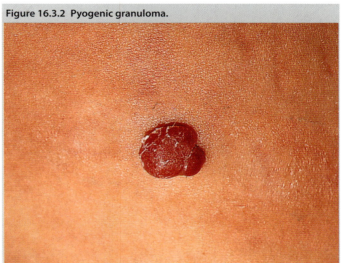

Figure 16.3.2 Pyogenic granuloma.

Distinguishing features

	Metastatic renal cell carcinoma	Pyogenic granuloma
Physical examination		
Morphology	Variable colored: flesh, red, blue, or black Dermal or subcutaneous nodules or plaques Ulceration and bleeding possible Single or multiple lesions	Red-colored Exophytic papules and nodules Ulceration and bleeding common Single lesion (rarely satellite lesions)
Distribution	Anywhere	Anywhere, but more common on fingers or mucosal surface
History		
Symptoms	History of renal carcinoma Weight loss, malaise	No history of carcinoma No weight loss or malaise
Exacerbating factors	None	Pregnancy Trauma
Associated findings	Hypertension, hypercalcemia, amyloidosis, and polycythemia are occasionally noted	No associated hypertension or hypercalcemia
Epidemiology	Adults	More common in children
Biopsy	Yes Neoplasm composed of lobules of clear- staining malignant cells with surrounding vascular stroma	Occasionally Neoplasm composed of lobules of uniform round blood vessels surrounded by a collarette of epithelium and inflammatory cells
Laboratory	Work-up for metastatic disease Serum calcium	None
Outcome	Poor	Excellent

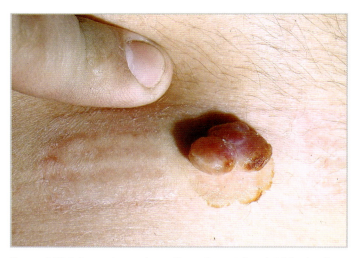

Figures 16.3.3 Pyogenic granuloma. *Clue to diagnosis:* 'band aid' sign (outline of band aid that patient was wearing) due to frequent bleeding.

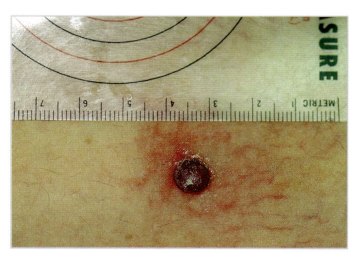

Figure 16.3.4 Pyogenic granuloma.

4. KAPOSI'S SARCOMA VERSUS HEMANGIOMA

Features in common: red vascular-appearing papules, nodules and plaques

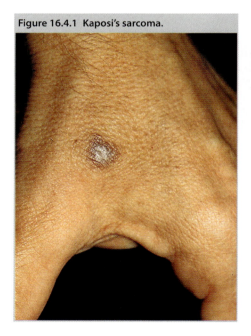

Figure 16.4.1 Kaposi's sarcoma.

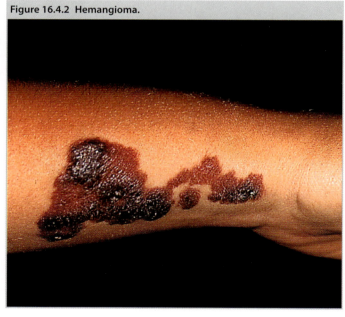

Figure 16.4.2 Hemangioma.

Distinguishing features

	Kaposi's sarcoma	Hemangioma
Physical examination		
Morphology	Pink, purple, to brown colored Patches, plaques, nodules Truncal lesions may follow skin lines May Koebnerize	Red colored Papules, nodules Does not follow skin lines Does not Koebnerize
Distribution	Classic: lower legs HIV associated: face, trunk, extremities and mucosa	Trunk and extremities
History		
Symptoms	Asymptomatic	Bleeds with trauma
Exacerbating factors	Immunosuppression	Trauma
Associated findings	Occasionally pulmonary or gastrointestinal symptoms due to systemic involvement	Occasionally thrombocytopenia or disseminated intravascular coagulation
Epidemiology	Classic: adult Mediterranean men HIV associated	Children Various hemangioma variants common in adults
Biopsy	Yes Blood-filled slitlike spaces with surrounding spindle cell proliferation	No Uniform round-appearing capillaries organized in lobules Infantile hemangiomas are glut-1 positive
Laboratory	Work-up for systemic disease as indicated by symptoms Experimental: herpesvirus type 8 DNA	Platelet, prothrombin and partial thrombo-plastin times if clinical symptoms of bleeding present
Outcome	Classic: chronic slowly progressive disease HIV related: poor prognostic indicator	Good: may spontaneously involute during childhood

Differential diagnosis of Kaposi's sarcoma

- Common causes
    - Dermatofibroma
    - Hemangioma
        - Angiokeratoma
        - Capillary hemangioma
        - Cavernous hemangioma
        - Targetoid hemosiderotic hemangioma
    - Hemorrhage trauma (talon noire)
    - Lichen planus
    - Melanocytic nevus
    - Postinflammatory hyperpigmentation
    - Pyogenic granuloma
    - Stasis dermatitis (acroangiodermatitis)
- Rarer causes
    - Angiosarcoma
    - Bacillary angiomatosis
    - Glomangioma
    - Pityriasis rosea
    - Psoriasis
    - Verruga peruana

MALIGNANT DERMAL NEOPLASMS

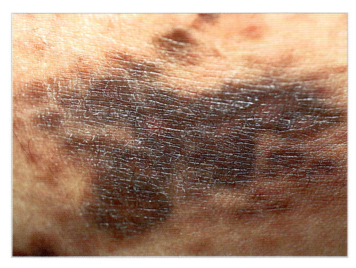

Figure 16.4.3 Kaposi's sarcoma. *Clue to diagnosis:* purple color, location, and clinical history.

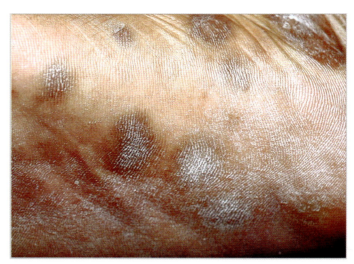

Figure 16.4.4 Kaposi's sarcoma.

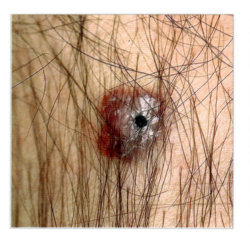

Figure 16.4.5 Kaposi's sarcoma.

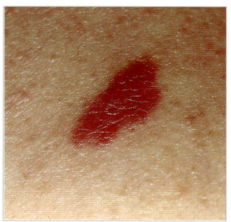

Figure 16.4.6 Kaposi's sarcoma.

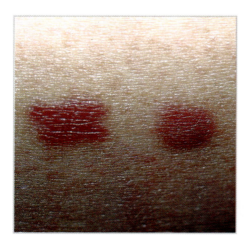

Figure 16.4.7 Kaposi's sarcoma.

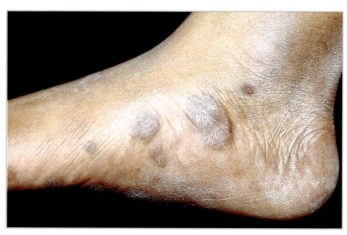

Figure 16.4.8 Kaposi's sarcoma.

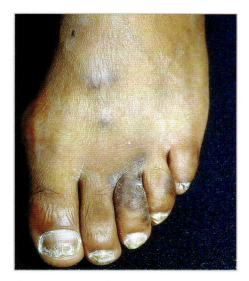

Figure 16.4.9 Kaposi's sarcoma.

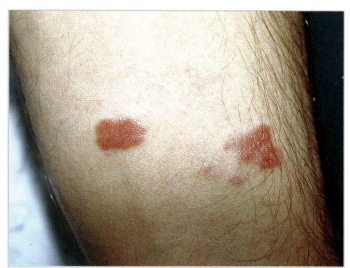

Figure 16.4.10 Kaposi's sarcoma.

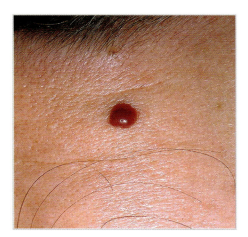

Figure 16.4.11 Hemangiomas.

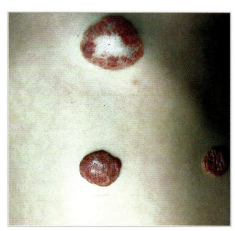

Figure 16.4.12 Hemangiomas.

5. CUTANEOUS B-CELL LYMPHOMA VERSUS PSEUDOLYMPHOMA

Features in common: red-to-plum-colored dermal nodules

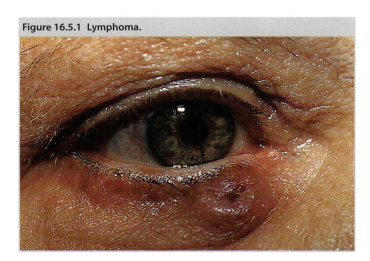

Figure 16.5.1 Lymphoma.

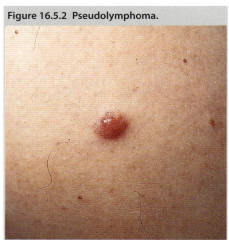

Figure 16.5.2 Pseudolymphoma.

Distinguishing features

	Cutaneous B-cell lymphoma	Pseudolymphoma
Physical examination		
Morphology	Identical appearance: red to plum-colored nodules Lesions tend to be large (golf-ball-sized) Ulcerated nodules occasionally present	Identical appearance: red to plum-colored nodules Lesions tend to be smaller than lymphoma Ulcerated nodules rare
Distribution	More common on trunk but can occur on head and neck	Head and neck, rarely truncal
History		
Symptoms	Occasionally prior or concurrent history of systemic lymphoma Fever, weight loss, and night sweats if systemic involvement	No history of systemic lymphoma No systemic symptoms
Exacerbating factors	Immunosuppression	Insect bites Lyme disease Medications
Associated findings	Lymphadenopathy or hepatosplenomegaly when systemic involvement is present	No lymphadenopathy or hepatosplenomegaly
Epidemiology	Adults	Any age
Biopsy	Yes Nodular infiltrate is usually predominantly located in bottom of dermis or subcutaneous tissue with atypical cells	Yes Nodular infiltrate composed of benign lymphocytes predominantly located in middle to upper dermis; eosinophils are frequently numerous
Laboratory	Immunophenotypic and gene rearrangement studies clarify the diagnosis in histological indeterminate cases by demonstrating a clonal cell population Systemic work-up: computed tomography, chest X-ray	Immunophenotypic and gene rearrangement studies in histological indeterminate lesions, no clonal cell population
Outcome	Curable if localized to skin	Excellent

Differential diagnosis of lymphocytic infiltrates in the skin

- Benign lymphocytic infiltrate of Jessner
- Cold panniculitis
- Cutaneous lupus erythematosus
- Drug eruption
- Insect bite reaction
- Lymphoma
- Pernio (chilblains)
- Polymorphous light eruption
- Pseudolymphoma

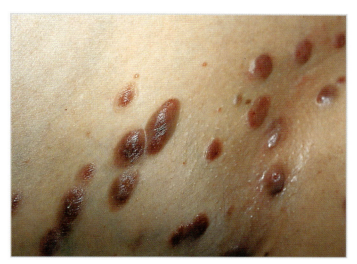

Figure 16.5.3 Lymphoma. *Clue to diagnosis:* numerous nodules.

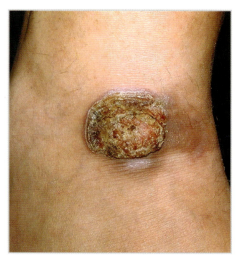

Figure 16.5.4 T-suppressor cell lymphoma.

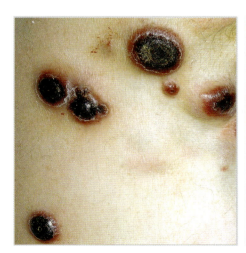

Figure 16.5.5 T-suppressor cell lymphoma.

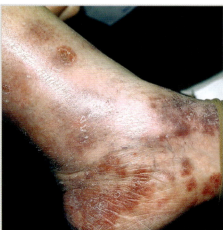

Figure 16.5.6 Lymphoma.

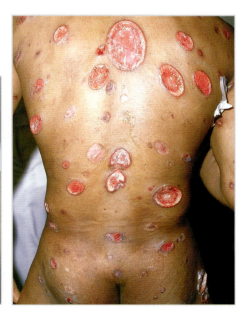

Figure 16.5.7 Lymphoma.

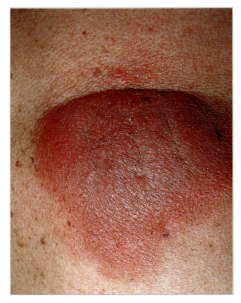

Figure 16.5.8 Lymphoma.

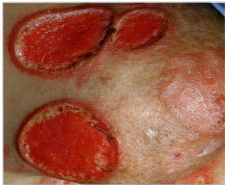

Figure 16.5.9 Lymphoma.

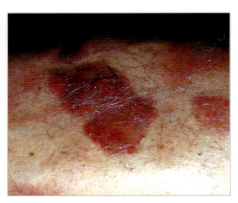

Figure 16.5.10 Mycosis fungoides: tumor stage.

DISEASE DISCUSSION

Primary cutaneous B-cell lymphoma

Definition and etiology
Primary cutaneous B cell lymphoma represents a heterogenous group of lymphomas which by definition originally are limited to the skin. By definition, diagnosis of primary cutaneous B-cell lymphoma requires the exclusion of systemic lymphoma that has spread to the skin. Most patients with the common types of primary cutaneous B-cell lymphomas have an excellent long term prognosis.

Clinical features
Patients with lymphoma involving the skin may present with either single or multiple dermal or subcutaneous nodules. Clinical findings are nondiagnostic, and the sudden onset of nodule(s) in a patient with non-Hodgkin's lymphoma or in patients with systemic symptoms requires a biopsy. If there is systemic involvement proximal lymph nodes frequently may be enlarged, and patients may also complain of fever, night sweats, and weight loss.

The two most common types of primary cutaneous B-cell lymphoma are cutaneous follicle center lymphoma, and cutaneous marginal zone lymphoma. Rare types include cutaneous diffuse large B-cell lymphoma leg type, and intravascular large cell lymphomas. Cutaneous follicle center lymphoma usually occurs in adults. Common site of involvement is the head, neck, and trunk and patients present with red papules, plaques, nodules and tumors. Cutaneous marginal zone lymphomas occur in young male adults with predilection for the upper extremities and trunk. Usually only a solitary nodule is present, but occasionally several lesions which may be clustered are present.

Primary cutaneous B-cell lymphoma needs to be differentiated from a benign reactive lymphocytic infiltrate such as pseudolymphoma (lymphocytoma). Accurate diagnosis requires a skin biopsy. The biopsy results reveal a dense infiltrate composed of atypical lymphocytes. The infiltrate is denser in the deep dermis and subcutaneous tissue. Immunophenotypic and gene rearrangement studies demonstrate a clonal population of lymphocytes.

In some cases, in spite of having done a biopsy, the diagnosis may be uncertain, since there are reports of pseudolymphoma evolving into lymphoma. The development of nodules after an insect bite or after the start of a new medication provides evidence in favor of a benign reactive lymphocytic infiltrate rather than lymphoma. In all cases, work-up involves complete physical examination, screening laboratory tests, and radiologic studies in addition to biopsy.

Treatment (Table 16.1)
Patients with systemic involvement suffer significant morbidity and mortality.

Aggressive treatment with radiation therapy or chemotherapy or both, is required.

The prognosis for patients with cutaneous B-cell lymphoma limited to the skin is excellent, and lesions can be treated solely with radiation therapy.

Cyst

Definition and etiology
A cyst is a sac lined by an epithelial layer. The two most common cysts are epidermal inclusion and pilar cysts (see Chapter 15).

Table 16.1 Treatment of primary cutaneous B cell lymphoma

Treatment	Precautions
Universal	
Exclude systemic disease	
Solitary lesion or minimal disease	
No treatment necessary except follow up for change	
Intralesional steroids	Skin atrophy
Topical corticosteroids bid	Skin atrophy, steroid induced rosacea
Surgical excision	Scar, infection
Localized radiation therapy	Radiation dermatitis, atrophy, cancer
Extensive disease	
Anti-cd20 antibody (rituximab)	Numerous side effects: fatal infusion reactions, hepatitis B reactivation, progressive multifocal leukoencephalopathy
Interferon-alpha	Flu-like symptoms
Chemotherapy	Numerous complications

Clinical features
Cysts are easily recognized as mobile, well-circumscribed, rubbery dermal and subcutaneous nodules. The ultimate classification of a cyst requires microscopic examination of its lining epithelium. Certain clinical clues may also help in differentiation. Epidermal inclusion cysts are by far the most common type of cyst encountered in clinical practice. They occur most frequently on the trunk, face, and scalp. Sometimes a central umbilication in the overlying epidermis is present. The second most common type of cyst is the pilar cyst. Pilar cysts (also known as isthmus catagen cysts) are cysts with a lining epithelium resembling hair. They occur most commonly on the scalp. Dermoid cysts are a type of hamartoma. They occur most commonly lateral to the eyebrows and are most often detected at birth. Thyroglossal duct and bronchogenic duct cysts should be suspected with cystic lesions in the midline area of the neck and are usually first noted in infancy. In adults, the sudden onset of multiple firm 'cystic' nodules should lead to the suspicion of metastatic disease. Metastatic nodular cutaneous lesions are easy to overlook or ignore. If a patient with a history of a prior malignancy develops a new cutaneous nodule, a biopsy is mandatory. The degree of suspicion is heightened if numerous 'cysts' develop suddenly. Metastatic lesions are firmer than epidermal inclusion cysts. They are frequently irregularly shaped and fixed to the surrounding skin. Occasionally, metastatic nodules can be the presenting sign of an underlying malignancy. For any dermal or subcutaneous lesions for which the diagnosis is not certain, a biopsy should be done. If lesions are firm and tender, the differential diagnosis includes the so-called ANGEL tumors (benign tumors commonly associated with pain): angiolipoma, neurilemmoma, glomus tumor, eccrine spiradenoma, and leiomyoma.

Treatment (Table 16.2)
Since cysts are benign, no treatment is necessary. For larger or cosmetically bothersome lesions, the treatment of choice is surgery with removal of the entire lining epithelium to prevent recurrence. If the lining epithelium is not removed, the cyst is likely to recur. Incision

Table 16.2 Treatment of cysts

Treatment	Precautions
Universal	
Biopsy if diagnosis is uncertain	Do not miss a malignant neoplasm
Reassurance	No treatment necessary if asymptomatic
Excision if tender or bothersome	Scar, infection and recurrence if not completely excised
Intralesional methylprednisolone 10 mg to 20 mg/mL if inflamed	Risk of atrophy
Oral antibiotics if infected	

and drainage with curettage to remove the cyst wall is done for ruptured or infected cysts.

Erysipelas

Definition and etiology

Erysipelas is a cutaneous infection caused by *Streptococcus pyogenes*.

Clinical features

Patients present with fever, anorexia, headache, and even vomiting. There is a cellulitic rash. Erysipelas most commonly involves the face or lower extremities in older children or adults and the trunk in infants. The skin is bright red, hot, and painful and early on has a sharply defined and slightly raised margin. With time, edema, vesicles, and bullae may develop. The margin becomes less well demarcated.

The major differential diagnostic considerations are contact dermatitis, carcinoma erysipeloids, an early lesion of herpes zoster, and cellulitis due to *Staphylococcus* and other organisms. In contact dermatitis, fever is absent, pruritus is present, and history or patch testing will implicate a triggering antigen. The lesions of herpes zoster occur in a dermatomal distribution, and patients usually have prodromal hyperesthesia and complain of a prickly or lacerating pain. Eventually grouped vesicles will develop in areas of pain. The rash of carcinoma erysipeloids occurs in the vicinity of an underlying malignancy and does not spread as rapidly as erysipelas. Fever is not present, although the skin feels warm. Nodules and indurated areas are found on palpation. Blisters do not occur.

Treatment (Table 16.3)

The treatment of erysipelas includes oral or intravenous antibiotics like penicillin that cover streptococcal organisms.

Table 16.3 Treatment of erysipelas

Treatment	Precautions
Universal	
Look for predisposing factor such as tinea pedis	
Mild disease	
Oral antibiotics such as cephalexin (Keflex) 500 mg bid or doxycycline 100 mg bid	Allergic reaction, rash, photosensitivity with doxycycline
Severe disease	
IV antibiotics	Numerous

Hemangioma

Definition and etiology

A hemangioma is a benign neoplasm of blood vessels. Hemangiomas can be further classified into different subtypes, such as infantile, cherry angioma, targetoid hemosiderotic hemangioma, strawberry nevus, cavernous hemangioma, and arteriovenous hemangioma, based on clinical and histologic appearance. Rarer variants include epithelioid, verrucous, glomeruloid, elastotic, microvenular, and tufted hemangiomas.

Clinical features

Cherry angioma and strawberry nevus derive their names from their clinical appearance: bright red papules and plaques resembling cherries and strawberries. Histologic examination reveals lobular proliferation of uniform round capillaries.

Cavernous hemangiomas are larger, massive, deep-dermal red nodules and plaques that are several centimeters in size, and most likely are arteriovenous malformations. Pathologic examination demonstrates large, dilated, thick-walled blood vessels. Targetoid hemosiderotic hemangiomas, primarily present in children and young adults, are small red angiomas with surrounding ecchymosis, which produces a targetoid appearance. Biopsy findings demonstrate irregularly shaped blood vessels that can be mistaken for Kaposi's sarcoma by unaware pathologists. Arteriovenous hemangiomas, collections of thick-walled arteries and veins, are red to skin-colored papules most commonly located on the face or on acral sites.

The major differential diagnostic considerations include pigmented nevi (see Ch. 14) and Kaposi's sarcoma. Usually, because of the bright red color, the diagnosis is relatively straightforward. Kaposi's sarcoma (discussed later) primarily occurs in adults and presents with violaceous, not red-colored, patches and plaques.

Treatment (Table 16.4)

Treatment of hemangioma is usually not necessary. Infantile hemangiomas in children usually involute over a period of 5–10 years. The treatment of choice for cosmetically unacceptable rapidly growing lesions or those that interfere with vision, eating, or breathing is laser surgery. Small lesions can also be destroyed with light electrodesiccation or can be removed with scalpel or scissors excision.

Kaposi's sarcoma

Definition and etiology

Kaposi's sarcoma is a malignant neoplasm of blood vessels. Recently, Kaposi's sarcoma has been linked to herpesvirus-8 infection in some individuals.

Clinical features

A variety of different clinical forms of Kaposi's sarcoma exist. The classic adult form is found primarily in elderly Mediterranean, Jewish, or eastern European men.

An endemic form is seen in Africa, and the immunosuppression-related form is most commonly seen in men with acquired immunodeficiency syndrome (AIDS). The cutaneous manifestations correlate with each of these clinical variants. In classic Kaposi's sarcoma, lesions are localized to the lower legs and can be confused with stasis dermatitis. The lack of pitting edema, the presence of violaceous-colored

Disease discussion

Table 16.4 Treatment of hemangiomas

Treatment	Precautions
Universal	
Exclude systemic involvement or syndrome	
In many cases, no treatment necessary	
Infantile hemangiomas	
Infantile hemangiomas which are on the face, large, ulcerated, or interfering with feeding and vision may require treatment such as topical timolol, systemic propranolol, or topical, intralesional or systemic corticosteroids	With propranolol: monitor of hypoglycemia, hypotension, bronchospasm
Excision very rarely if bleeding, or for residual, unacceptable scar	Scar and infection
Pulsed dye laser for ulcerated hemangioma, or incomplete resolution	Pain, pigmentary changes, scar
Hemangiomas in adults	
Pain, hemorrhage	
Pain, scar	
Surgical excision	Scar, infection

Table 16.5 Treatment of Kaposi's sarcoma

Treatment	Precautions
Universal	
Stage the disease	
Localized or generalized skin involvement	Patients with generalized skin, systemic, and low CD4 count have worse prognosis
Pure cutaneous or systemic involvement	
Low or high CD4 count (> or <200)	
Mild localized disease	
If asymptomatic, no treatment necessary	
Localized radiation therapy	Potential radiation dermatitis
Excision	Scar, infection, recurrence
Cryotherapy	Pain, blister, scar
Electrodessication and curettage	Pain, ulcer, scar, poor wound healing, infection
Alitretinoin gel 0.1% bid up to 4× a day 2–14 weeks	Dermatitis, pruritus, edema, stinging, pain, and photosensitivity
Generalized and systemic disease	
HAART or antiviral therapy in HIV patients	Numerous side effects
Chemotherapy with cytotoxic agents	Numerous side effects

nodules, and the genetic and ethnic background of the patient will indicate the need for a skin biopsy, which confirms the diagnosis. The African endemic form commonly presents in children with generalized lymphadenopathy. The lesions in the immunosuppressed and AIDS-related forms are scattered and can involve the entire integument plus the oral mucosa. The tumor evolves through macule-patch, papule-plaque, and nodular stages. The macule patches are small, oval, round, non-scaly, and reddish-purple. Isolated lesions can be confused with dermatofibromas or hemangiomas. Dermatofibromas do not have purple color, however, are usually smaller, and umbilicate upon squeezing. Large hemangiomas are bright red (not purple) and are primarily seen in young infants and children. The smaller cherry angiomas in adults are red, small, and symmetric and only a few millimeters in size.

Lesions of Kaposi's sarcoma follow skin lines when present on the trunk and may be confused with pityriasis rosea. Unlike in pityriasis rosea, the lesions lack scale and there is no preceding herald patch. The lesions have a purple hue and last indefinitely. The papular lesions of Kaposi's sarcoma can be confused with pyogenic granuloma and bacillary angiomatosis. Pyogenic granulomas occur in young healthy children and adults, are isolated exophytic lesions, and bleed profusely when traumatized. Bacillary angiomatosis, an infection due to *Rochalimaea henselae*, occurs in immunocompromised patients, resembles pyogenic granuloma and Kaposi's sarcoma, and may be correctly diagnosed with a skin biopsy and a Warthin-Starry stain, which reveals the infectious organisms. Plaquelike and nodular lesions of Kaposi's sarcoma can be confused with angiosarcoma. Angiosarcoma, however, develops most commonly on the scalp or in areas of chronic lymphedema. Ultimately, any lesion suspected to be Kaposi's sarcoma should undergo biopsy. Findings will reveal a proliferation of spindle cells, erythrocytes in slitlike spaces, and irregularly shaped blood vessels.

Treatment (Table 16.5)

Many treatment modalities exist for Kaposi's sarcoma. For a few isolated lesions, excision, laser therapy, sclerotherapy, intralesional chemotherapy, radiation therapy, cryosurgery, or intralesional interferon can be used. For widespread and systemic disease, chemotherapy, radiation therapy, retinoids, and interferon-α are of benefit.

In patients with Kaposi's sarcoma who have other risk factors for AIDS, human immunodeficiency virus test should be done. The sarcoma may also improve with anti-retroviral therapy.

Metastatic carcinoma

Definition and etiology

Metastasis is the spread of a malignant tumor beyond its primary site of origin to a discontinuous area. The spread can occur through vascular or lymphatic pathways. The majority of patients with cutaneous metastases have a known underlying primary malignancy, but cutaneous lesions may sometimes be the first sign of malignancy.

Clinical features

Cutaneous metastases can occur at any age. They are most common in elderly adults. Excluding melanoma, the majority of cutaneous metastases are from lung, breast (in women), or gastrointestinal tract tumors. Metastatic tumors can have a variety of different morphologies:

1. Nodules
2. Inflammatory metastases (carcinoma erysipeloids)
3. Cicatricial metastases
4. Carcinoma en cuirasse
5. Zosteriform metastases

Each of these different types can be confused with a variety of other diseases.

Nodules of metastatic carcinoma are usually firm and vary in color from flesh-colored to red or purple. They can easily be confused with cysts, lipomas, or adnexal neoplasms. Therefore, the sudden development of a new nodule in a patient with known malignancy mandates a skin biopsy. A firm nodule that does not feel cystic and cannot be definitively classified should also undergo biopsy even if the patient does not have a history of underlying malignancy. Metastatic nodules in patients with renal cell carcinoma have a red vascular color and can easily be confused with hemangioma or pyogenic granuloma. Pyogenic granulomas occur in young adults and children and are exophytic papules. A pyogenic-granuloma-like lesion in an adult should undergo biopsy. Similarly, because most hemangiomas (cherry angiomas) in adults are small papules, a large hemangioma-like lesion should undergo biopsy.

Inflammatory metastases appear as red plaques mimicking erysipelas and have been called carcinoma erysipeloids. Unlike erysipelas, fever is absent, the lesions progress at a slower rate, and an indurated and nodular component may be present.

The lesions also most commonly occur in an area overlying a prior malignancy. Of note is that occasionally after surgical excision, some patients may also present with transient erythema lasting a few months to years in the site of surgery due to obstructed lymphatic vessels.

Cicatricial metastases appear as sclerotic plaques and can be mistaken for scars or sclerosing basal cell carcinoma. On the scalp, alopecia may be present (alopecia neoplastica). Therefore, cutaneous scar appearing without a prior history of injury or surgery should undergo biopsy, especially if the 'scar' is enlarging. Carcinoma en cuirasse refers to extensive metastatic involvement of the chest, which produces a circumferential fibrotic plaque. The tumor gives the patient the appearance of being encased in a breastplate of armor (en cuirasse). Metastatic nodules that involve a dermatome are referred to as zosteriform metastases. This pattern may be confused with herpes zoster. The presence of nodules rather than vesicles leads to a correct diagnosis.

Treatment (Table 16.6)

The prognosis for patients with cutaneous metastases is poor but depends on the type of malignancy. Chemotherapy or immunotherapy is the treatment of choice.

Pseudolymphoma

Definition and etiology

Pseudolymphoma (also known as lymphocytoma) is a benign proliferation of lymphocytes that is often confused with lymphoma. The cause is unknown, but pseudolymphoma can be triggered by insect bites, medications, and *Borrelia burgdorferi* infection.

Clinical features

Pseudolymphoma primarily occurs in children and young adults. There is a slight predilection for females. The skin examination shows a single or occasionally multiple subcutaneous blue-red nodules on the earlobes, face, chest, and scrotum. The presence of large lesions that ulcerate and predominantly involve the trunk should, however,

Table 16.6 Treatment of cutaneous metastasis

Treatment	Precautions
Determine the origin of primary	Not always possible
Chemotherapy or immunotherapy based upon primary site of tumor	Most treatments in future will be based upon the molecular characteristics of the patients tumor and will be individualized

raise suspicion of the presence of an underlying lymphoma. A chest x-ray and complete blood count with differential should be ordered, and patients should be examined for lymphadenopathy and hepatosplenomegaly when the diagnosis is not certain. Conversely, the history of occurrence of the lesions after an insect bite or onset of new medication would indicate a benign process. Phenytoin (Dilantin) has been associated with a pseudolymphoma-like reaction.

Clinically, the lesions cannot be differentiated from cutaneous lymphoma. If an etiologic agent cannot be ascertained with certainty, a biopsy is required for accurate diagnosis. Ultimately, all persistent lesions should undergo biopsy. Findings show a proliferation of lymphocytes in germinal centers mimicking a lymph node.

Because of occasional histologic resemblance to lymphoma, ancillary tests such as gene rearrangement or phenotypic studies are necessary to confirm the reactive nature of the infiltrate. Lesions of lymphocytoma cutis can also be confused with benign lymphocytic infiltrate of Jessner-Kanof, which is another reactive lymphocytic infiltrate. Clinically, however, the lesions of lymphocytic infiltrate of Jessner-Kanof usually are annular, and histologically the infiltrate is less dense without germinal center formation.

Treatment (Table 16.7)

A variety of different treatment modalities have been used. None is entirely effective. Topical and intralesional steroid injections are most commonly used. Lesions associated with *Borrelia burgdorferi* respond to penicillin or doxycycline therapy.

Any possibly associated medications should be discontinued. Cryotherapy and radiation therapy are also effective. Any lesion that does not respond to therapy should be followed carefully, since evolution of pseudolymphomas into true lymphomas has been reported.

Pyogenic granuloma

Definition and etiology

Pyogenic granuloma is a benign vascular proliferation. Whether the proliferation of blood vessels is reactive or neoplastic is yet to be determined.

Clinical features

Pyogenic granuloma can occur at any age but most commonly is found in young children. Pyogenic granuloma develops rapidly over a period of weeks with predilection for the head, neck, and arms. In pregnant women, mucosal lesions can occur. The skin examination reveals bright red, round, exophytic papules and nodules that bleed easily. Rarely, satellite lesions can occur after prior treatment or excision.

Table 16.7 Treatment of pseudolymphoma

Treatment	Precautions
Eliminate drug or other potential inciting agent Consider testing for Lyme disease Periodic follow up	Occasionally pseudolymphomas can evolve into primary cutaneous B cell lymphomas
Asymptomatic nodule: no treatment necessary	
Topical or intralesional steroid	Skin atrophy, scarring
Localized radiation therapy	Radiation dermatitis and scar
Excision if small	Scar, infection, recurrence
Cryotherapy	Blister, scar, pain

The differential diagnosis of pyogenic granuloma includes hemangioma, Kaposi's sarcoma, bacillary angiomatosis, primary cutaneous neoplasms such as Spitz nevus, atypical fibroxanthoma, amelanotic melanoma, and metastatic carcinoma. Hemangiomas usually start as macules and gradually grow into nodules in young children. They usually are larger, more lobulated masses as compared with the small, round, exophytic papules of pyogenic granulomas. A pyogenic-granuloma-like lesion in an immunocompromised patient, especially one with AIDS, requires a biopsy to differentiate the lesion from both Kaposi's sarcoma and bacillary angiomatosis, since both tumors can be exophytic vascular papules. The additional presence of flat purple patches or plaques would be indicative of Kaposi's sarcoma. Some primary cutaneous malignancies such as amelanotic melanoma and atypical fibroxanthoma can appear as red papules or nodules. If the lesion is asymmetric and only parts of it bleed, and if it exhibits a dermal component on palpation, a malignancy rather than pyogenic granuloma should be suspected. Although a Spitz nevus can appear red, be perfectly symmetric, and develop rapidly, usually a Spitz nevus is more dome- or sessile-shaped, is nonulcerated, and has a more tan-colored appearance. Metastatic carcinoma, especially metastatic renal cell carcinoma, can also present as a red, rapidly growing dermal nodule. Asymmetry, a palpable dermal component, or occurrence in elderly adults should arouse suspicion. A biopsy of pyogenic granuloma should be done to confirm the diagnosis. It shows an exophytic lobular proliferation of uniform round appearing blood vessels surrounded by edematous inflamed stroma and a collarette of epithelium.

Table 16.8 Treatment of pyogenic granulomas

Treatment	Precautions
Universal	
Consider biopsy to confirm diagnosis	Do not mistake metastatic carcinoma (especially renal) or melanoma/Spitz tumor for pyogenic granuloma
Excision	Scar, infection, recurrence
Electrocautery and curettage	Scar, infection, recurrence
Cryotherapy	Pain, blister, scar

Treatment (Table 16.8)

Pyogenic granuloma can be excised, removed with curettage and electrodesiccation, or treated with liquid nitrogen cryosurgery. Spontaneous resolution may also occur.

Section 4

SELF-ASSESSMENT

Chapter 17: Self-assessment

INTRODUCTION

This chapter is designed to provide practice using the algorithms at the beginning of each chapter of the text to arrive at a diagnosis. Review the figure followed by the multiple choice answers. Utilize the decision trees from the corresponding chapter to arrive at an answer. For dermatology, the morphology drives the diagnosis in most cases, so a history for the patient is not provided. The correct answers are provided on page 324–335, each one including a discussion guided by the appropriate algorithm. This exercise will increase your visual diagnostic skills.

QUESTIONS

Question 1

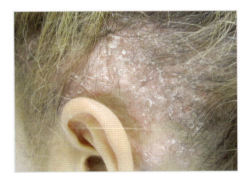

Pre-treatment.

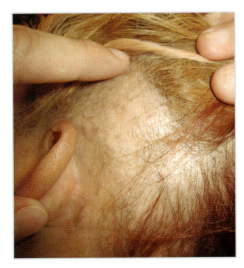

Post-treatment.

Which of the following is the correct diagnosis?
A. Alopecia areata
B. Psoriasis vulgaris
C. Tinea capitis
D. Discoid lupus erythematosus (DLE)
E. Seborrheic dermatitis

Question 2

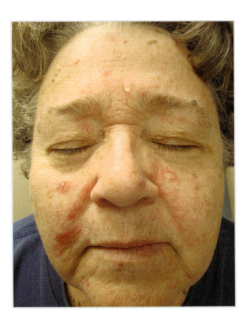

Which of the following is the correct diagnosis?
A. Cutaneous lupus erythematosus
B. Acne rosacea
C. Contact dermatitis
D. Polymorphous light eruption
E. Seborrheic dermatitis

Which of the following is the correct diagnosis?

Question 3

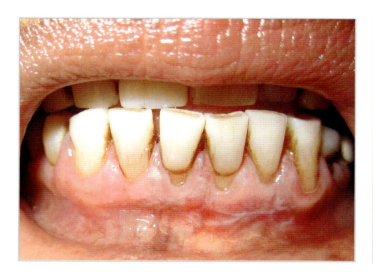

A. Oral candidiasis
B. Lichen planus
C. Aphthous ulcers
D. Herpes simplex
E. Pemphigus vulgaris

Question 4

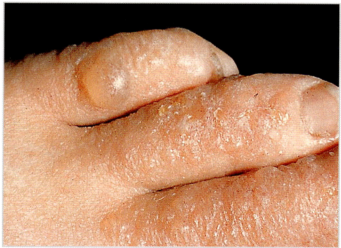

Which of the following is the correct diagnosis?
A. Psoriasis
B. Pustular psoriasis
C. Atopic dermatitis
D. Tinea pedis
E. Dyshidrotic eczema

Question 5

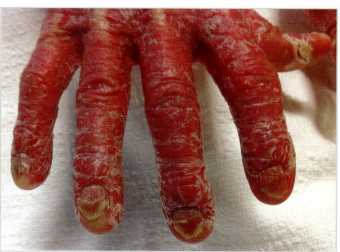

Which of the following is the correct diagnosis?
A. Psoriasis
B. Lichen planus
C. Onychomadesis
D. Onychomycosis
E. Onychophagia

Question 6

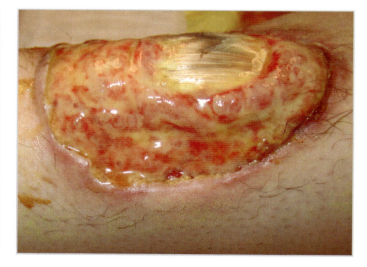

Which of the following is the correct diagnosis for this lesion on the shin?
A. Stasis ulcer
B. Leukocytoclastic vasculitis
C. Erythema nodosum
D. Polyarteritis nodosa
E. Pyoderma gangrenosum

Question 7

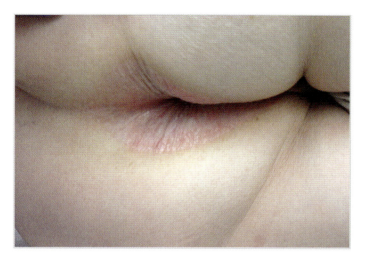

Which of the following is the correct diagnosis?
A. Condyloma acuminata
B. Lichen sclerosus et atrophicus
C. Tinea cruris
D. Extramammary Paget's disease
E. Contact dermatitis

Question 8

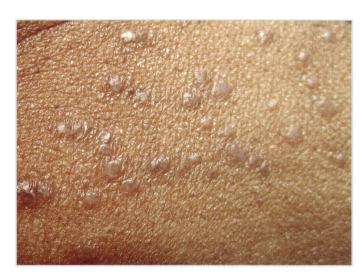

Which of the following is the correct diagnosis?
A. Lichen nitidus
B. Cutaneous T-cell lymphoma
C. Secondary syphilis
D. Lichen planus
E. Nummular dermatitis

Question 9

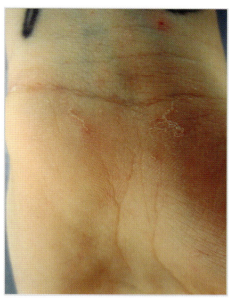

Which of the following is the correct diagnosis?
A. Winter itch
B. Dermatitis herpetiformis
C. Scabies
D. Contact dermatitis
E. Neurodermatitis

Question 10

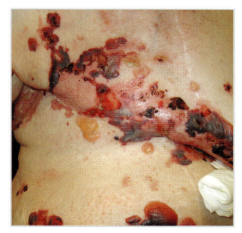

Which of the following is the correct diagnosis (anatomy distorted by mastectomy)?
A. Pemphigus vulgaris
B. Staphylococcal scalded skin
C. Herpes zoster
D. Contact dermatitis
E. Bullous pemphigoid (BP)

Question 11

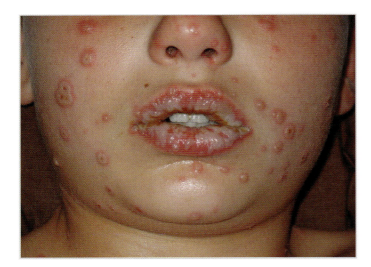

Which of the following is the correct diagnosis?
A. Viral exanthem
B. Angioedema
C. Insect bite reaction
D. Urticaria
E. Erythema multiforme

Question 12

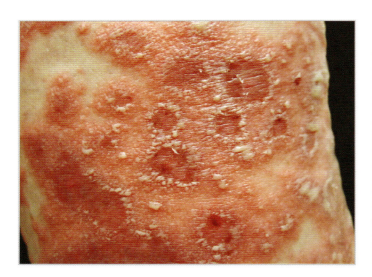

Which of the following is the correct diagnosis for this generalized eruption (shin pictured)?
A. Pustular psoriasis
B. Miliaria
C. Bacterial folliculitis
D. Eosinophilic pustular folliculitis
E. Meningococcemia

Question 13

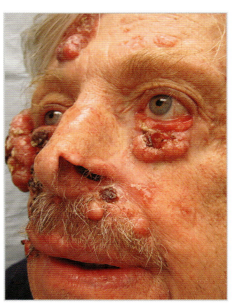

Which of the following is the correct diagnosis?
A. Basal cell carcinoma
B. Keratoacanthoma
C. Warts
D. Actinic keratoses
E. Chondrodermatitis nodularis chronica helicis

Question 14

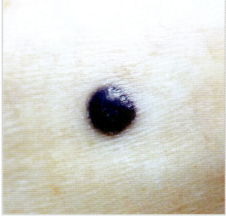

Which of the following is the correct diagnosis?
A. Cherry angioma
B. Solar lentigo
C. Malignant melanoma
D. Blue nevus
E. Seborrheic keratosis

Question 15

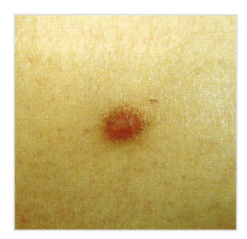

Which of the following is the correct diagnosis?
A. Pilar cyst
B. Lipoma
C. Neurofibroma
D. Dermatofibroma
E. Dermatofibrosarcoma protuberans

Question 16

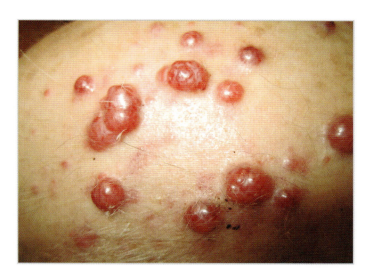

Which of the following is the correct diagnosis for these firm, fixed scalp lesions?
A. Cherry angioma
B. Pyogenic granuloma
C. Warts
D. Carcinoma erysipeloides
E. Metastatic carcinoma

ANSWERS

Answer 1: D. Discoid lupus erythematosus (DLE)

The photograph captures a patient with a defined patch of alopecia. In the pre-treatment photo, we can see that the alopecia is inflammatory, pink and scaly, and the posttreatment photo demonstrates that the alopecia is scarring. The hair in the affected region that remains is sparse, and unbroken, but there are areas of intervening skin that are smooth, lacking follicular ostia. Following the algorithm, we arrive at the correct answer. At the inferior aspect of the posttreatment photo, a classic example of active DLE, an atrophic plaque with an erythematous active border is present.

Unlike DLE, alopecia areata does not produce scale, nor is it inflammatory (pink). After resolution, DLE leaves areas of hyper and hypopigmentation (visible in the post treatment photograph). There are no exclamation point hairs in either photograph. Alopecia areata does not scar, and would not produce smooth areas of skin lacking follicular ostia.

Psoriasis may include sharply defined scaly pink plaques on the scalp. Unlike DLE, scalp psoriasis does not commonly produce alopecia, and would not result in the scarring visible in the posttreatment photograph.

Tinea capitis can manifest as scaly alopecia, and may be erythematous. However, there are no broken or "black dot" hairs present in the photographs to suggest this fungal infection. Tinea capitis does not scar.

Seborrheic dermatitis may involve the scalp, and may demonstrate erythema and scale which is usually not well demarcated. However, seborrheic dermatitis does not produce alopecia.

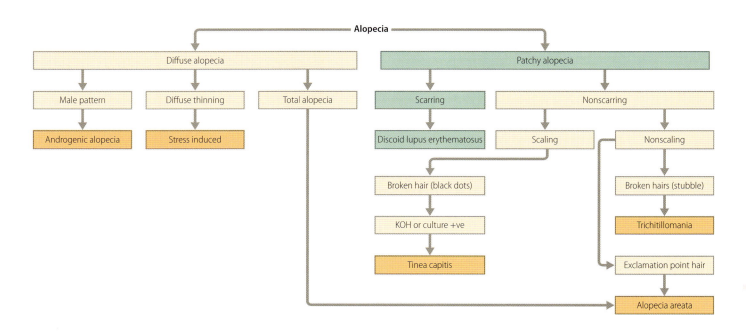

Answer 2: E. Seborrheic dermatitis

Here a patient presents with redness and scaling on the face. Disfiguring scarring is not present, and the rash is accentuated in the nasolabial folds, glabella, eyebrows and forehead, and extends toward the scalp. Following the algorithm, the presence of scaling and accentuation in nasolabial folds makes seborrheic dermatitis the best fit.

Acute cutaneous lupus (malar or butterfly rash) manifests as photodistributed pink or violet pink macules or plaques, and may be scaly. It characteristically spares the nasolabial folds, as well as areas of the face shaded from light such as the upper eyelids, the chin, the submandibular region, and behind the ears. This patient shows accentuation of the nasolabial folds, and involvement of the upper eyelids. Furthermore, cutaneous lupus is more likely to present in younger women. Discoid lupus presents with discrete pink or red plaques with thick scale that eventually become atrophic and scarring.

Acne rosacea more characteristically presents with either papules and pustules, or red macules rife with telangiectases. Neither telangiectases, nor papules and pustules are visible in the photograph above.

Contact dermatitis typically features a sharply geographic border on the face, and would be expected to appear less patchy. It is unlikely that the patient is coming in contact with an allergen or irritant in such a limited facial distribution.

As with lupus, polymorphous light eruption favors areas exposed to direct light, and would not be expected to involve the eyelids, eyebrows and chin.

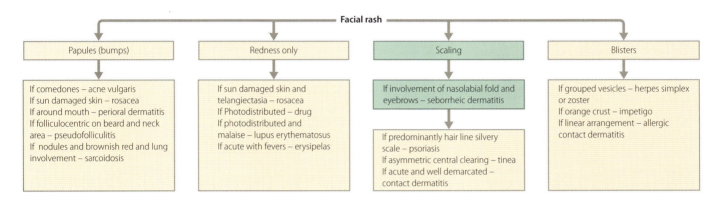

Answer 3: B. Lichen planus

In this picture, the gingival mucosa is affected by inflammatory plaques resulting in recession of the gum line. The inflammation is generalized across all visible gingival mucosa. Lacey or reticulated white plaques (Wickham's striae) are visible just inferior to the mandibular incisors, and prominently at the junction of the gingival and buccal mucosa. These striae are characteristic of oral lichen planus, and allow for clinical diagnosis. Due to the presence of inflammation, the patient reported burning pain.

Oral candidiasis typically presents as white plaques much thicker than those of lichen planus and without erosion. Candidal plaques are loosely adherent and easily removed by gentle scraping with a tongue depressor. Examination of the plaques with KOH preparation and microscopy would show fungal elements. Oral candidiasis is most commonly asymptomatic, and may be associated with a number of conditions including glucocorticoid or antibiotic use, poorly controlled diabetes, immunodeficiency, lymphomas and many others.

Aphthous ulcers appear as discrete ulcers with a white to yellow base, and are classified based on their size. Minor aphthae are a few millimeters in diameter and heal within a week, while major aphthae are more than a centimeter in diameter, and may scar. The patient photographed above has generalized gingival inflammation, inconsistent with the solitary appearance of aphthous ulcers.

The herpes simplex virus can cause herpetic gingivostomatitis. Like lichen planus, HSV can cause painful inflammation and ulceration. Unlike lichen planus, the ulcerations are preceded by vesicles, are clustered, and have a punched-out appearance with scalloped borders. Wickham's striae are not present in herpetic gingivostomatitis.

Pemphigus vulgaris invariably affects the oral mucosa (though clinical severity varies). Patients affected by pemphigus vulgaris manifest generalized erosion and ulceration of the oral mucosa. The erosions and ulcerations expand with application of trivial shearing force (Nikolsky sign). The patient may or may not have disease activity on the skin, depending upon which antibody profile the patient has developed. Wickham's striae will not be present in pemphigus vulgaris. If pemphigus is considered in the differential, biopsy for histopathologic and immunofluorescent evaluation should be performed.

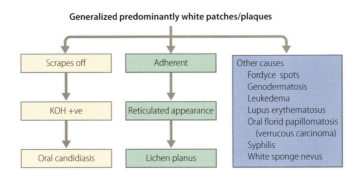

Answer 4: E. Dyshidrotic eczema

The algorithm first tasks the reader to determine whether this rash is sharply or poorly demarcated. Unlike psoriasis, it is difficult to say where the edge of this eruption lies (compare to **Figure 4.3.3** for an example of psoriasis' sharp borders). Thus, is it poorly demarcated. Faint scale is present on the toes. Absent are the serpiginous and scaly borders of tinea pedis, though it is always reasonable to perform KOH preparation on scaling rashes of the feet. Finally the numerous small vesicles (blisters <1cm) dotting the toes, with emphasis on the lateral aspects, cement the diagnosis of dyshidrotic eczema.

The proper application of morphologic terms is important in diagnosing skin disorders. The small blisters filled with clear fluid on this patient's toes are vesicles. Pustular psoriasis features small blisters filled with pus, aptly called pustules. The presence of vesicles rather than pustules in the photograph argues against pustular psoriasis and psoriasis vulgaris.

Dyshidrotic dermatitis is restricted to the hands and feet. Atopic dermatitis uncommonly features vesicles, but should also include scaly pink patches on flexural surfaces, often with a history of other atopic disorders such as allergic rhinitis or asthma.

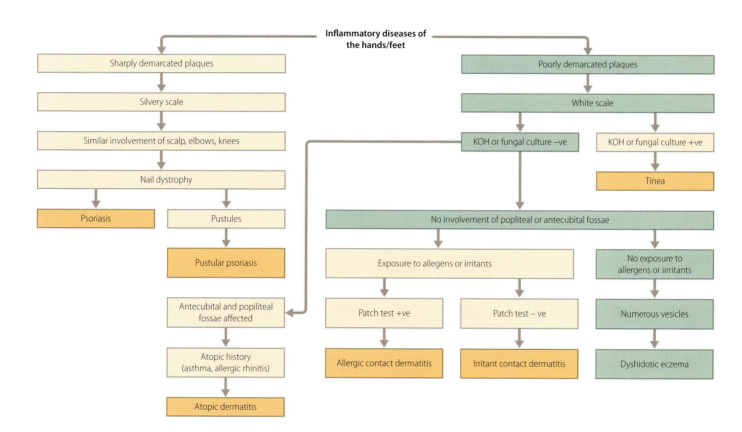

Answer 5: A. Psoriasis

Significant nail dystrophy and erythroderma are presented in the photograph above. Even in the most striking clinical presentations, the algorithm above is still helpful. In this particular case, the appearance of the patient's nails was the clue to diagnosing his erythroderma. Examination of the nails reveals thickened plates (onychodystrophy), pitting and the presence of oil spots (yellow brown discoloration of the nail). Red plaques with silver-white lamellar scale are present over all visible skin in the photograph. These findings are characteristic of psoriasis.

A small percentage of patients with lichen planus will develop nail changes (about 10%), with variable appearance. The most representative change is called ventral pterygium, a scarring of the nail matrix that results in an atrophic, tapered or v-shaped appearance to the nail (pictured in **Figures 5.2.4** and **5.2.5**). Nail pitting and oil spots are not found in lichen planus. The rash of lichen planus is characterized by purple, flat topped papules, often arrayed in a linear fashion, unlike the red, scaly plaques pictured above.

Onychomadesis describes shedding of the nails. This can be secondary to trauma, viral infection (coxsackie virus in children), or idiopathic. It may be isolated, or may occur periodically. It does not result in onychodystrophy nor oil spotting.

Onychophagia results from biting or chewing the nail plate and would not present with erythroderma, oil spots and pitting.

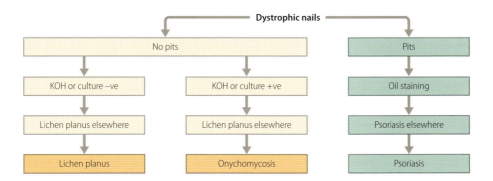

Answer 6: E. Pyoderma gangrenosum

Presented above is a full thickness ulcer on the inferior aspect of the left shin. The border is violet and has an undermined appearance. The skin around the ulcer is healthy in appearance without rash, necrosis, purpura, or prominent vessels. Following the algorithm, pyoderma gangreonsum is the best answer. A biopsy performed at the medial aspect (not pictured) formed a second ulcer consistent with pathergy. The patient reports that the lesion started as a solitary pustule that expanded rapidly. At the center of the ulcer, the exposed tendon of the extensor digitorum longus is visible.

While leukocytoclastic vasculitis can result in small necrotic ulcerations, affected patients will also demonstrate palpable purpura in the surrounding skin. Neither purpura nor necrosis are pictured above.

Erythema nodosum does occur most commonly on the shins, but is not expected to ulcerate, and certainly not to the degree in the photograph. Typically, erythema nodosum presents as tender and warm, pink to dusky nodules on the shin. Erythema nodosum is associated with a bevy of other conditions including medications, pregnancy, infections, malignancy, autoimmune disease and inflammatory bowel disease.

Polyarteritis nodosa is a medium sized vasculitis that may affect the skin of the lower legs. Most often patients with cutaneous involvement exhibit tender dusky nodules or necrotic stellate ulcerations. Systemic symptoms such as fever, weight loss, abdominal pain, and neuropathy may also be present, but there is a cutaneous-only variant. The borders of the ulcer above are undermined, and do not demonstrate necrosis or a stellate appearance.

Stasis ulcers are common on the lower leg, but more typically affect the medial malleolus. Patients usually exhibit stasis related changes to skin around the ulcer, such as dermatitis, ectatic tortuous veins, or lipodermatosclerosis.

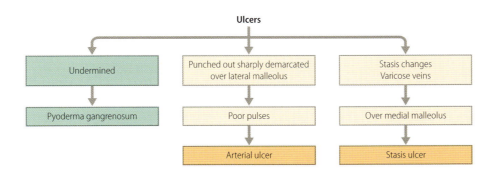

Answer 7: B. Lichen sclerosus et atrophicus

Here, a patient experiences a symmetric confluent perianal plaque, extending across the perineum to the vulva (not pictured). There are no ulcers, erosions nor papules present. The white discoloration of the plaques is a strong clue toward the diagnosis, and the fine wrinkling of the plaque results from atrophy of the epidermis (atrophic skin). Lichen sclerosus et atrophicus is clearly the best (and correct) diagnosis.

Condyloma acuminata, or the common genital wart, may develop in the perianal region, but would appear as verrucal papules. As this patient has atrophic plaques, condyloma are ruled out.

Tinea cruris, a dermatophyte infection commonly referred to as jock itch, does develop as plaques in the groin. Like most variants of dermatophyte infection, tinea cruris will show scaly plaques with a serpigenous border, in contrast to the atrophic plaques with a smooth regular border pictured above. Tinea cruris often has has central clearing, which also distinguishes it from lichen sclerosus et atrophicus. Patients with tinea cruris usually have concomitant tinea pedis.

Extramammary Paget's (EMPD) disease can be a challenge to diagnose, as it may mimic or be mistaken for other disorders such as dermatitis, tinea or Bowen's disease. In its classic appearance, EMPD appears as an asymmetric red plaque, with sharp clear borders, sometimes with a white crusting (the red and white colors are termed 'strawberries and cream'). Generally, if a rash in the groin is not responding as expected to therapy, biopsy should be considered to evaluate for EMPD.

Rather than the white and atrophic plaqe in this patient, contact dermatitis typically manifests a geometric red to pink plaque with scale. Atrophy is not a key feature of contact dermatitis.

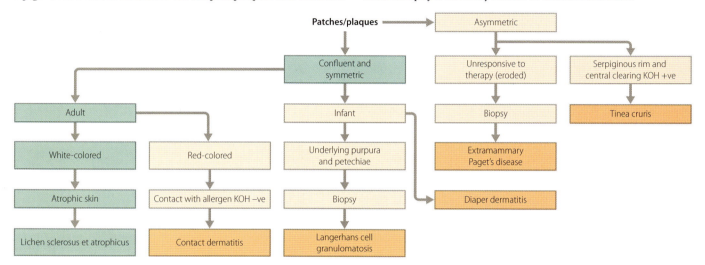

Answer 8: D. Lichen planus

This photograph represents a rash on the low back. The rash is comprised predominantly of papules, and provides an entry point to the algorithm. The papules are purple, with polygonal borders, and are flat topped (planar). Following the decision tree, lichen planus is the correct choice. Note that in the photograph, some of the papules are arranged in a linear fashion. This represents koebnerization (the isomorphic response), or the tendency for a rash to occur in traumatized areas (such as those injured by scratching). This is a common feature of lichen planus.

Cutaneous T-cell lymphoma (CTCL) can have a variety of presentations, including macules, patches, plaques and tumors. Plaque stage CTCL typically has an irregular border, or may be serpiginous or annular in appearance with some degree of scale, atrophy or poikiloderma present. Regardless, T-cell lymphoma does not appear as purple planar papules with a monomorphic appearance.

Secondary syphilis occurs between 8 weeks to 2 years after untreated primary infection. It erupts as scaly red-pink plaques and papules primarily on the trunk which follow skin tension lines. Because of this pattern it can mimic pityriasis rosea. Unlike pityriasis rosea, the rash of secondary syphilis usually involves the palms and soles. Lichen planus is usually easily distinguished from syphilis by color (purple), and morphology (polygonal koebnerizing papules). However, if the palms and soles are affected, think of syphilis.

Nummular dermatitis presents as pink or red scaly round, plaques with indistinct borders and may include vesicles or crusting. The coin shaped plaques are typically larger than the small papules of lichen planus.

Lichen nitidus appears as tiny grouped monomorphic flesh colored papules. The individual papules of lichen nitidus are considerably smaller than the papules of lichen planus. Both are well described to exhibit koebnerization.

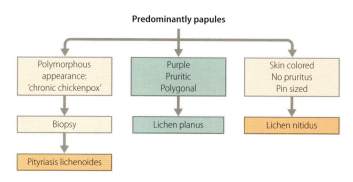

Answer 9: C. Scabies

The wrist and palm of a patient with significant pruritus is photographed. An excoriated papule, and scale are present on the volar wrist. On the hypothenar eminence, a serpiginous tract of scale is present surrounded by thin pink erythema, and terminating at a tiny brown dot at its distal aspect. This is a classic example of a burrow. Mineral oil or KOH preparation of scrapings from this burrow revealed a sarcoptes scabiei mite. Preparation of scrapings must include the black dot, which represents the mite. Typical distribution of excoriations, papules and burrows includes wrists, breasts, abdomen and genitals.

Winter itch, or asteatotic dermatitis usually manifests with serpiginous scaly fissured patches that are much more inflammatory (red or pink), and much more densely arrayed than typical burrows.

Dermatitis herpetiformis is another intensely pruritic condition. Rather than burrows, dermatitis herpetiformis typically presents as erosions resulting from excoriated thin vesicles on the elbows, knees, shoulders and low back or buttocks.

Contact dermatitis is an eczematous eruption usually with geographic borders as opposed to papules or burrows.

Neurodermatitis presents as excoriations without primary lesions. The excoriations are characteristically linear, and relegated to areas the patient can reach.

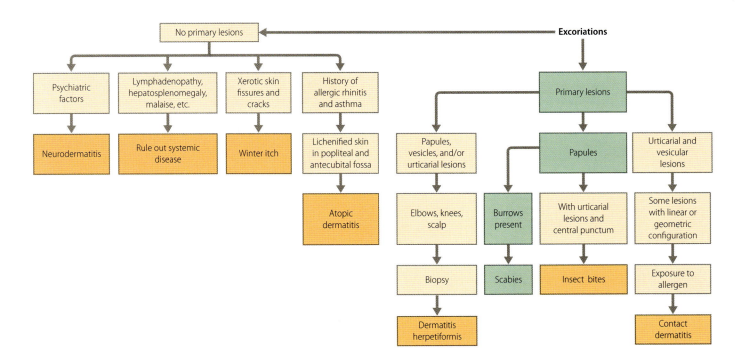

Answer 10: E. Bullous pemphigoid (BP)

This woman is experiencing a wide-spread eruption featuring erosions and intact bullae (blisters >1cm in diameter). Tense blisters are indicative of a subepidermal pathology. When acquired and generalized, as in this case, the bullae are most likely due to bullous pemphigoid (or closely related but uncommon disorders). Medication history is important, as a significant proportion of BP is drug related. Bullous pemphigoid may affect the oral mucosa in roughly 1/3rd of cases, but clinical features of mucosal disease are difficult to differentiate from other blistering conditions.

Pemphigus vulgaris (PV) is another immunobullous disorder. Understanding the pathogenic features of pemphigus can help the clinician differentiate PV from BP. In PV, autoantibodies target desmogleins on the surface of keratinocytes. These proteins help keratinocytes in the superficial layers of the epidermis adhere to one another. Disruption of the desmogleins interferes with keratinocyte adhesion, resulting in skin separation in the upper layers of the epidermis (intra-epidermal). Thus, patients will develop erosions or fragile vesicles. BP's antibodies target components of the hemidesmosomes, which are present only at the interface of the epidermis and dermis. Loss of hemidesmosome function results in a split underneath the full thickness of the epidermis (sub-epidermal). In these patients, clinicians will observe tense blisters or bullae. Thus, the presence of intact bullae can help distinguish BP from PV. PV patients always have some degree of immunoreactivity of the oral mucosa, with or without symptoms. The astute clinician may detect erosions of the oropharynx that the patient was aware of.

Herpes zoster presents with pain, itching or burning, along with clusters of vesicles (blisters < 1cm) arrayed along a dermatomal region of skin. The woman in the photograph has a generalized eruption of bullae and erosions (not clustered vesicles), and her eruption is present across several thoracic dermatomes.

Desquamation and erosion are most prominent in staphylococcal scalded skin syndrome (SSSS). Bacterial toxins disrupt the same adhesion molecules as those affected in pemphigus family disorders, resulting in superficial erosions or fragile vesicles. SSSS erosion and sloughing accentuate in the flexures (neck, axillae, antecubital fossae), and around the eyes and mouth. The facial involvement is characteristic, and results in a typical 'sad facies'.

Contact dermatitis can cause vesicles or bullae in any combination, but is not usually generalized. Rather, the borders of the eruption are typically strikingly geographic, related to the area of skin contact. In the case of poison ivy (rhus dermatitis), bullae or vesicles are often found in linear arrangements where sap was deposited as the plant brushes past the skin.

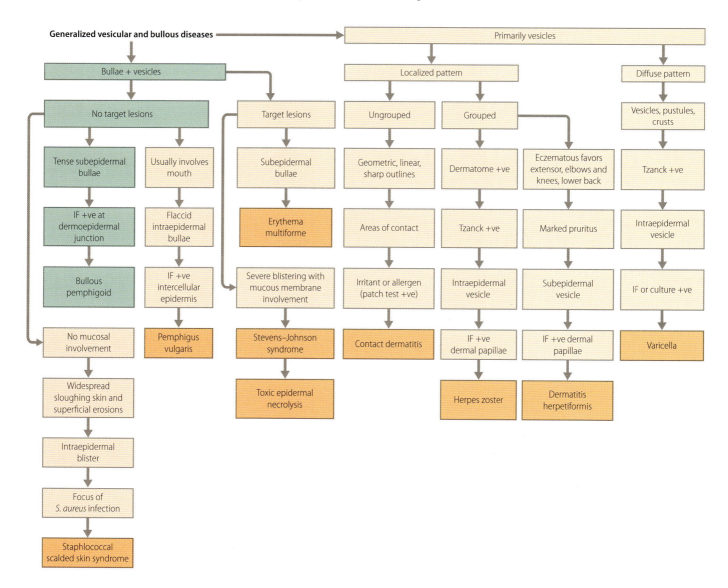

Answer 11: E. Erythema multiforme

Looking at the algorithm, the first decision branch asks whether the patient has maculopapular rash, or an urticarial eruption. No macules are present. Rather, edematous papules and plaques are present on the face, lips and oral mucosa of this child. Thus, the urticarial eruption tree is best. Even without taking a history, it can be reasonably established that these lesions are fixed. With as much inflammation and edema as pictured, it is unlikely that the papules would resolve quickly or without sequelae. As no post-inflammatory changes are present in unaffected skin, and the papules demonstrate inflammation and edema enough to persist, they must not be transient. Closer inspection of the papules on the cheeks reveals targetoid morphology, and the reader is directed toward the correct diagnosis, erythema multiforme. This patient has mucosal involvement, which is commonly, but not always, seen.

Viral exanthems are a prototypical maculopapular rash. These patients exhibit pink hyperemic macules, and fine pink papules which may coalesce to plaques. Rather than fine papules or macules, this patient experiences edematous urticarial papules and plaques.

Angioedema presents as non-pitting edema, often affecting large portions of the lips, tongue, mouth face, or other body parts. It does not involve discrete urticaria, and should not cause vesiculation of the oral mucosa.

Reactions to insect bites will develop as discrete fixed urticarial papules. However, they would not be expected to cause vesiculation of the lips or oral mucosa. Rather than a targetoid shape, insect bites may include a central punctum.

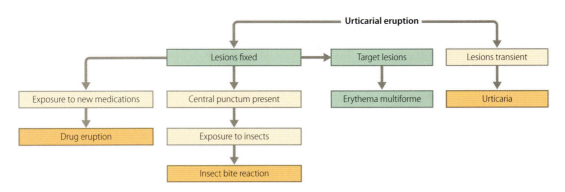

Answer 12: A. Pustular psoriasis

Pustular eruptions can be distressing to both the patient and the provider as the presentation is often striking. Patients may appear toxic. This case is challenging, but the algorithm can help rule out all but the correct response. Generalized pustules are present (as described in the stem), but they are not follicular based. Folliculocentric implies that each individual pustule is centered on a follicle, with a hair shaft at its center. The lack of folliculocentricity rules out bacterial and eosinophilic pustular folliculitides (answers C and D). Since the photograph is from the shin, miliaria is unlikely as this condition favors areas of occlusion, typically on the trunk (e.g. a critical care patient lying on a plastic mattress for an extended period of time). Pustular psoriasis and pustular drug eruption cannot be distinguished easily on exam, and both can feature fever. Detailed history taking is the key to securing the diagnosis, including past history of psoriasis, or new medications.

Meningococcemia can feature pustules, but typically also includes purpura in an acutely ill patient.

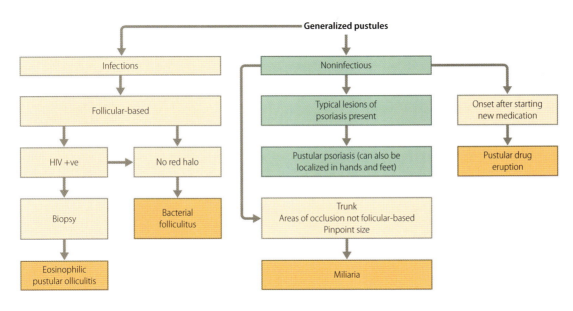

Answer 13: A. Basal cell carcinoma

Here is another extreme example of a common problem. Such a dramatic presentation can be intimidating at first examination, but appropriate application of morphologic terms, and of the chapter's algorithm allow for diagnosis. Inspection of the lesion under the patient's left eye reveals a crusted pearly tumor, with a rolled border and telangiectasia: a perfect description of a basal cell carcinoma. This patient has a mutation in his PTCH (patched 1 human homologue) gene resulting in basal cell nevus syndrome. Among other features, patients develop myriad basal cell carcinomas.

Keratoacanthoma can be easily confused with a classic basal cell carcinoma. Keratoacanthoma features a central keratin filled crater, rather than the central erosion or ulceration that a basal cell might exhibit. This central keratinization can develop the appearance of a plug or horn. The crust in the ulceration of this patient's basal cell is composed of dried blood and serous fluid (a scab), not keratin. In addition, keratoacanthomas usually develop quickly in 1-2 months in contrast to basal cell carcinomas which take many months to years to become large. A biopsy will ready distinguish the two entities.

While some of the patient's tumors may have a verrucal appearance, warts do not typically ulcerate, nor do they feature telangiectasia and rolled borders. Warts tend to exhibit a cauliflower like surface texture that interferes with skin lines. Close inspection may reveal dark puncta in the substance of the wart representing thrombosed vessels.

Actinic keratoses are typically scaly pink patches or macules with a sandpaper texture. While these precancerous lesions may be come hyperkeratotic appearing as a horn, they do not develop into tumors. Any fleshy substance around a suspected actinic keratosis suggests malignancy and should be biopsied for histopathologic evaluation.

Chondrodermatitis nodularis chronica helicis appears on the ear, resulting from chronic pressure and cartilage degeneration. It does not occur on the face.

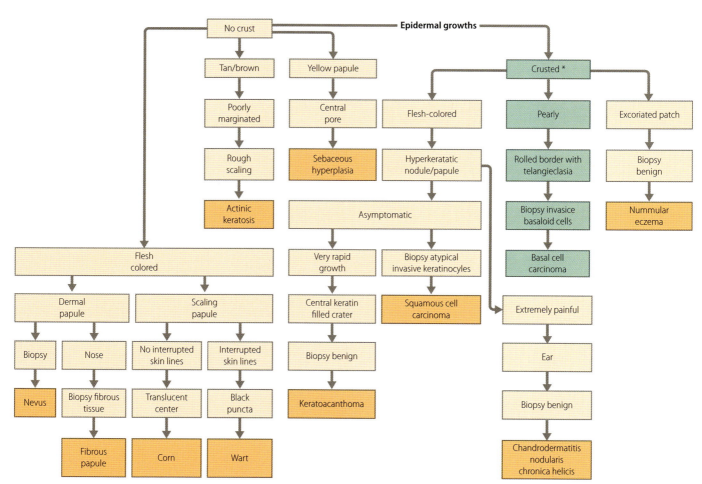

*Basal cell and squamous cell carcinoma may not be crusted when small

Answer 14: D. Blue nevus

Following the algorithm, the photograph includes a pigmented papule. The papule is uniform in its color, which is deep blue to black. The border of the papule is smooth and regular, and there is no asymmetry present to suggest malignancy. Dermoscopy of a blue nevus will demonstrate uniform blue black pigmentation. Because of the presence of black coloration, it would not be unreasonable to biopsy this papule, which would secure its diagnosis as a blue nevus.

Solar lentigines appear as macules on sun exposed skin, with regular brown pigmentation. Lentigines do not form papules, like the one present in the photograph.

Discerning malignant melanoma from a blue nevus can be challenging. Melanoma can take on a variety of clinical appearances, and often includes blue or black coloration. Blue nevi are usually small, with a history of stable appearance over many years. Since early or developing nodular malignant melanoma may be difficult to distinguish from a blue nevus, biopsy plays a valuable role in establishing the correct diagnosis. This is especially true if the patient was not aware of the presence of the lesion, or if they report that the papule has developed recently. Since blue nevi are dermal collections of melanocytes, excisional or punch biopsy is often best.

Cherry angiomas appear as small papules with uniform color much like a blue nevus. Most typically, angiomas are bright crimson red, but may appear blue to purple. Close inspection of an angioma with dermoscopy will reveal small vascular saccules called lacunae comprising the papule.

Seborrheic keratoses are epidermal benign growths with brown discoloration resulting from keratin rather than melanin pigment in most cases. They develop as waxy plaques with a pasted-on appearance. Keratin filled pits resembling black heads may dot the surface of the plaques, or they may have a cerebriform or fissured texture.

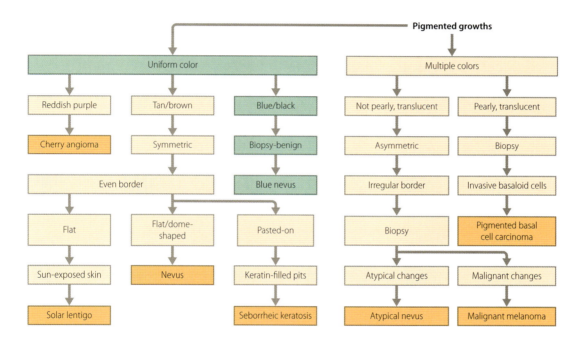

Answer 15: D. Dermatofibroma

A small, regularly shaped pink papule with surrounding tan brown discoloration is presented on the leg of this patient. Following the algorithm, we can see that it is small, and includes tan brown coloration. It is not pedunculated. While the photograph does not show umbilication with lateral pressure, it appears as a firm discrete nodule. This leaves dermatofibroma as the most likely, and correct, answer. The peripheral brown coloration and a more hypopigmented center are also characteristic features of a dermatofibroma.

Pilar cysts are uncommon anywhere other than the scalp, removing this answer choice from consideration. They appear as well circumscribed round firm nodules that feel cystic when palpated.

Lipomas generally do not have superficial features other than slight outward deformation of the epidermis. One would not expect to see pigmentary changes overlying these benign fatty tumors. Typically lipomas are soft rubbery subcutaneous tumors that are mobile, with poorly defined borders.

Neurofibromas, as the algorithm suggests, are usually larger, soft, exophytic papules or tumors. They are readily compressible, and often give the impression that they can be reduced back into the skin (button-holing).

Dermatofibrosarcoma protuberans (DFSP) is a scar-like malignancy, which can have a similar consistency to the dermatofibroma when examined. However, DFSP are typically larger than dermatofibromas, with an irregularly shaped outline. Biopsy and special staining techniques can help to distinguish the two where necessary.

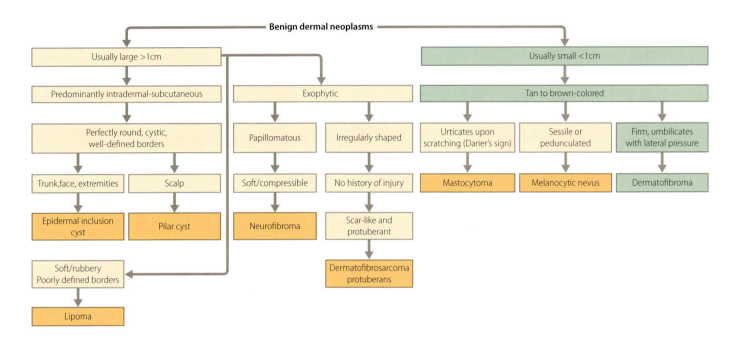

Answer 16: E. Metastatic carcinoma

The nodules on this gentleman's scalp were diagnosed as Merkel cell carcinoma on biopsy. The firm, fixed features of these dermal nodules led to strong clinical suspicion for metastatic disease. That there were multiple lesions argues against a benign process.

These tumors are pink to red, and might at first blush be confused for a vascular process such as a cherry angioma. Visible on the surface of several of these lesions are telangiectasia. Vascular appearing tumors such as cherry angiomata, renal cell carcinoma and pyogenic granulomas, have a more saccular appearance, representing vascular lacunae rather than vessels. Further, true vascular lesions are much more bright red (due to blood) to purple (if thrombosed). Pyogenic granulomas are typically solitary.

Warts are typified by flesh colored papules which interfere with skin lines, a cauliflower like surface texture, and small dark punctae representing thrombi. The tumors above are smooth because they are dermal processes, unlike warts which derive from the epidermis leading to textural changes.

Carcinoma erysipeloides, despite being a malignant process, mimics a cellulitic rash. This gentleman has developed tumors.

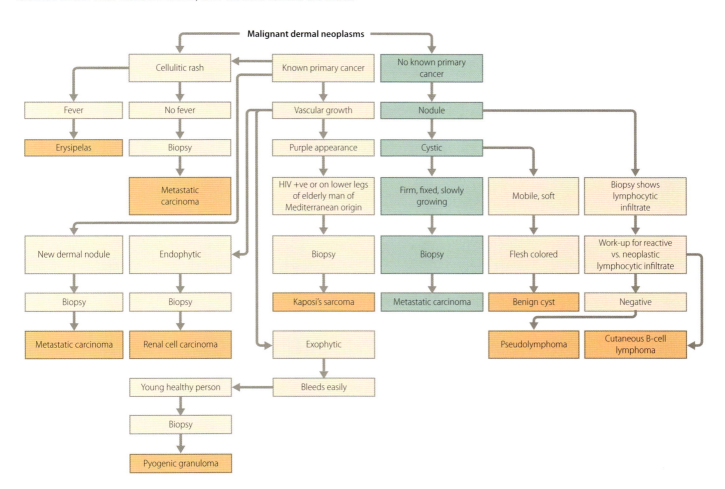

Index

Note: Page numbers in **bold** or *italic* refer to tables or figures respectively.

A

Acneiform drug eruptions 211, **211**
Acne rosacea 43, 325
    acne vulgaris vs. 28, 28–29, *29*
    clinical stages 43–44
    papules and pustules 31
    systemic lupus erythematosus vs. 30, 30–31, *31*
    treatment 44, **44**
Acne vulgaris 43
    acne rosacea vs. 28, 28–29, *29*
    adenoma sebaceum mimicking 29
    clinical features 43
    comedones *29*, 43
    cysts 29
    pseudofolliculitis vs. 32, *32*
    treatment 43, **43**
Acrodermatitis enteropathica *121*, 125
Actinic keratosis 221–222, 248, 332
    seborrheic keratosis vs. 220–221, *220–222*
    squamous cell carcinoma vs. 223–224, *223–225*
    treatment 248, **248**
Acute generalized exanthematous pustulosis 213
    pustular psoriasis vs. *210*, 210–211
    treatment 213, **213**
Acute generalized pustular psoriasis of von Zumbusch type 213, 214
Allergic contact dermatitis 66–68
    from artificial nails 84
    irritant contact dermatitis vs. 66, *66*, 67
Alopecia 3, 22, 324 see also specific type
    diffuse 3
    patchy 3
Alopecia areata 3, *5*, *6*, 23
    clinical features 23
    discoid lupus erythematosus vs. *13*, 13–14, *14*
    exclamation point hairs *5*, 23
    loss of eyebrow and eyelashes *6*, *12*
    tinea capitis vs. *4*, 4–5, *5*, *6*
    treatment **23**, 23–24
    trichotillomania vs. *11*, 11–12, *12*
Alopecia neoplastica 299, 314
Alopecia totalis *5*, 23
Alopecia universalis 23
Anagen effluvium secondary to chemotherapy 19
Androgenic alopecia *16*, 23
    clinical features 23
    stress-induced alopecia vs. *15*, 15–16, *16*
    treatment 23, **23**
ANGEL tumors 296, 311
Angioedema 331
Angiosarcoma 313

Aphthous ulcers 60, 325
    differential diagnosis 60
    herpetiform lesions 60
    major 60
    minor 60
    pemphigus vulgaris vs. *52*, 52–53, *53*
    treatment 60, **60**
Aplasia cutis 22
Arsenical keratosis 247
Arterial ulcers 105, 109
    stasis ulcer vs. 100, *100*, *101*
    treatment 105, **105**
Arteriovenous hemangiomas 312
Asteatotic dermatitis see Winter itch
Atopic dermatitis 72, 125, 166, 326
    contact dermatitis vs. 162, *163*
    dermatitis herpetiformis vs. *160*, 160–161, *161*
    lichenified antecubital fossa *163*
    lichenified skin *161*
    major and minor features 166
    major criteria for diagnosis of 71
    psoriasis vs. 70–71, *70–72*
    treatment 166, **166**
Atopic hand-and-foot dermatitis 75
    differential diagnosis 75
    eczematous eruption in 75
    treatment 75, **75**
Atypical nevus 278
    malignant melanoma vs. 261, *261*

B

Bacillary angiomatosis 313
Bacterial folliculitis 211–212
    eosinophilic pustular folliculitis vs. *206*, 206–207, *207*
    follicular-based abscess 207
    hot tub use 207
    miliaria rubra vs. *208*, 208–209, *209*
    sites of 211
    treatment 212, **212**
Balanitis xerotica obliterans *115*, 127
Basal cell carcinoma 248, 278–279, *322*, 332
    differential diagnosis 248
    fibrous papule vs. 241, *241*
    morpheaform 248
    nodular 248
    pigmented 248
    sebaceous hyperplasia vs. *239*, 239–240, *240*
    superficial *242*, 242–243, 248
    treatment 248–249, **249**
Basal cell carcinoma (nodular)
    intradermal nevus vs. *237*, 237–238, *238*
    squamous cell carcinoma vs. 233–234, *233–236*

Becker's nevus 275
Black hairy tongue (lingua nigra) 59
Blastomycosis-like pyoderma 245
Blue nevus 278, *322*, 333
    malignant melanoma vs. *267*, 267–268, *268*
Bowenoid papulosis 123
    condyloma acuminatum vs. *112*, 112–113, *113*
    differential diagnosis 123
    treatment **123**, 123–124
Bronchogenic duct cyst 296
Brown reclose spider bite 199
Bullous acute cutaneous lupus erythematosus 187
Bullous impetigo 186
Bullous pemphigoid (BP) 187, *321*, 330
    contact dermatitis vs. 172–173, *172–174*
    differential diagnosis 187
    erythema multiforme vs. 178, *178*, *179*
    pemphigus vulgaris vs. 175–176, *175–177*
    treatment 187, **188**
Buttonhole sign 297

C

Candida albicans 60
Carcinoma en cuirasse 314
Carcinoma erysipeloides 299, 335
    erysipelas vs. 302, *302*
Cavernous hemangiomas 312
Cellulitis 105, *200*
    differential diagnosis 105
    stasis dermatitis vs. 104, *104*
    treatment 105, **105**
Central centrifugal cicatricial alopecia 20
Chancroid 117, 126, 128
Cherry angioma 277, 312, 333, 335
    malignant melanoma vs. *271*, 271–272, *272*
    treatment 277, **277**
Chickenpox see Varicella
Cholesterol emboli 94
Chondrodermatitis nodularis helicis 249, 332
    squamous cell carcinoma vs. *231*, 231–232, *232*
    treatment 249, **249**
Cicatricial metastases 314
Cicatricial pemphigoid 22, 59
Collagenoma 294
Comedo 43 see also Acne vulgaris
Common baldness see Androgenic alopecia
Condyloma acuminatum 123, 124, 328
    bowenoid papulosis vs. *112*, 112–113, *113*
    treatment 124, **124**
Condyloma latum (syphilis) 124
Conradi–Hunermann syndrome 19

337

INDEX

Consort dermatitis 44
Contact dermatitis 34, 42, 44, 69, 75–76, 124, 166–167, 187–188, 325, 329, 330
    acute 187
    allergic 44, 75, 167
    atopic dermatitis vs. 162, 163
    bullous pemphigoid vs. 172–173, *172–174*
    chronic 187–188
    contact with poison ivy 74
    differential diagnosis 44
    dyshidrotic eczema vs. 68, 68–69, *69*
    erythema in 41
    hand cream and 74
    lichen sclerosus et atrophicus vs. 114, 114–115, *115*
    linear vesicles 163
    perioral dermatitis vs. 41, 41–42, *42*
    positive patch tests 163
    seborrheic dermatitis vs. 33, 33–34, *34*
    tinea vs. 73, *73*, *74*
    treatment 44, **44**, 124, **125**, 167, **167**, 188, **188**
Corn 249
    plantar wart vs. 218, 218–219, *219*
    treatment 249, **249**
Cradle cap 48
Crohn's disease 124
Cutaneous amebiasis 124
Cutaneous B-cell lymphoma 299, 311
    pseudolymphoma vs. 308–309, *308–310*
    treatment 311, **311**
Cutaneous lupus erythematosus 149
Cutaneous T-cell lymphoma (CTCL) 144, 150, 328
    clinical stages 150
    dermatitis vs. 143, *143*, 144
    treatment 150, **150**
Cylindroma 244
Cyst 311
    epidermal inclusion 311
    pilar 311
    treatment 311–312, **312**

D

Darier's disease 84
Darier's sign 296
Dermatitis herpetiformis 161, 167, 188–189, 329
    atopic dermatitis vs. 160, 160–161, *161*
    gluten-sensitive enteropathy in 188
    IgA in dermal papillae 183
    treatment 167, **168**, 189, **189**
    varicella vs. 182, *182*, *183*
Dermatofibroma 273, 281, 295, *323*, 334
    dermatofibrosarcoma protuberans vs. 284, 284–285, *285*
    melanocytic nevus (intradermal) vs. 282, 282–283, *283*
    treatment 295, **295**
Dermatofibrosarcoma protuberans (DFSP) 295, 334
    dermatofibroma vs. 284, 284–285, *285*
    treatment 295, **295**
Dermatographism 200
Dermatomyositis 20
Dermoid cysts 296, 298
Desquamative gingivitis 59
Diabetic ulcers 105
Diaper dermatitis 124, 125
    candidal 125
    chafing 125
    differential diagnosis 125
    Langerhans cell granulomatosis vs. 120–121, *121*
    treatment 125, **125**
Diffuse alopecia 3 *see also* Androgenic alopecia; Stress-induced alopecia
Digital mucous cyst 244
Discoid lupus erythematosus (DLE) 3, 14, 24, *319*, 324
    alopecia areata vs. 13, 13–14, *14*
    clinical features 24
    treatment 24, **24**
DRESS (drug reaction with eosinophilia and systemic symptoms) 213
Drug eruption 202
    treatment 202, **203**
    viral exanthem vs. 194, 194–195, *195*
Dyshidrotic dermatitis 326
Dyshidrotic eczema 69, 76, *320*, 326
    contact dermatitis vs. 68, 68–69, *69*
    differential diagnosis 76
    treatment 75, 76
Dystrophic nails 79, 84, 327
    Darier's disease 84
    differential diagnosis 81
    dyskeratosis congenita 85
    epidermolysis bullosa 85
    ingrown toenails 86
    median canal of Heller 86
    mucocutaneous candidiasis 86
    nail tic 86
    pachyonychia congeniata 85
    pseudomonas infection 86
    scabies 86
    tuberous sclerosis 85

E

Eccrine poroma 244, 276
Eccrine spiradenoma 276
Ectodermal dysplasia 20
Eczema craquelé 169
Elephantiasis verrucosa nostra 99
Eosinophilic cellulitis 201
Eosinophilic granuloma 126
Eosinophilic pustular folliculitis 205, 212
    bacterial folliculitis vs. 206, 206–207, *207*
    treatment 212, **212**
Epidermal cysts 298
Epidermal growths 217, 243–244
Epidermal inclusion cyst 296
    lipoma vs. 291, 291–292, *292*
    pilar cyst vs. 293, *293*
    treatment 296, **296**
Epidermal nevus 243
Epidermolysis bullosa acquisita 22
Erysipelas 105, 312
    carcinoma erysipeloides vs. 302, *302*
    treatment 312, **312**
Erythema elevatum diutinum 107
Erythema induratum 106
    differential diagnosis 106
    erythema nodosum vs. 90, 90–91, *91*
    treatment 106, **107**
    and tuberculosis 106
Erythema migrans (Lyme disease) 199
Erythema multiforme 57, 61, 189, 202–203, *322*, 331
    bullous pemphigoid vs. 178, *178*, *179*
    major 61, *179*, 203
    target lesion 179
    and toxic epidermal necrolysis 61
    treatment 61, **61**, 189, **189**, 203, **203**
    urticaria vs. 196, 196–197, *197*
Erythema nodosum 106, 327
    Bruise-like appearance 91
    causes of 96
    differential diagnosis 106
    erythema induratum vs. 90, 90–91, *91*
    polyarteritis nodosa vs. 95, 95–96, *96*
    treatment 106, **106**
Erythroplakia 62
Exclamation point hairs 5, 23
Excoriations 157, 329
    differential diagnosis 159
Extramammary Paget's disease (EMPD) 119, 125, 328
    tinea cruris vs. 118, *118*, *119*
    treatment 125, **126**
Eyelid dermatitis 44

F

Facial flushing, causes of 31
Facial rashes 27, 325 *see also specific rash*
    macular 31
Factitial dermatitis 22
Familial atypical mole and melanoma syndrome 278
Fibroma 245
Fibrous papule 250
    basal cell carcinoma vs. 241, *241*
    treatment 250, **250**
Fitzpatrick's sign 295
Fixed drug eruption 201
Fogo selvagem 63
Folliculitis decalvans 21

G

Genital papules, differential diagnosis of 113
Genital warts 252
Geographic tongue 59
Giant condyloma of Buschke-Löwenstein 124
Gingival hyperplasia, dilantin and 59
Glomus 274
Gougerot–Blum syndrome 107
Graft *versus* host disease 21, 200
Granuloma fissuratum 245
Granuloma inguinale 126, 128
Grover's disease 212
Guttate psoriasis 154
    pityriasis rosea vs. 138, *138*

H

Hailey–Hailey disease 115, 124
Hair loss *see* Alopecia
Hair pull test 25
Halo nevus 274
Hand and foot eruptions 65
Hand-foot-and-mouth disease 59
Hand–Schüller–Christian disease 126
Hemangioma 312, 315
    Kaposi's sarcoma vs. 304, 304–305, *306*, *307*
    subtypes 312
    treatment 312, **313**
Henoch–Schönlein purpura (HSP) 107
Herpes genitalis 117, 125–126
    differential diagnosis 126
    syphilitic chancre vs. 116, *116*, *117*
    treatment 126, **126**

Herpes labialis 45, *57*
 differential diagnosis 45
 treatment 45, **45**
Herpes simplex
 grouped vesicles *36*
 impetigo contagiosa vs. 35, *35*, *36*
Herpes zoster *185*, 189, 330
 dermatomal involvement *185*
 post-herpetic scarring *185*
 treatment 189–190, **190**
 varicella vs. 184, *184*, *185*
Herpetic gingivostomatitis 61, 325
 erythema multiforme vs. 56, 56–57, *57*
 treatment 62, **62**
Hidrocystoma 294
High grade squamous intraepithelial lesion (HSIL) 123
Histiocytosis X *see* Langerhans cell histiocytosis
Hives *see* Urticaria
Hydatoid sting 201
Hypersensitivity vasculitis *see* Leukocytoclastic vasculitis

I
Impetigo contagiosa *36*, 44–45
 erosions and blisters in *45*
 and herpes simplex 45
 herpes simplex vs. 35, *35*, *36*

 treatment 45, **45**
Ink-spot lentigo 275
Insect bite reaction 203, 331
 urticaria vs. *198*, 198–199, *199*
Inverse psoriasis 154
Irritant contact dermatitis *66*, 66–67
 allergic contact dermatitis vs. 66, *66*, *67*

J
Juvenile xanthogranuloma 296

K
Kaposi's sarcoma 273, 274, 299, 312–313, 315
 differential diagnosis. 305
 hemangioma vs. *304*, 304–305, *306*, *307*
 treatment 313, **313**
Keloid 294
Keloidal folliculitis 21
Keratoacanthoma *230*, 250, 332
 squamous cell carcinoma vs. *229*, 229–230, *230*
 treatment **250**, 250–251
 types of 230
Keratosis pilaris 151
Kerion *5*, 26
Koebner's phenomenon 127, 252
Koplik's spots 204

L
Langerhans cell granulomatosis *121*, 125
 diaper dermatitis vs. 120–121, *121*
Langerhans cell histiocytosis *19*, 126
 treatment 126, **126**
Lentigo 275
 Crowe's sign 275
Lentigo maligna melanoma
 solar lentigo vs. *269*, 269–270, *270*
Letterer–Siwe disease 126
Leukocytoclastic vasculitis *93*, 106–107, 327

differential diagnosis 107
 pigmented purpura vs. 92–93, *92*–*94*
 treatment 107, **107**
Leukoedema 60
Leukoplakia 60, 62
 differential diagnosis 51, 55, 62
 lichen planus vs. *54*, 54–55, *55*
 squamous cell carcinoma in 55
 treatment 62, **62**
Lichen aureus 107
Lichen nitidus *146*, 151, 328
 ball and claw pattern 151
 lichen planus vs. *145*, 145–146, *146*, 151
 treatment 151, **151**
Lichenoid drug eruption due to gold 149
Lichen planopilaris 20
Lichen planus 51, 60, 62, *103*, 123, 126–127, 131, 142, *146*, 151, *320*, *321*, 325, 327, 328
 biopsy of 151
 condyloma acuminatum vs. *122*, 122–123, *123*
 drug-induced 62
 Koebner's phenomenon 151
 leukoplakia vs. *54*, 54–55, *55*
 lichen nitidus vs. *145*, 145–146, *146*
 morphologic variants 151
 oral candidiasis vs. *50*, 50–51, *51*
 psoriasis vs. *141*, *141*, *142*
 treatment 62–63, **63**, 127, **127**, 151, **152**
 Wickham's striae 151
Lichen planus of nails 87
 differential diagnosis 87
 psoriatic nails vs. *83*, 83–84, *84*
 treatment 87, **87**
Lichen sclerosus et atrophicus 127, *321*, 328
 contact dermatitis vs. *114*, 114–115, *115*
 treatment 127, **127**
Lichen scrofulosorum 151
Lichen simplex chronicus 165
Lichen spinulosus 151
Linear IgA disease 186
Linear scleroderma 21
Lipoma 281, 296, 334
 epidermal inclusion cyst vs. *291*, 291–292, *292*
 treatment 296, **296**
Livedoid vasculitis 94
Loose anagen syndrome 20
Lupus erythematosus 38, 45–46
 acne rosacea vs. *30*, 30–31, *31*
 criteria for diagnosis of 46
 discoid 45, 46
 malar redness *31*, *39*
 polymorphous light eruption vs. *37*, 37–38, *38*
 seborrheic dermatitis vs. *39*, *40*
 subacute cutaneous *40*, 45, 46
 systemic 45, 46
 treatment 46, **47**
 white atrophic plaques of *58*
Lymphangioma 275, 294
Lymphocytoma *see* Pseudolymphoma
Lymphoma *19*, 244, 308–309, *308*–*310*

M
Maculopapular and urticarial rashes 193
Maculopapular drug eruption
 viral exanthem vs. *194*, 194–195, *195*
Majocchi's disease 107
Malignant melanoma 277
 ABCD signs of 277
 acral lentiginous 277

atypical nevus vs. 261, *261*
 blue nevus vs. *267*, 267–268, *268*
 cherry angioma vs. *271*, 271–272, *272*
 lentigo maligna 277
 melanocytic nevus vs. 254–255, *254*–*260*
 metastatic 259, *260*
 nodular melanoma 277
 pigmented basal cell carcinoma vs. *265*, 265–266, *266*
 superficial spreading 277
 treatment 277–278, **278**
 vitiligo surrounding *260*
Malignant tumors 299
Mastocytoma 281, 296–297
 Darier's sign 290
 melanocytic nevus (intradermal) vs. *289*, 289–290, *290*
 treatment 297, **297**
Melanocytic nevus 251, 278, 297
 compound nevus 255
 congenital nevus 255, *257*
 dermatofibroma vs. *282*, 282–283, *283*
 differential diagnosis 278
 malignant melanoma vs. 254–255, *254*–*260*
 mastocytoma vs. *289*, 289–290, *290*
 neurofibroma vs. *286*–287, *286*–*288*
 seborrheic keratosis vs. *262*–263, *262*–*264*
 treatment 251, **251**, 278, **278**, 297, **297**
Meningococcemia 331
Meningomyelocele 296
Merkel cell carcinoma 244
Metastatic carcinoma 313–314, *323*, 335
 treatment 314, **314**
Metastatic renal cell carcinoma
 pyogenic granuloma vs. *303*, *303*, *304*
Microsporum canis 25, 26
Miliaria 212–213
Miliaria crystalline 209
Miliaria pustulosa *209*, 212
Miliaria rubra
 bacterial folliculitis vs. *208*, 208–209, *209*
 treatment **213**
Molluscum contagiosum 245
Morsicatio buccarum 60
Mucosa hyperpigmentation, minocycline and *59*
Mycobacterium chelonae 247
Mycobacterium marinum 246
Mycosis fungoides 310 *see also* Cutaneous T-cell lymphoma

N
Nail pigmentation 276
Nails 79 *see also* Dystrophic nails
Necrobiosis lipoidica *103*, 105
Necrotizing vasculitis *see* Leukocytoclastic vasculitis
Neurodermatitis 167–168, 329
 scabies vs. *158*, 158–159, *159*
 treatment 168, **168**
Neurofibroma 281, 287, 297, 334
 button hole sign 287
 crow's sign 288
 melanocytic nevus (intradermal) vs. *286*–287, *286*–*288*
 multiple 288
 treatment 297–298, **298**
Neurofibromatosis 297
 diagnostic criteria for 287
 Riccardi's classification of 287

Nevus sebaceus 243
Nevus spilus 274
Nikolsky sign 325
Nodular metastatic disease, cutaneous cyst vs. 300, 300–301, 301
Nodular vasculitis see Erythema induratum
Nonscarring patchy alopecia 3
Nummular dermatitis 131, **135**, 151–152, 328
    differential diagnosis 152
    oval pruritic plaques in 152
    psoriasis vs. *134*, 134–135, *135*
    treatment 152, **152**
Nummular eczema 249
    basal cell carcinoma (superficial) vs. *242*, 242–243
    treatment 249–250, **250**

O

Ofuji's disease see Eosinophilic pustular folliculitis
One hand, two feet syndrome 73, 77
Onychomadesis 327
Onychomycosis **80**, 87
    potassium hydroxide test and culture 81
    psoriasis of nails vs. 80–81, *80–82*
    with superficial white infection 81
    treatment 87, **87**
Onychophagia 327
Oral candidiasis 60, 325
    lichen planus vs. *50*, 50–51, *51*
    in patient with graft vs. host disease 51
    systemic diseases associated with 60
    treatment 60–61, **61**
Oral florid papillomatosis 60
Oral hairy leukoplakia 58
Oral lesions 49 see also specific lesions
Oral thrush see Oral candidiasis
Oral ulcers, differential diagnosis of 53

P

Papulosquamous diseases 131 see also specific disease
    differential diagnosis 13
Paraneoplastic pemphigus 63
Patchy alopecia 3
    differential diagnosis 5, 14
    nonscarring 3 (see also Alopecia areata; Tinea capitis; Trichotillomania)
    scarring 3 (see also Discoid lupus erythematosus)
Pearly penile papules 113
Pemphigus erythematosus 44
Pemphigus vegetans 63
Pemphigus vulgaris (PV) 63, *176*, 190, 325, 330
    and aphthous stomatitis 63
    aphthous ulcers vs. *52*, 52–53, *53*
    bullous pemphigoid vs. 175–176, *175–177*
    chronic unremitting oral ulcers 53
    differential diagnosis 63, 190
    Nikolsky's sign 63, *176*, 190
    treatment 63, **63**, 190, **190**
Periocular dermatitis 46
Perioral dermatitis 41, 46
    contact dermatitis vs. *41*, 41–42, *42*
    treatment 46, **47**
Peutz–Jeghers syndrome 276
Photodistributed rashes, differential diagnosis of 38
Pigmented basal cell carcinoma 278–279
    malignant melanoma vs. *265*, 265–266, *266*
    treatment 279, **279**

Pigmented growths 253, 255, 333
Pigmented purpura 107
    cayennepepper-like appearance 93
    differential diagnosis 93, 107
    leukocytoclastic vasculitis vs. 92–93, *92–94*
    lichen aureus variant of 94
    treatment 107, **108**
    variants 107
Pilar cyst 296, 298, 334
    epidermal inclusion cyst vs. *293*, 293
    treatment 298, **298**
Pilomatrixoma 244
Pityriasis lichenoides *148*, 152–153
    acuta 153
    chronica 153
    psoriasis vs. *147*, 147, *148*
    treatment 153, **153**
Pityriasis rosea 131, 137, 153
    differential diagnosis 153
    guttate psoriasis vs. *138*, 138
    herald plaque of 139
    secondary syphilis vs. *136*, 136–137, *137*
    tinea corporis vs. *139*, 139, *140*
    treatment 153–154, **154**
Pityriasis rubra pilaris *132–133*
    psoriasis vs. *132*, 132–133, *133*
Pityrosporum folliculitis 212
Plantar wart 219, *228*, 252
    in cardiac transplant patient 219
    corn vs. *218*, 218–219, *219*
Plasmacytoma 19
Poison ivy (rhus dermatitis) 330
Polyarteritis nodosa 96, 107, 108, 327
    erythema nodosum vs. *95*, 95–96, *96*
    treatment 108, **109**
Polymorphous light eruption 46–47, 325
    differential diagnosis 47
    lupus erythematosus vs. *37*, 37–38, *38*
    treatment 47, **48**
    urticarial-like papules 38
Pompholyx see Dyshidrotic eczema
Porokeratosis 245
Poroma 294
Pressure ulcers 105
Pretibial myxedema 108–109
    stasis dermatitis vs. *102*, 103
    treatment 109, **109**
Propionibacterium acnes 43
Prurigo nodularis 165
Pruritic urticarial papules and plaques of pregnancy 201
Pruritus of systemic disease 168
    treatment 168, **168**
    winter itch vs. *164*, 164–165, *165*
Pseudofolliculitis barbae 47–48
    acne vulgaris vs. *32*, 32
    treatment 48, **48**
Pseudolymphoma 314
    cutaneous B-cell lymphoma vs. 308–309, *308–310*
    treatment 314, **314**
Pseudomembranous candidiasis see Oral candidiasis
Psoriasis 18, 24, 71, 76, *133*, 135, 154, 213–214, *320*, 324, 327
    atopic dermatitis vs. 70–71, *70–72*
    clinical features 24
    clinical variants 154
    Koebner's reaction 135
    lichen planus vs. *141*, 141, *142*
    of nail 87–88, **88**

    nummular dermatitis vs. *134*, 134–135, *135*
    pityriasis lichenoides vs. *147*, 147, *148*
    pityriasis rubra pilaris vs. *132*, 132–133, *133*
    psoriatic arthritis 72
    pustular 72, 213
    seborrheic dermatitis vs. *17*, 17–18, *18*
    tent sign 18
    treatment 24, **25**, 76, **77**, 154, **155**, 214, **214**
Psoriatic arthritis 72
Psoriatic nails 87–88
    lichen planus vs. *83*, 83–84, *84*
    onychomycosis vs. 80–81, *80–82*
    treatment 88, **88**
Pustular eruptions 205–214
Pustular hand dermatoses, differential diagnosis of 71
Pustular psoriasis 213, *322*, 326, 331
    acute generalized exanthematous pustulosis vs. *210*, 210–211
PUVA lentigines 275
Pyoderma gangrenosum 98–99, 105, 107–108, *320*, 327
    stasis ulcer vs. *97*–98, *97–99*
    systemic diseases associated with 107
    treatment 108, **108**
Pyogenic granulomas *273*, 313, 314–315, 335
    band aid sign 304
    metastatic renal cell carcinoma vs. *303*, 303, 304
    treatment 315, **315**

S

Scabies 159, *169*, *321*, 329
    neurodermatitis vs. *158*, 158–159, *159*
    treatment 169, **169**
Schamberg's disease 107
Sebaceous hyperplasia 251
    basal cell carcinoma vs. *239*, 239–240, *240*
    treatment 251, **251**
Seborrheic dermatitis 8, 18, 34, 24, 48, *319*, 325
    clinical features 24
    contact dermatitis vs. *33*, 33–34, *34*
    involvement of chest, axilla and groin 39
    lupus erythematosus vs. *39*, 40
    in neonates 48
    psoriasis vs. *17*, 17–18, *18*
    of scalp, differential diagnosis of 25
    tinea capitis vs. *7*, 7–8, *8*
    treatment 25, **25**, 48, **48**
Seborrheic keratosis 124, *221*, 251, *263*, 279, 333
    actinic keratosis vs. *220*–221, *220–222*
    melanocytic nevus vs. *262*–263, *262–264*
    treatment 251, **251**, 279, **279**
Secondary syphilis 131, 154, 328
    moth-eaten alopecia 137
    palmar lesions 137
    pityriasis rosea vs. *136*, 136–137, *137*
    treatment 154–155, **155**
Shagreen patch, in tuberous sclerosis 294
Skin tag 124, *276*
Small plaque parapsoriasis 149
Sneddon–Wilkinson disease 187
Solar lentigines 333
Solar lentigo 279
    lentigo maligna melanoma vs. *269*, 269–270, *270*
    treatment 279, **279**
Spitz nevus *273*, 315
Sporotrichosis 246
Squamous cell carcinoma 60, *232*, 224, 248, 252

actinic keratosis vs. 223–224, *223–225*
basal cell carcinoma (nodular) vs. 233–234, *233–236*
chondrodermatitis nodularis helicis vs. *231*, 231–232, *232*
differential diagnosis 252
keratoacanthoma vs. *229*, 229–230, *230*
in situ Bowen's disease *225*, 252
of tongue 55
treatment 252, **252**
types of 227
wart vs. 226–227, *226–228*
Staphylococcal scalded skin syndrome (SSSS) 190–191, 330
intraepidermal blister *181*
positive Nikolsky's sign *181*
toxic epidermal necrolysis vs. *180*, 180–181, *181*
treatment 191, **191**
Stasis dermatitis 109
cellulitis vs. *104*, *104*
differential diagnosis 109
pretibial myxedema vs. *102*, *103*
and ulcer 109, **109**
Stasis ulcer 105, 327
arterial ulcer vs. *100*, *100*, *101*
eczematous skin surrounding ulcer *98*
pyoderma gangrenosum vs. *97–98*, *97–99*
Still's disease 200
Strawberry nevus 312
Stress-induced alopecia 25
androgenic alopecia vs. *15*, 15–16, *16*
clinical features 25
differential diagnosis 25
treatment 25, **25**
Stucco keratosis 222
Subcorneal pustular dermatosis 214
Sunburn 186
Syphilis 127–128, 131, 154
primary 127–128
secondary *117*, 128
tertiary 128
treatment 128, **128**
Syphilitic chancre 126
herpes genitalis vs. *116*, *116*, *117*
Syringocystadenoma papilliferum 243
Syringoma 294

T
Targetoid hemosiderotic hemangiomas 312
Telogen effluvium *see* Stress-induced alopecia
Thrombophlebitis 96
Thyroglossal duct cyst 296
Tick bite *199*
Tinea amiantacea 48 *see also* Seborrheic dermatitis
Tinea capitis 6, 9, 25, 324
alopecia areata vs. *4*, 4–5, *5*, *6*
clinical features 26
differential diagnosis 26
kerion *5*, *6*, 26
seborrheic dermatitis vs. *7*, 7–8, *8*
treatment 26, **26**
trichotillomania vs. *9*, 9–10, *10*
Tinea corporis 131, 140, 155
differential diagnosis 155
pityriasis rosea vs. *139*, *139*, *140*
potassium hydroxide test *140*
treatment 155, **155**
Tinea cruris *119*, 124, 125, 128, 328
differential diagnosis 128
extramammary paget's disease vs. *118*, *118*, *119*
treatment 128, **128**
Tinea faciei 44
Tinea manuum *74*, 77, **77**
Tinea pedis *74*, 77, **77**
Tinea unguium *see* Onychomycosis
Tinea versicolor 149
hyper and hypopigmentation *149*
Toxic epidermal necrolysis (TEN) 61, 191, 203
staphylococcal scalded skin syndrome vs. *180*, 180–181, *181*
subepidermal blister and necrotic epidermis *181*
treatment 191, **191**
Traction alopecia 19
Trichilemmal cyst *see* Pilar cyst
Trichoepithelioma 243
Trichophyton tonsurans 25, 26
Trichotillomania 9, 26
alopecia areata vs. *11*, 11–12, *12*
clinical features 26
Friar Tuck sign 26
tinea capitis vs. *9*, 9–10, *10*
treatment 26, **26**
T-suppressor cell lymphoma 309

U
Urticaria 202
erythema multiforme vs. *196*, 196–197, *197*
insect bite reaction vs. *198*, 198–199, *199*
treatment 202, **202**
Urticarial vasculitis 201
Urticaria multiforme 203
Urticaria pigmentosa 290

V
Varicella *183*, 191
dermatitis herpetiformis vs. *182*, *182*, *183*
herpes zoster disseminated vs. *184*, *184*, *185*
treatment 191, **191**
Ventral pterygium 327
Verruca vulgaris *see* Wart
Verrucous hemangioma 274
Vesicular and bullous diseases 171
Viral exanthems 204, 331
maculopapular drug eruption vs. *194*, 194–195, *195*
treatment 204, **204**
Vitiligo 127

W
Wart 248, 252, 332, 335
cryotherapy, treatment with 228
filiform 228
flat 227
genital 228
in immunosuppressed patients 252
plantar 228
squamous cell carcinoma vs. 226–227, *226–228*
treatment 252, **252**
Wegener's granulomatosis 107
White sponge nevus 60
Wickham's striae 127, 325
Winter itch 169, 329
pruritus of systemic disease vs. *164*, 164–165, *165*
treatment 169, **169**

Z
Zosteriform metastases 314